Autism Spectrum Disorders from Theory to Practice

Autism Spectrum Disorders from Theory to Practice

Assessment and Intervention Tools Across the Lifespan

Belinda Daughrity, Ph.D., CCC-SLP

Assistant Professor, California State University
Long Beach, CA, USA

and

Ashley Wiley Johnson, Ph.D., CCC-SLP

Vice President, LA Speech and Language Therapy Center
Los Angeles, CA, USA

WILEY Blackwell

The right of Belinda Daughrity and Ashley Wiley Johnson to be identified as the authors of the editorial material in this work has been asserted in accordance with law.

Registered Office
John Wiley & Sons Ltd, The Atrium, Southern Gate, Chichester, West Sussex, PO19 8SQ, UK

Editorial Office
9600 Garsington Road, Oxford, OX4 2DQ, UK

For details of our global editorial offices, customer services, and more information about Wiley products visit us at www.wiley.com.

Wiley also publishes its books in a variety of electronic formats and by print-on-demand. Some content that appears in standard print versions of this book may not be available in other formats.

Library of Congress Cataloging-in-Publication Data
Names: Daughrity, Belinda, 1984– author. | Johnson, Ashley Wiley, 1985– author.
Title: Autism spectrum disorders from theory to practice : assessment and intervention
    tools across the lifespan / Belinda Daughrity and Ashley Wiley Johnson.
Description: First edition. | Hoboken, NJ : Wiley-Blackwell, 2023. |
    Includes bibliographical references and index.
Identifiers: LCCN 2022019638 (print) | LCCN 2022019639 (ebook) | ISBN
    9781119819561 (paperback) | ISBN 9781119819578 (adobe pdf) | ISBN
    9781119819585 (epub)
Subjects: MESH: Autism Spectrum Disorder
Classification: LCC RC553.A88 (print) | LCC RC553.A88 (ebook) | NLM WS
    350.8.P4 | DDC 616.85/882–dc23/eng/20220613
LC record available at https://lccn.loc.gov/2022019638
LC ebook record available at https://lccn.loc.gov/2022019639

Cover image: © Tony Anderson/Getty Images; © Klaus Vedfelt/Getty Images
Cover design by Wiley

Set in 10.5/13pt STIXTwoText by Straive, Pondicherry, India

SKY10073756_042524

Contents

About the Authors

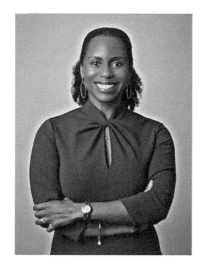

Dr. Belinda Daughrity is a California state-licensed and American Speech–Language–Hearing Association (ASHA) certified bilingual speech–language pathologist (SLP) with more than 20 years of experience working with individuals with autism. She earned her BA in English and Spanish from Spelman College. She earned her MA in speech–language pathology and audiology from New York University before earning her doctorate at University of California, Los Angeles (UCLA), where she worked in the world-renowned Center for Autism Research and Treatment. During her training at UCLA, she worked on cutting edge research for autism intervention and furthered her expertise in evaluation procedures via clinical and research training in the Autism Diagnostic Interview – Revised and the Autism Diagnostic Observation Schedule, second edition, often considered the "gold standard" of autism assessment.

Belinda has presented at national and international conferences about autism spectrum disorder (ASD) including: the ASHA, the National Black Association of Speech–Language and Hearing, the California Speech–Language–Hearing Association, the Illinois Speech–Language and Hearing Association, the ASHA Connect Conference, and the International Society of Autism Research Regional International Meeting for Autism Research. She has teaching experience at New York University, UCLA, and Chapman University. Currently, she serves as an assistant professor at California State University, Long Beach in the speech–language pathology department.

Her clinical experience includes assessment, individual and group intervention, and social skills in the home, private practice, schools, and telepractice settings. She has led social skills groups for children with autism in preschool, elementary, middle, and high school. Bilingual in Spanish, she has worked with families from culturally and linguistically diverse backgrounds to promote caregiver training and education. Additionally, Belinda serves as a clinical supervisor to train speech–language pathologists and SLP assistants. She hopes that this textbook helps current and future clinicians working with children with autism and their families.

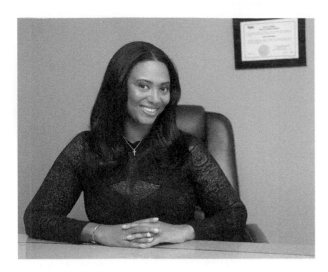

Dr. Ashley Wiley Johnson is Vice President of Los Angeles Speech and Language Therapy Center, a family-owned small business founded over 41 years ago, which is at the forefront of working with people with autism and other special needs across the lifespan. A second-generation speech pathologist, Ashley manages licensed speech pathologists, therapists, and behaviorists serving clients in early intervention programs, social skills classes, summer programs, employment readiness programs, and typical and therapeutic preschool programs across five sites within Los Angeles County. As part of her practice, she consults with school districts and charter schools to help improve their delivery of speech and language-based services to students with special needs. She has focused on the over-identification of African-American and Latino students classified for special education services, has created innovative pathways to service delivery for people with autism across the lifespan, forged partnerships between public school systems and private practice setting, and brought traditional speech therapy methods into the classroom setting to encourage facilitation and increased development in students with speech and language delays.

Ashley began her professional career in the public school system serving as a bilingual SLP and ultimately as the lead preschool district-wide assessor. During her tenure, she developed a passion for working to decrease and build awareness of disparity in provision of services for Black and Hispanic students with autism. Using her fine arts background, Ashley developed Drama Kings and Queens (DKQ), a six- to eight-week summer program and weekly social skills class focused on developing pragmatics and creativity for students ages 5–15 years with autism through the arts.

Ashley is a proud graduate of the University of North Carolina at Chapel Hill. She obtained her Masters of Arts from San Josè State University in Communication Sciences and Disorders and her PhD from Claremont Graduate School in Educational Studies with an emphasis on urban education and special education.

As a bilingual SLP, Ashley is a sought-after national trainer, lecturer and presenter addressing a range of topics around service delivery innovation, effective social skills treatment models, and arts advocacy for children with autism and their families. Ashley also is active in leadership in the ASHA, where she most recently held the title of Topic Chair for the 2021 ASHA Convention. She currently sits on the board of directors of Child 360, a statewide organization at the forefront of providing access to quality early childhood education for children across California.

Ashley is married to Alex Martin Johnson Esq., and they are the proud parents of a precocious and adorable daughter, Alexa Danielle and son, Alain.

Introduction

This textbook is the product of two interventionists with more than 40 years of combined experience working with individuals with autism and their families. In each chapter, we share personal anecdotes from our own clinical practices to help illustrate the application of theoretical approaches. It is our intent, that this book will be used as a bridge to support an interventionist's ability to think of the theories surrounding autism and then put them into actual practice.

Additionally, several chapters end with a *reflection letter* from individuals from various perspectives and backgrounds: autism researchers, speech–language pathologists, developmental psychologists, adapted physical education teachers, professors, celebrity advocates like Holly Robinson Peete, and, most importantly, adults living and thriving with autism each day of their lives.

Further, we are delighted to have a special contributor to write Chapter 7: Autism Spectrum Disorder in Adulthood. Dr. Pamela Wiley, founder and president of Los Angeles Speech and Language Therapy Center, Inc., and the Wiley Center for Speech and Language Development. She has more than 50 years of clinical experience treating individuals with autism and their families from all over the world. Her wealth of clinical knowledge on autism spectrum disorder (ASD) intervention throughout the lifespan includes developing cutting-edge programs to serve young adults with ASD during the transition out of high school. Her manualized approach, Autism, Attacking Social Interaction Problems (*AASIP*), has been used in social skills treatment in her centers and throughout the world. She holds the title of American Speech–Language–Hearing Association Honors, the highest award in our profession. We are grateful that she has taught us much of what we know today.

This textbook is meant to bridge the divide between theory and practice for students and/or new interventionists from any discipline who work with clients with ASD. Throughout the chapters, you will notice repeated references to terms like *cultural competence* and *culturally responsive intervention practices*. As speech–language pathologists of color, we believe strongly that cultural competence should be repeatedly considered in discourse about assessment and intervention with our clients and their families, who come from a myriad of diverse backgrounds.

We encourage you to continue learning long after you read this textbook. You should be informed by your professional discipline, clinical experiences, and continuing education as you use your clinical judgment to inform your best practices. To guide your reading, we have used a few different symbols and headings throughout the book:

Active Learning Task: This is a point where you and/or your instructor will look to promote active learning via activities designed to prompt your direct engagement with the material. This might include doing research, completing a brief activity, or writing a reflection. We encourage you to complete these tasks to interact with the textbook and deepen your learning.

Goal Spotlight: This symbol indicates a sample intervention goal you might use with a future client with autism. These are good opportunities to practice writing your own goals and/or developing treatment activities that might address the goal.

Therapy Golden Nugget: This indicates a practical suggestion for you to use in intervention. We include several of these ideas because many of our students and interns over the years have simply asked, "But what should I do?!" These examples are intended to get you thinking so you can begin to develop your own ideas for treatment activities to engage clients with autism across the lifespan.

Therapy Viewpoint

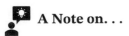 **A Note on. . .**

It is our hope that this piece of work is cherished and will help to support a client with autism as they go *beyond the label*.

CHAPTER 1

Historical Perspectives of Autism Spectrum Disorder

Learning Objectives

By reading this chapter, interventionists will be able to:

1. Compare and contrast diagnostic criteria for autism spectrum disorder (ASD) from the fourth edition of the *Diagnostic and Statistical Manual of Mental Disorders* (DSM-IV) to the fifth edition (DSM-V).
2. Identify a reason why girls with autism may be overlooked in comparison to their male counterparts.
3. Define the neurodiversity movement and ableism.
4. Compare the medical and social model of disability.

Before You Begin, Think About These Questions

- What do I know about autism?
- How did I first learn about autism?
- What do I want to know about autism?

While criteria and descriptions have certainly evolved, ASD as we know it today is not vastly different from the way we knew it nearly 100 years ago when a psychiatrist,

---

Autism Spectrum Disorders from Theory to Practice: Assessment and Intervention Tools Across the Lifespan, First Edition. Edited by Belinda Daughrity and Ashley Wiley Johnson.
© 2023 John Wiley & Sons Ltd. Published 2023 by John Wiley & Sons Ltd.

Leo Kanner, first wrote about his experiences with children with the disorder, all younger than age 11, beginning in 1938 (Kanner 1943). He published his longitudinal study as his counterpart Hans Asperger was writing of the same phenomenon, hence the former diagnostic term, "Asperger's Syndrome". His seminal paper titled "Autistic disturbances of affective contact" described his experiences of 11 cases of children. Similar to the gender disparity we see today, Kanner included more boys than girls in his study.

As Kanner's study title suggests, the primary impairment of those children was social engagement, as all the children demonstrated deficits in key social domains including functional play skills and reciprocal social interaction. One case describes a child who "always worked and played alone" with "no manifestation of friendliness or interest in persons" and "no display of affection." The descriptions clearly outline social communication deficits, in spite of typical IQ scores.

Cases often described various restricted and repetitive behaviors, a hallmark feature of ASD. Though written in 1943, descriptions could be included in diagnostic reports of the present day. For example, one case included the descriptions "stereotyped movements," "repetitions carried out in exactly the same way," and "verbal rituals," which all could be used to describe common restricted and repetitive behaviors observed in individuals with ASD today.

What are the diagnostic categories for autism? In past years, a formal diagnosis according to the DSM-IV had to involve three distinct categories:

- Impairments in social interactions
- Impairments in communication
- Restricted, repetitive, and/or stereotyped patterns of behavior
- Interests, and/or activities (Table 1.1).

Each category had to be identified to qualify for a diagnosis. Notably, the social interaction domain had to be identified twice as much as the other two diagnostic domains, highlighting the importance of social interaction deficits in the diagnosis of ASD.

Active Learning Task

Think, Pair, Share

Review Kanner's 1943 publication. What were some of the descriptions of the cases of ASD in Kanner's seminal work?

How do those descriptions compare with our current knowledge of ASD?

Beginning in 2013, the DSM-V collapsed the three diagnostic domains to just two domains: (i) deficits in social communication and social interaction, and (ii) restricted, repetitive patterns of behavior, interests, or activities. Essentially, the newest edition collapsed the social interaction and communication impairments into just one domain, rather than two independent categories, while maintaining the criteria for restricted and repetitive behaviors (Figure 1.1).

TABLE 1.1   DSM IV categories used in the formal diagnosis of ASD

Social interaction impairments	Communication impairments	Restricted and repetitive behaviors
• Marked impairment in the use of multiple nonverbal behaviors, such as eye-to-eye gaze, facial expression, body postures, and gestures to regulate social interaction. • Failure to develop peer relationships appropriate to developmental level. • A lack of spontaneous seeking to share enjoyment, interests, or achievements with other people (e.g. by a lack of showing, bringing, or pointing out objects of interest). • Lack of social or emotional reciprocity.	• Delay in, or total lack of, the development of spoken language (not accompanied by an attempt to compensate through alternative modes of communication such as gesture or mime). • In individuals with adequate speech, marked impairment in the ability to initiate or sustain a conversation with others. • Stereotyped and repetitive use of language or idiosyncratic language. • Lack of varied, spontaneous make-believe play or social imitative play appropriate to developmental level.	• Encompassing preoccupation with one or more stereotyped and restricted patterns of interest that is abnormal either in intensity or focus. • Apparently inflexible adherence to specific, nonfunctional routines or rituals. • Stereotyped and repetitive motor mannerisms (e.g. hand or finger flapping or twisting or complex whole-body movements). • Persistent preoccupation with parts of objects.

So why was this change made? Researchers and clinicians alike readily identified social impairments and restricted and repetitive behaviors as defining features of ASD. However, readily identifying communication impairments was a challenging area even for professionals with significant experience with the population, particularly for diagnosing highly verbal individuals with little to no expressive and/or receptive language delays and typical IQ. These highly verbal individuals were often diagnosed with Asperger's, considered a "high-functioning" version of autism. Even more controversial was a diagnosis of pervasive developmental disorder – not otherwise specified (*PDD-NOS*), a label used to describe individuals who may have presented with autism-like symptomology, but not enough characteristics to clearly receive an autism or Asperger's diagnosis.

Essentially, even the most experienced professionals were having difficulty reaching a consensus on these three diagnostic categories, with potential for one individual to receive three different diagnoses if evaluated by three different clinicians. This acknowledgment led to a shift in the perception of diagnosis and the idea of an autism spectrum, rather than a singular diagnosis. In fact, many current clinicians now more commonly use the term ASDs, indicating that autism is not just one single disorder, but actually several different types of disorders, each with a different presentation based upon symptom severity and expression. (Figure 1.1).

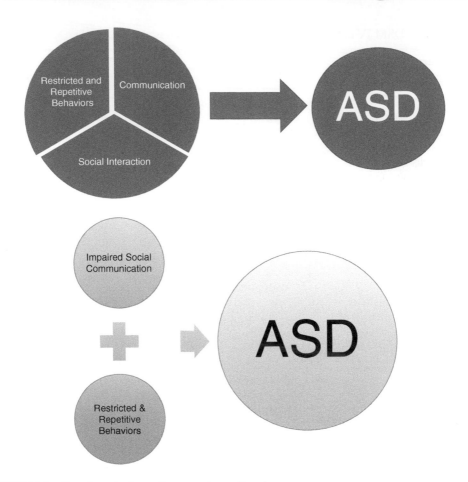

FIGURE 1.1   One domain for autism spectrum disorders.

Why does this matter? As we discuss a bit later, appropriate, differential diagnosis is critical for individuals to be able to access appropriate services and to receive targeted interventions to best address their unique needs. The common refrain from Dr. Shore of: "If you have met one person with autism, then you have met one person with autism" remains accurate due to the vast heterogeneity of ASD. Research scientists in autism work to explore gene mutations in the disorder and recognize the likelihood of several different genetic markers, given the vast differences found in the heterogeneous disorder (Geschwind 2008). Of course, autism is not simply a genetic disorder. If it were, we could clearly test and identify it early on much like we do for other gene mutations, such as Down Syndrome, which we can identify in utero. Complexly, autism is thought to be a combination of pre-existing genetic risk coupled with environmental factors. However, there still exists an element of the unknown that fails to explain the presentation of autism. For example, if there were only genetic and environmental factors, we might expect to see sets of twins both diagnosed and presenting similarly. That is not the case, despite siblings being at higher risk for diagnosis.

One of my most interesting patients was a four-year-old boy with autism who was nonverbal and had significant communication difficulties. He presented with ASD symptomology like hand flapping, difficulty with changes in routine, and significant

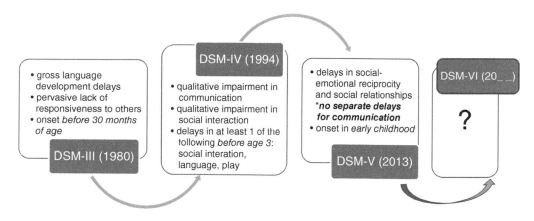

FIGURE 1.2   Changes in the diagnosis of autism in successive editions of the Diagnostic and Statistical Manual of Mental Disorders.

social communication delays. His twin brother was the exact opposite. He was very social and loved to engage in play, often lamenting that he wanted to go to "speech class" because it looked fun and he never got a turn. They were a great example of siblings who shared the same genetic code and gestational environment as identical twins. It could largely be assumed that their environments after birth were also near identical. Yet, they did not both present with autism. The hardest question we are asked by parents is "What causes autism?" It is not hard because we are not well versed in the topic; it is hard because, like most clinicians, researchers, and scientists, it is difficult to say, "We do not completely know."

It is important to consider that diagnostic criteria can change over time, often to create greater specificity and more standards for diagnosticians. Note how the criteria for a diagnosis for autism has changed over the past 40 years (Figure 1.2). Despite changes, note that the key elements remain stable over time: deficits in interaction skills with or without delays in language, and early presentation of delays.

CLINICAL CONSIDERATION

Some clinicians may have a fixed view of restricted and repetitive behaviors, which can prevent appropriate referral and diagnosis. Consider restricted and repetitive behaviors along a continuum that can include restricted and intense interests as well as verbal rituals, in addition to more commonly discernable presentations such as hand flapping. Consider the following examples:

- Lining up toy cars
- Intensely investigating objects at eye level
- Difficulty adjusting to changes in routine
- Insistence on discussing a particular subject with little regard for other topics

- Immediate or delayed echolalia
- Verbal rituals performed with the same script and intonation patterns
- Hand or finger mannerisms.

Active Learning Task

Ask five different people, "What is autism?" Compare their responses. Do your respondents have any personal connections to ASD (do they know a person with autism)? How accurate is their response? What do they think the cause of autism is? Where did they get their information? Based on your findings, how can you go about better educating the general public on autism?

Clinical Anecdote

As a teenager in high school, I worked at a summer camp for children with special needs. One of the campers was a four-year-old boy who I adored. He was very chatty and loved riding bikes. One afternoon, I had him and two other campers in my car to head to a local park for a field trip day. As usual, I had taken a wrong turn and gotten lost (this was pre-GPS, Waze, or Google Maps ☺). I pondered what to do aloud when suddenly my favorite camper in the backseat said, "Turn right on Centinela. Then make a left on Jefferson and a right on Bristol Parkway." I chuckled, but then realized *that was actually the way to get there*. I mentioned it to his father later that day and his dad replied, "Oh he *loves* maps. He can honestly tell you how to get just about anywhere in the city. He doesn't play that great with other kids, but he is amazing at directions." I later learned that the boy was diagnosed with autism. Subsequently, he became my permanent passenger on all camp field trips, with his penchant for maps camouflaging my horrible sense of direction.

A NEURODEVELOPMENTAL DISORDER: AUTISM AND THE BRAIN

Active Learning Task

Recall your studies in neuroanatomy. What are the key areas of the brain for:

- Language?
- Motor functioning?

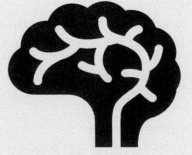

Although we do not have an exact answer about what causes autism, we do know that individuals with ASD can demonstrate atypical neurological presentations in comparison with their typically developing peers and evidence suggests multiple interacting genetic factors (Muhle et al. 2004). While there is not a single, specific, genetic marker of ASD, evidence indicates that there are several different potentially impacted genes, which supports the theory of there being several autisms.

Research suggest that Purkinje cells, located in the cerebellum and thought to be responsible for motoric inhibition, are limited in individuals with autism (Whitney et al. 2008). Neurological deficits causing motor communication deficits have been explored as a factor for poor speech production in individuals with ASD (Mody and McDougle 2019). Studies indicate abnormal brain growth and enlarged cerebral gray and white matter in toddlers with ASD (Schumann et al. 2010). Further research into white matter indicates that children with ASD may rely more on visuospatial processing networks than their neurotypical peers (Sahyoun et al. 2010). Additionally, research suggests atypical function and organization in brain hemispheres among individuals with ASD, which may contribute to language delays (Kleinhans et al. 2008).

While most parents are less interested in the etiology and more interested in direct supports to promote communicative and social success for their children, it is important for interventionists to at least have an understanding of potential causes for autism. Inevitably, a parent will ask,

What causes autism?

How did this happen?

We should be able to counsel parents with accurate information and with empathy. It is important to note to parents that it is not anyone's fault. Autism is highly heterogeneous and differences in genetic factors and neural circuitry, along with environmental influences, all play a role in autism presentation (Rylaarsdam and Guemez-Gamboa 2019). While we have yet to definitively identify all of the genes involved, research clearly points to the significance of the interaction of both genetic and environmental factors that contributes to autism risk (Chaste and Leboyer 2012).

THE CLINICAL TEAM: WHO AND WHAT

In working with individuals with ASD, it is critical to take a team-based approach to promote holistic care that optimizes clinical strengths to promote achievement of optimal outcomes. The most important members of the treatment team, aside from the individual, are the primary caregivers, such as parents who are the first point of contact. Although there are several interventions available in the treatment of individuals with autism, it should be stressed that primary caregivers spend the most significant amount of time with their children, significantly more than any interventionist. As such, the importance of caregiver education cannot be stressed enough. All interventionists should incorporate caregiver education as a critical component of their intervention so that caregivers can continue to employ successful strategies in the home environment.

Interventionists serve as specialists within their respective domains. While each has a particular area of expertise, interventionists should strive for an interdisciplinary and collaborative approach in order to best treat autism from a holistic perspective. Collaboration is addressed in Chapter 11. The ultimate goal of treatment should be to promote communication and skills that permit the individual to live a fulfilling and independent life Figure 1.3.

Active Learning Task

What Is *Your* Scope of Practice?

Understanding the scope of practice outlined by your national organization is important when working with individuals with autism. The scope of practice tells interventionists what one should and should not be working on in your profession when working with individuals with autism. Using this document, write a one-page reflection on the top three scope of practice areas you found interesting and/or never considered. Discuss these findings with your peers. Below you will find information surrounding scope of practice for specific professions working with individuals with autism. This list includes but is not limited to:

American Speech and Hearing Association	https://www.asha.org/practice-portal/clinical-topics/autism
American Journal of Occupational Therapy	https://ajot.aota.org/article.aspx?articleid=1865177
American Physical Therapy Association	https://www.apta.org/patient-care/evidence-based-practice-resources/clinical-summaries/autism-spectrum-disorder-in-children
American Association of Pediatrics	https://pediatrics.aappublications.org/content/145/1/e20193447
American Psychological Association	https://www.apa.org/topics/autism-spectrum-disorder/diagnosing
Centers for Disease Control and Prevention	https://www.cdc.gov/ncbddd/autism/hcp-dsm.html

Interventionists working with young children are encouraged to work with the end in mind. Be mindful that individuals spend significantly more time as adults than they do as children. Addressing maladaptive behaviors that significantly prevent individuals from learning and engaging with others around them should be targeted early using a direct approach, rather than a "wait and see" method. Developing and fostering unique skills that may be marketable as viable future job skills should be explored long before individuals are preparing to transition out of high school. This point is discussed extensively in Chapter 7.

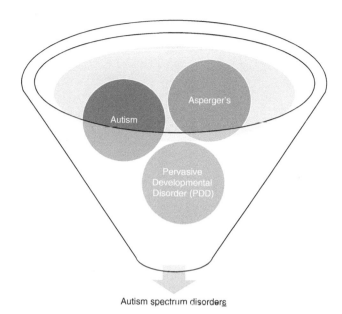

FIGURE 1.3   Autism Spectrum Disorders.

NEURODIVERSITY

In consideration of adults, consideration should be given to self-perception of individuals with autism. The **neurodiversity movement** challenges the deficit-based approached of viewing autism and other neurodevelopmental disorders. Having grown over the last decades, proponents argue that autism is a variation along the spectrum of human differences, aligning autistics to other marginalized cultural groups (Jaarsma and Welin 2012). Scholars acknowledge that disability itself is a socially constructed concept, with the social model of neurodiversity arising as an alternative to the traditional **medical model of disability** (Figure 1.4; Krcek 2013). For a better understanding, see the "Social Model Animation," which can be found on YouTube (Adams-Spink 2011) to help increase understanding about how disability can be framed as a social construct. **Ableism**, which intersects with other systems of oppression, is defined as attitudes that discriminate and devalue people with disabilities; this includes the language we use to describe such individuals (Bottema-Beutel et al. 2021). Interventionists working with individuals with autism and their families should be mindful of the language used to discuss clients and their areas of need, while also considering various perspectives of disability.

Rather than viewing the individual with autism as someone in need of intervention to better adapt to societal conventions, leaders of the neurodiversity movement, such as those with autism and others, implore neurotypical stakeholders to get involved and champion changes that may better accommodate the needs of individuals with autism by normalizing autistic experiences (den Houting 2019). Supporters of this movement champion the rights of individuals with autism to speak for themselves. Additionally, the neurodiversity movement seeks to recognize neurological differences as variances that require more understanding, rather than treatment.

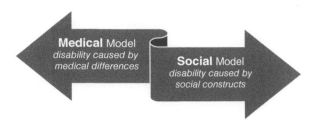

FIGURE 1.4   Medical and social models of autism.

Active Learning Task

Consider the following scenarios through the approach of a medical model vs. that of a neurodiversity paradigm. Discuss how to address these challenges first through a medical lens (What kind of intervention would you employ?) and then through a social lens (What about the environment would you change?).

- John is 13 years old and has significant difficulty in public spaces due to sensory sensitivity to noise, and bright lights.
- Melanie is seven years old and has difficulty attending birthday parties. She loves blowing out candles and tantrums when she is not permitted to blow out the candle at peers' parties.

Importantly, this movement cites the need for individuals with autism to have a central voice in research. For example, in research led by individuals with ASD, Kapp et al. (2019) reframe the perspective of repetitive motor movements as an important adaptation and coping mechanism, rather than as a behavior to be eliminated. Such perspectives are important in considering that many interventions for autism are behavioral; scholars note the controversy between traditional behavioral therapies and the need for a more humanistic approach for interventions for ASD (Shyman 2016).

Highlighted in the movement are notable individuals with autism who have made significant societal contributions such as climate change activist Greta Thunberg, scientist Temple Grandin, and Kent State Division I basketball player Kalin Bennett. Autism itself is viewed as a strength, rather than as a disability. As such, many in this community prefer identity-first language rather than person-first language. This concept is usually the antithesis of what students are taught in schools, as most training programs would advocate for "person with autism," rather than "autistic person" to use person-first language. This difference in wording can be easily addressed by asking clients and their families what language they prefer or listening to how they identify themselves and then using language that respects their choice (Dorsey et al. 2020).

A NOTE ON LANGUAGE

Should I use person with autism or autistic person with my client? – Understand that both parents and clients can become offended if you use language inconsistent with their beliefs and/or self-perception. While many professions advocate person first language, if unsure, *ask your client and use their preferred language!*

Some individuals with ASD who support the neurodiversity movement take issue with groups that support autism research, citing that research funding disproportionately supports efforts to find causes of autism and effective treatments, rather than funding efforts to support individuals themselves to make an active difference in their lives. Currently, much of the public efforts have begun to shift from solely autism awareness to autism acceptance, signaling the change to a more inclusive perspective. As a whole, established researchers have questioned if the neurodiversity movement will shift the full concept of disorders and intervention practices such as in psychiatry and other fields (Baron-Cohen 2017).

Language describing individuals with autism has also changed. In the past, common terms to describe abilities included "low functioning" and "high functioning," while current practices support describing abilities in reference to support and need such as "high support needs" or "low symptom severity." Alternatively, some researchers may use "highly verbal" as opposed to "high functioning." Similarly, many opt for "minimally verbal" instead of "nonverbal" to acknowledge those individuals who might have significantly limited verbal output but who still may present with some kind of verbal productions. Appropriate language is often evolving and interventionists should be mindful of current practices and reflect appropriate trends in light of changing information and preferences.

Additionally, many agencies have moved away from the use of imagery associated with autism, like the puzzle piece, as individuals with ASD have disputed the idea of autism as a puzzle or mystery to be solved rather than a person to be accepted and welcomed. Some current imagery may reflect other images such as an infinity symbol to represent the range of abilities and challenges in autism. Future imagery may consist of something completely different than what we see now. Overall, it is important to consider how our ideas and language about autism have transformed over the years and will likely continue to shift over time.

Research centered on reframing the social deficits in autism focus on evidence cited as the **double empathy problem**, which offers a counternarrative to common theory of mind deficits with findings that autistic people relate to each other much in the same way that neurotypical people relate to each other, despite the difficulty of interrelatedness between the two groups (Milton 2012; Mitchell et al. 2021). This idea presents the concept of autistic people as a minority group deemed "other" by a neurotypical majority. Such perspectives challenge ableist views that serve as the foundation of much of the medical community. Rather than solely considering ableist perspectives, the neurodiversity movement encourages people to consider diversity in social interaction skills rather than a binary right and wrong way of interacting with people. We encourage clinicians to consider this approach as all interventionists continue to evolve our understanding of autism and other neurodevelopmental disorders.

A NOTE ON TERMS

Aspie or Aspergian	This term may be used to refer to individuals formally diagnosed with **Asperger's syndrome**. Although this term is no longer used in current diagnostic criteria as of 2013 in favor of autism spectrum disorder<u>s</u> with accompanying levels of severity, many individuals who were first diagnosed with Asperger's Syndrome may still refer to themselves as such.
Autistic	Some clients might prefer **identity-first language** (e.g. autistic person) as opposed to **person-first language** (e.g. person with autism). If unsure, ask your client about their language preferences.
Masking	This term may refer to the **camouflaging** behaviors that some autistic people report doing in an attempt to fit in and/ or make their autistic traits less noticeable. Often, clients report this masking behavior is tiring and requires considerable effort.
Neurodivergent	This term may be used to refer to individuals with autism and other disorders, while the term **neurotypical** may be used to refer to individuals without such disorders.
Stimming	This term often refers to **self-stimulatory behaviors** credited as a restricted and/or repetitive behavior in the diagnostic criteria of ASD. Examples may include hand and/or finger mannerisms. Some autistic people report this behavior serves as a calming function to self-soothe when anxious.

One fact that is not lost on us is that individuals with moderate to severe symptomology are not fully represented in the neurodiversity conversation as these clients who continue to struggle with independent communication may very well have their own opinions that remain unknown. However, we applaud the autonomy of individuals with autism having a strong voice in their own care, a right we do not believe that educators or allied health professionals would deny any client. As clinicians, we have received the neurodiversity movement as yet another way of conceptualizing of autism and we support the shift away from the deficit narrative. Emerging research support the concept of celebrating deficits as differences, a perspective that is more welcomed by those who self-identify as autistic as well as those who report familiarity with the neurodiversity movement (Kapp et al. 2013). Some have warned of divisions spurred by the neurodiversity movement between those supporting autistic cultural identify and those with a perspective of the medical model of disability (Baker 2006). As future clinicians working with clients with ASD, we encourage you to consider the needs of your clients and their families, while not being tempted to view your clients from a deficit only approach.

SUMMARY

ASD is a complex neurodevelopmental disorder that centers around social communication challenges and includes the presence of restricted and repetitive behaviors. Causes of autism include genetic and environmental factors, although the complete cause remains unknown. The DSM-IV had three diagnostic domains required to meet diagnostic criteria for diagnosis: restricted and/or repetitive behaviors, communication, and social interaction challenges. The DSM-V reduced the diagnostic criteria to two domains and collapsed the domains of communication and social interaction to form the criteria of social communication. Current views support the idea of several disorders classified as an autism spectrum rather than former separate diagnostic categories such as PDD-NOS and Asperger's. Optimal treatment of ASD includes a collaborative approach between several disciplines with respective expertise. Treatment of ASD should focus on promoting communication and independence. The neurodiversity movement offers a perspective that includes more acceptance of neurological variance. The voices of individuals with autism should be included in their own care. This can be accomplished in part by valuing first-hand accounts, centering the scholarship of researchers with autism, and reconceptualizing the ideas of autism to prioritize strengths of individuals, rather than deficits.

REFLECTIONS ALONG THE PATH

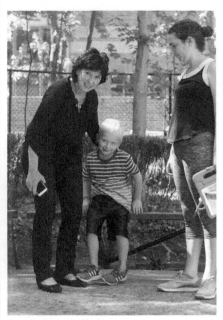

Connie Kasari, Ph.D.

I began working with children with disabilities in the late 1970s/early 1980s. We were just starting to work with severely delayed children, who had limited services and support. I was very involved in Child Find efforts, because at the time, school-aged children with disabilities were not given an opportunity to attend public school programs. That changed in the late 1970s with the passage of PL 94-142 (the Education for All Handicapped Children Act of 1975). Now that all children could gain access to school, we worked hard to locate children, often with the most severe disabilities, and to bring them into school settings. As educators, we also began working with infants and toddlers with disabilities, who previously were only seen by medical professionals. It was an exciting time of developing services for children with disabilities, and connecting families and children to these needed services.

I started out in a metropolitan area in the southern United States, working primarily with low-income, minority families and their severely disabled infants under the age of two years. All of these children and families were amazing, but one child in particular stood out to me. It was a little girl just under two years of age. Her developmental profile was very perplexing. She was not interested in toys or engaging with people. We could teach her something one day, but she would not show the skill again; or she learned something in one setting but could not demonstrate it across settings (like home and school). I now recognize that the child likely had autism, but at the time, I knew very little about this condition. Our team was very unprepared to help this child and her family, and I often think back to her now that we know so much more about interventions for children with autism.

I have spent my career trying to understand the core social communication difficulties of these children, and I have developed interventions to address their needs. Thirty years ago, when I began, three-quarters of children entering kindergarten were minimally verbal; today only about 30% of children remain minimally verbal. The field has made tremendous progress, and yet, we still have much more to learn. Today, I am involved in the combination and sequencing of interventions, to better personalize interventions for individual children. One thing we have learned is that a single intervention is not effective for all children, and that many children will benefit from several different interventions that are more or less intense during different phases of their development.

This recognized heterogeneity in autism also propels us to think about the children who are often left out of research studies, including minimally verbal children, and those with intellectual disability, females, low income, and ethnic-minority children. We need to do a better job of developing interventions that fit their needs. To do this work well, we also need to have a more diversified work force, one that reflects the cultural and linguistic needs of our population. I hope we can attract a broad and diverse new group of therapists who will see the potential in each and every child, and work to systematically personalize effective interventions.

Connie Kasari, Ph.D.
Professor of Human Development and Psychology and Professor of Psychiatry
University of California Los Angeles

TEST QUESTIONS

1. According to the DSM-IV, an ASD diagnosis was evaluated by ___ domains.
   A. 2
   B. 3
   C. 4
   D. 5

2. According to the DSM-V, the diagnostic criteria for ASD include the following categories except:
   A. Restricted and repetitive behaviors
   B. Social communication
   C. Social interaction
   D. All of the above

3. According to the DSM-V, an ASD diagnosis includes ___ key domains.
   A. 2
   B. 3
   C. 4
   D. 5

4. Which of the following is true about sex differences in ASD diagnostic rates?
   A. Boys are diagnosed more than girls
   B. Girls are diagnosed more than boys
   C. Boys and girls are diagnosed at the same rate
   D. Gender data about ASD diagnostic rates are unknown

5. Leo Kanner authored his seminal work about ASD in what year?
    A. 1984
    B. 1954
    C. 2002
    D. 1943

6. Restricted and repetitive behaviors may include all of the following except:
    A. Verbal rituals
    B. Difficulty disrupting routines
    C. Self-injury behaviors
    D. Difficulty maintaining eye gaze

7. In the autistic community, some clients may prefer identity-first language (autistic person) as opposed to person-first language (person with autism).

8. _____ are camouflaging behaviors that some autistic individuals may use to better fit in with neurotypical people.
    A. Masking
    B. Stimming
    C. Echolalia
    D. Facial grimaces

REFERENCES

Adams-Spink, G. (2011). Social model animation. *YouTube*, 7 November. Available at https://www.youtube.com/watch?v=9s3NZaLhcc4 (accessed 4 February 2022).

Baker, D. (2006). Neurodiversity, neurological disability and the public sector: notes on the autism spectrum. *Disability and Society* 21 (1): 15–29.

Baron-Cohen, S. (2017). Editorial perspective: neurodiversity – a revolutionary concept for autism and psychiatry. *Journal of Child Psychology and Psychiatry* 58 (6): 744–747.

Bottema-Beutel, K., Kapp, S., Lester, J. et al. (2021). Avoiding Ableist language: suggestions for autism researchers. *Autism in Adulthood* 3 (1): 18–29.

Chaste, P. and Leboyer, M. (2012). Autism risk factors: genes, environment, and gene-environment interactions. *Dialogues in Clinical Neuroscience* 14 (3): 281–292.

Dorsey, R., Crow, H., and Gaddy, C. (2020). *Putting Autistic Voices at the Forefront of Care.* The ASHA Leader.

Geschwind, D. (2008). Autism: many genes, common pathways? *Cell* 135 (3): 391–395.

den Houting, J. (2019). Neurodiversity: an insider's perspective. *Autism* 23 (2): 271–273.

Jaarsma, P. and Welin, S. (2012). Autism as a natural human variation: reflections on the claims of the neurodiversity movement. *Health Care Analysis* 20: 20–30.

Kanner, L. (1943). Autistic disturbances of affective contact. *The Nervous Child* 2: 217–250.

Kapp, S., Gillespie-Lynch, K., Sherman, L., and Hutman, T. (2013). Deficit, difference, or both? Autism and neurodiversity. *Developmental Psychology* 49 (1): 59–71.

Kapp, S., Steward, R., Crane, L. et al. (2019). 'People should be allowed to do what they like' autistic adults' views and experiences of stimming. *Autism* 23 (7): 1782–1792.

Kleinhans, N., Muller, R., Cohen, D., and Courchesne, E. (2008). Atypical functional lateralization of language in autism spectrum disorders. *Brain Research* 1221: 115–125.

Krcek, T. (2013). Deconstructing disability and neurodiversity: controversial issues for autism and implications for social work. *Journal of Progressive Human Services* 24: 4–22.

Milton, D. (2012). On the ontological status of autism: the 'double empathy problem'. *Disability and Society* 27 (6): 883–887.

Mitchell, P., Sheppard, E., and Cassidy, S. (2021). Autism and the double empathy problem: implications for development and mental health. *British Journal of Developmental Psychology* 39: 1–18.

Mody, M. and McDougle, C. (2019). Getting the word "out": a role for the motor system in autism spectrum disorder. *Perspectives of the ASHA Special Interest Groups* 4 (6): 1221–1228.

Muhle, R., Trentacoste, S., and Rapin, I. (2004). The genetics of autism. *Pediatrics* 113 (5): e472–e486.

Rylaarsdam, L. and Guemez-Gamboa, A. (2019). Genetic causes and modifiers of autism spectrum disorder. *Frontiers in Cellular Neuroscience* 13: 385.

Sahyoun, C., Belliveau, J., and Mody, M. (2010). White matter integrity and pictorial reasoning in high-functioning children with autism. *Brain and Cognition* 73 (3): 180–188.

Schumann, C., Bloss, C., Barnes, C. et al. (2010). Longitudinal magnetic resonance imaging study of cortical development through early childhood in autism. *Journal of Neuroscience* 30 (12): 4419–4427.

Shyman, E. (2016). The reinforcement of ableism: normality, the medical model of disability, and humanism in applied behavior analysis and ASD. *Intellectual and Developmental Disabilities* 54 (5): 366–376.

Whitney, E., Kempter, T., Bauman, M. et al. (2008). Cerebellar Purkinje cells are reduced in a subpopulation of autistic brains: a stereotypical experiment using calbindin-D28k. *Cerebellum* 7 (3): 406–416.

FURTHER READINGS

Cosentino, L., Vigli, D., Franchi, F. et al. (2019). Rett syndrome before regression: a time window of overlooked opportunities for diagnosis and intervention. *Neuroscience and Biobehavioral Reviews* 107: 115–135.

Geschwind, D.H. and Constantino, J.N. (2010). Brief report: under-representation of African Americans in autism genetic research: a rationale for inclusion of subjects representing diverse family structures. *Journal of Autism and Developmental Disorders* 40 (5): 633–639.

Hilton, C.L., Fitzgerald, R.T., Jackson, K.M. et al. (2016). Hispanic immigrant mothers of young children with autism spectrum disorders: how do they understand and cope with autism? *American Journal of Speech-Language Pathology* 25: 200–213.

Jiang, X., Matson, J., Cervantes, P. et al. (2017). Gastrointestinal issues in infants and children with autism and developmental delays. *Journal of Developmental and Physical Disabilities* 29: 407–417.

Kayama, M. (2010). Parental experiences of children's disabilities and special education in the United States and Japan: implications for school social work. *Social Work* 55 (2): 117–125.

Keller-Bell, Y. (2017). Disparities in the identification and diagnosis of autism spectrum disorder in culturally and linguistically diverse populations. *Perspectives of the ASHA Special Interest Groups* 2 (Part 3): 68–81.

Lovaas, O. (1987). Behavioral treatment and normal educational and intellectual functioning in young autistic children. *Journal of Consulting and Clinical Psychology* 55 (1): 3–9.

Lovaas, O., Schaeffer, B., and Simmons, J. (1965). Building social behavior in autistic children by use of electric shock. *Journal of Experimental Research in Personality* 1 (2): 99–109.

Mandell, D., Ittenbach, R., Levy, S., and Pinto-Martin, J. (2010). Disparities in diagnoses received prior to a diagnosis of autism spectrum disorder. *Journal of Autism and Developmental Disorders* 37 (9): 1795–1802.

Nguyen, C.T., Krakowiak, P., Hansen, R. et al. (2016). Sociodemographic disparities in intervention service utilization in families of children with autism spectrum disorder. *Journal of Autism and Developmental Disorders* 46 (12): 3729–3738.

Sannar, E., Palka, T., Beresford, C. et al. (2018). Sleep problems and their relationship to maladaptive behavior severity in psychiatrically hospitalized children with autism spectrum disorder (ASD). *Journal of Autism and Developmental Disorders* 48: 3720–3726.

Sokolova, E., Oerlemans, A., Rommelse, N. et al. (2017). A casual and mediation analysis of the comorbidity between attention deficit hyperactivity disorder (ADHD) and autism spectrum disorder (ASD). *Journal of Autism and Developmental Disorders* 47: 1595–1604.

Walker, N. and Raymaker, D. (2020). Toward a neuroqueer future: an interview with Nick Walker. *Autism in Adulthood* 3 (1): https://doi.org/10.1089/aut.2020.29014. njw.Connie Kasari, Ph.D.

CHAPTER 2

Indications for Assessment

Learning Objectives

By reading this chapter, interventionists will be able to:

1. Identify at least five indications for assessment for autism spectrum disorder (ASD).
2. Name at least two different formal and informal assessment tools for ASD.
3. List common barriers for successfully diagnosing ASD in culturally and/or linguistically diverse populations.
4. Identify at least three key members on an assessment team and their roles.
5. Identify critical components of appropriate intervention goals.
6. Define the acronym SMART.

Appropriately assessing autism is critical to access appropriate evidenced-based practices that can promote optimal outcomes. Misdiagnosis and non-diagnosis are harmful to individuals and their families because they can miss essential early intervention services, which are important to help close the gap in skills prior to a child entering school. While it is clearly critical to accurately identify ASD, findings from recent studies indicate that only about half of professionals like speech–language pathologists (*SLPs*) accurately identify diagnostic criteria for autism to include both social communication deficits and the presence of restricted and/or repetitive behaviors (Beverly and

Matthews, 2021). Evidence suggests that early screening tools such as the Modified Checklist for Autism in Toddlers, Revised with Follow-up (M-CHAT-R/F), can be reliable in detecting autism in children less than two years of age (Robins et al., 2014). Despite autism symptomology being able to be reliably documented as early as age two, many children are not diagnosed until years later, which restricts access to appropriate intervention (Moore and Goodson, 2003). Those who work with young children, such as SLPs, SLP assistants, early education specialists, and others may play a critical role in helping to identify children exhibiting symptomology, referring those children to assessment, and advocating for those children to receive proper intervention services (Swineford, 2017). Overall, research is clear in the critical need to bridge early identification with early treatment (Crais and Watson, 2013).

So how does a child get assessed appropriately and who should do assessments? The exact 'how' can vary across settings, but appropriate assessment should include thorough evaluation using a variety of formal and informal assessment measures that confirm consistent symptomology across contexts and evaluators. Assessments should be conducted by professionals with particular expertise in child development and autism, as not all professionals are trained to evaluate for ASD. Qualified individuals should be able to specifically identify their credentials, licenses, and experiences that make them particularly capable of diagnosing autism.

As SLPs with more than 20 years of experience working with individuals with ASD, we often see one of two possibilities:

1. The parents themselves have concerns and are actively seeking answers, although they might not exactly suspect ASD. These caregivers may have noted a delay in speech and language or have another child with ASD or have a family history of communication delays.
2. The parents do not have direct concerns, but are seeking answers to dispute someone else's concerns. Maybe their pediatrician raised a few questions or their brother's wife, who is a preschool teacher, suggested an evaluation.

In our experience, these two groups will report their child's behavior very differently, although they may be describing the same acts using very different terminology and connotations. Recall from Chapter 1 that ASD is differentially marked by two key diagnostic criteria: (i) social communication deficits and (ii) restricted and repetitive behaviors. Symptoms must be present in early childhood, although they might not present as clinically significant until later in development with changing social communication demands. Autism can look *significantly* different from case to case, since it has historically been considered as a *spectrum* with a wide range of presentations. We depend on behavioral assessments and differential diagnosis to evaluate ASD. To properly diagnose, we rely on clinical observation and formal assessment, in conjunction with caregiver report. We also look holistically at other points of concern like early repetitive play with objects, low sensitivity to social cues, and atypical motor development, which may all be indicative of concern for autism (Zwaigenbaum et al., 2015).

Differences in parent report is where it can get tricky! Parents may describe behaviors in a variety of ways, which is why it is important to get a variety of caregiver reports in addition to clinical observation and standardized testing to confirm diagnosis. Some examples of points of concern reported by parents are shown in Figure 2.1.

AUTISM AND ASSESSMENT OF CULTURALLY, LINGUISTICALLY DIVERSE POPULATIONS

Differences in parent report become vital when it comes to appropriate diagnosis. Neurodevelopmental disorders like ASD rely on behaviorally defined diagnostic criteria that can be strongly influenced by cultural values and expectations (Norbury and Sparks, 2013). Culturally and/or linguistically diverse parents may have differences in parent report. Clinicians across all fields must demonstrate cultural competence in effectively distinguishing among differences in parent report to promote accurate diagnosis. Children of color are diagnosed with ASD later than their white counterparts. African-American children are frequently misdiagnosed as having behavior problems before later being diagnosed with ASD (Mandell et al., 2010). These diagnoses may reflect a combination of racial bias on behalf of evaluators, as well as a lack of cultural competence that may prevent evaluators from appropriately interpreting parent report. Misdiagnosis can prevent these children from receiving targeted therapy

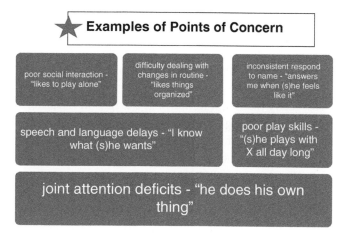

Examples of Points of Concern

poor social interaction - "likes to play alone"	difficulty dealing with changes in routine - "likes things organized"	inconsistent respond to name - "answers me when (s)he feels like it"

speech and language delays - "I know what (s)he wants"

poor play skills - "(s)he plays with X all day long"

joint attention deficits - "he does his own thing"

FIGURE 2.1   Examples of points of concern reported by parents.

Active Learning Task

How else might a caregiver describe common autism symptomology? Identify at least two other statements you might hear from a parent that can be a concern for autism.

services in early intervention that can promote optimal life outcomes. As such, it is critically important to educate all interventionists on cultural biases that might adversely impact their clinical judgment, while also promoting advocacy to help families effectively navigate access to services for their children with special needs.

There is evidence that race and ethnicity, in addition to other factors such as socioeconomic status and language background, are related to disparities in services for families impacted by autism (Nguyen et al., 2016; Wiley, 2016). Cultural differences may prevent parents from advocating for necessary services for their children. For example, Japanese culture places a high importance on blending in and respecting rules and seniority, which may prevent them from readily offering dissenting opinions on an intervention plan even if they disagree (Kayama, 2010; Seung, 2013). Researchers urge the importance of culturally appropriate assessment that can be effective in low-resource areas, in addition to increasing awareness of autism to reduce stigma (Wang et al., 2019).

Among Hispanic immigrant mothers, preconceptions about autism and developmental milestones may be barriers to early diagnosis and treatment (Ijalba, 2016). Latino parents have identified various barriers to ASD diagnosis including limited information about ASD, disability stigma in the Latino community, limited English proficiency, and poor access to healthcare services, in addition to an often confusing diagnostic process (Zuckerman et al., 2014). Disparities in ASD diagnosis for African-American and Hispanic populations, as well as differences in access to intervention services, have been clearly documented (Keller-Bell, 2017). Additionally, the absence of African-American representation in autism research such as the noted underrepresentation in ASD genetic research has been acknowledged (Hilton et al., 2010). Additionally, in many cultures, awareness and accurate knowledge of ASD may be limited. For example, survey research exploring awareness of ASD in Saudi Arabia found that many respondents know about autism, but reported limited knowledge and incorrectly likened it to mental retardation (Alsehemi et al., 2017).

Ethnographic interviewing may be the best approach for families from diverse backgrounds. This approach of using open-ended questions rather than questions that produce yes/no responses may yield more descriptive answers that gather more client participation (Westby et al., 2003). Furthermore, as assessment also involves counseling to families to begin the intervention process, it is important to consider cultural values in order to provide treatment plans that are culturally responsive and aligned with the family's views rather than only applying evidenced-based approaches often lauded as best practices, but with little application across diverse cultural groups (Ravindran and Myers, 2012).

Active Learning Task

Research a peer-reviewed journal article centered on the experience of a culturally, linguistically diverse group and autism. How might you adjust your future clinical practices to better meet the needs of culturally, linguistically diverse families impacted by ASD? Following the assignment, engage in small groups to discuss findings and clinical approaches.

Differential Diagnosis

It is important to be able to differentiate ASD from other disorders. Appropriate diagnosis is the key to appropriate intervention. Autism can often present with elements of symptoms of other disorders, which is why appropriate diagnosis will include a team of trained professionals who have extensive knowledge about typical developmental milestones and a variety of disorders to effectively rule out other diagnoses (Figure 2.2).

Key to a diagnosis of autism is that symptoms must not be better explained by a different diagnosis. As such, it is important to be aware of other disorders that may better explain symptoms other than a diagnosis of ASD. For example, pediatric hearing impairment can present similarly to ASD in poor response to name and reduced language skills so it would be important to rule out hearing impairment to help prevent misdiagnosis (Camarata, 2013).

Diagnoses Other than Autism

Attention-deficit/hyperactivity disorder (ADHD) is characterized by key diagnostic criteria of inattention and impulsivity. Further, it can present as predominantly inattention, predominantly impulsivity, or a combination of both. Overlapping characteristics can often be confused for autism, particularly in highly verbal individuals. For example, difficulties in autism of maintaining a topic in conversation may appear very similar to inattention in clients with ADHD who may appear not to listen during conversation or may appear easily distracted.

Developmental language delay is also indicated in early childhood by expressive language delays. These children can present similarly to children with ASD because both may demonstrate less interest in interaction and less integrated eye gaze; however, in comparison with ASD, children with developmental language delay demonstrate more pretend play skills and use of gesture (Paul et al., 2008).

Obsessive–compulsive disorder (OCD) has diagnostic criteria of the presence of obsessions or compulsions, or a combination of both. Examples of compulsions can be repetitive behaviors applied in a rigid way, which can be misinterpreted as restricted and/or repetitive behaviors present in ASD.

Rett syndrome is a neurological disorder typically characterized by cognitive, physical, and social deficits. Also unlike ASD, it predominantly impacts girls. Unlike autism, it is linked to a specific gene mutation, although its presentation is often described by autism like characteristics (Cosentino et al., 2019).

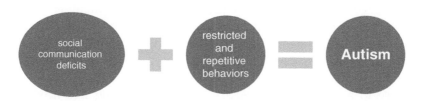

FIGURE 2.2   Recall the two key diagnostic criteria for ASD reviewed in Chapter 1.

Social pragmatic or *social communication disorder* is defined as persistent difficulties in the social use of verbal and nonverbal communication that results in functional limitations in effective communication, social participation, social relationships, academic achievement, and/or occupational performance. Similar to ASD, symptoms must be present in the early developmental period and symptoms should not be better explained by another disorder. This disorder presents highly similar to ASD, but remember, ASD must also include the presence of restricted and/or repetitive behaviors.

Active Learning Task

See the criteria below for a diagnosis of Social Pragmatic Disorder according to the DSM-V. How might this diagnosis differ from a diagnosis of autism? How might someone without sufficient knowledge in diagnostic criteria misdiagnose a client with autism with social pragmatic disorder?

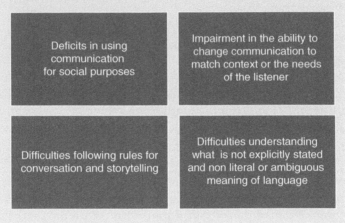

Autism Spectrum Disorder Diagnostic Team

There are a variety of professionals who may serve on the diagnostic team, which may be smaller than the clinical services team if assessment warrants intervention. Team based diagnosis aims to triangulate observations and reconcile differences in presentation. In an ideal assessment, all members of the team would note common presentations, such as lack of response to name, poor joint attention skills, reduced play skills, and poor social engagement. Here are some ideas of members to include:

Audiologists specialize in hearing by diagnosing hearing difficulties and providing support to compensate for hearing deficits. Many presentations of ASD, such as inconsistent response to name or apparent lack of social interaction, can be confused with hearing challenges (Camarata, 2013). An audiologist can help to rule out hearing difficulties and contribute to appropriate diagnosis. A child with hearing loss needs appropriate intervention that strongly differs from ASD intervention. Appropriate early intervention with hearing loss can lead to optimal outcomes with speech and language development.

Primary caregivers are the people who spend the most time with the child. They could be biological parents, grandparents, foster parents, or any adult who is primarily responsible for the child's overall warfare. Professionals may have expertise in their respective fields, but family members are experts on the child! Parents or primary caregivers provide critical background information on the child and family to contribute to differential diagnosis. Key information needs to be gathered during a thorough caregiver interview including client medical history (birth history, prior diagnoses, etc.), speech and language milestones (first words, play level, social interaction, etc.), gross motor development (crawling, walking, etc.), and current levels of functioning. The most important question you can ask during a caregiver interview is "What are your concerns?" Professionals must demonstrate cultural competence during the caregiver interview process, especially as it relates to appropriately interpreting parent report. Because this portion of the diagnostic process is so important, considerations must be made for caregivers who do not speak English as a first language. Using an interpreter or other linguistic and cultural broker is critical to obtaining accurate information to best inform assessment.

Speech-language pathologists (*SLPs*) specialize in communication disorders including receptive and expressive language skills and speech, as well as feeding and pragmatic skills. An evaluation for ASD must include a speech and language evaluation that includes formal and informal assessment. A SLP has extensive knowledge and training on typical speech and language milestones. An evaluation will assess: (i) if the child is demonstrating delays, (ii) whether those delays exhibit expressive or receptive language difficulties or both, and (iii) how extensive those delays are in comparison to typically developing peers. If the child is exposed to languages other than English, it is important to obtain a bilingual evaluation with a bilingual SLP, or appropriately trained SLP assistant, or interpreter to support during the evaluation to rule out language differences from disorders.

Neurodevelopmental pediatricians are medical doctors who have additional training in the subspeciality of developmental-behavioral pediatrics. This additional training and certification is different from a pediatrician, a medical doctor who is responsible for a child's physical health. A pediatrician may be concerned about typical development because The American Academy of Pediatrics recommends all children receive ASD screenings at their 18- and 24-month medical visits. Results from the screening may lead to a referral to a developmental pediatrician who has the expertise for differential diagnosis of ASD.

Neurodevelopmental psychologists with specific training and expertise in autism assessment are professionals well versed in child development. They are often trained in using ASD specific assessment tools such as the M-CHAT-R/S, Childhood Autism Rating Scale, second edition (CARS-2), Autism Diagnostic Interview, Revised (ADI-R), and the Autism Diagnostic Observation Schedule, second edition (ADOS-2). These professionals should have extensive experience in working with children and have a proper understanding of the range of typical development to appropriately identify atypical development.

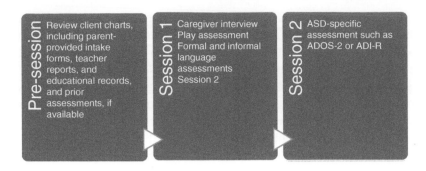

Pre-session Review client charts, including parent-provided intake forms, teacher reports, and educational records, and prior assessments, if available

Session 1 Caregiver interview Play assessment Formal and informal language assessments Session 2

Session 2 ASD-specific assessment such as ADOS-2 or ADI-R

FIGURE 2.3   Evaluation process for ASD assessment.

In additional to the professionals named above, a variety of other professionals may be involved to rule out other diagnoses and appropriately assess ASD. For example, if needed, an **interpreter** would be an important member of the assessment team so families can fully participate in the evaluation process Figure 2.3.

Therapy Golden Nugget
As an interventionist, your objective is to provide parents with appropriate information to help them be informed about the evaluation process. When seeking out an evaluation, especially if there are concerns about a diagnosis of autism, encourage families to directly ask evaluators about their experience with children with ASD. This experience should include graduate level education, training, certification, and clinical experience. All professionals should encourage families to advocate for transparency.

ASSESSMENT TOOLS

Autism Specific Formal Screeners and Evaluations

A list of some common formal and informal evaluations used in ASD assessment is provided in Table 2.1. This list is not exhaustive. Evaluation methods should include language samples, naming and imitation tasks, and thorough analysis of speech, language, and behavioral characteristics (Broome et al., 2017). Among screening tools, evidence suggests tools like the M-CHAT-R/F, First Years Inventory, and Quantitative-Checklist for Autism in Toddlers (*Q-CHAT*) are helpful for healthcare professionals for early indicators (Petrocchi et al., 2020). For young children at high risk, such as those with an older sibling already diagnosed with autism, screening tools like the Systematic Observation of Red Flags have demonstrated appropriate discrimination, specificity, and sensitivity to measure for ASD (Pileggi et al., 2021).

TABLE 2.1   Autism-specific tests.

Tool	Purpose
Screening tools	**Help determine the need for further assessment.**
Modified Checklist for Autism in Toddlers, Revised (MCHAT)	Presents questions about a child's behavior. It will provide an indicator of risk for autism to share with a professional and inform the need for a formal assessment. This screening is readily available for caregivers or anyone suspecting an autism diagnosis for their child.
Communication and Symbolic Behavior Scales Developmental Profile	Helps to determine the need for a formal developmental evaluation. The Infant Child Checklist is readily available and encouraged as a tool at an infant's first year check-up to help identify children at risk for ASD.
Standardized assessments	**Provide a component of a formal diagnosis.**
Autism Diagnostic Observation Schedule, 2nd edition (ADOS-2)	Administered with a client to characterize the severity of ASD symptoms and help determine treatment planning. Modules are available for minimally verbal to verbally fluent children and adults. There is also a toddler version of the assessment for younger children. Test-specific training is recommended for this assessment, which typically includes multi-day training.
Autism Diagnostic Interview Revised (ADI/R)	Administered to parents of a client being assessed for autism and information is wholly gathered from caregiver interview.
Childhood Autism Rating Scale, 2nd edition (CARS-2)	Helps to identify ASD and symptom severity.
Gilliam Autism Rating Scale, 3rd edition (**GARS-3**)	Helps to identify ASD, indicate severity, and determine appropriate intervention approaches.

Some of these tools are available in a number of different languages. Tools should be administered by a professional with appropriate training in administering standardized assessments, in addition to training language.

Holistic Formal Assessment

In addition to an autism specific assessment, other evaluations should be conducted to gather a full picture of the client's strengths and weaknesses. While guidelines vary across settings and locations, we strongly suggest using at least three different standardized measures, together with informal assessment to appropriately diagnose autism. When possible, formal assessments should be administered for speech and language to compare the child with age-matched peers. Such assessments will provide percentile ranks, age-equivalents, and standardized scores. Some of those assessments may include those shown in Table 2.2.

TABLE 2.2   Core areas tests.

Name	Purpose
Rossetti Infant–Toddler Language Scale	This criterion-referenced measure is not norm referenced so it does not compare children with age-matched peers, but it does allow the examiner to evaluate mastery of assessed behaviors. This measure assesses communication and interaction skills for children up to age three and includes subtests for: interaction attachment, pragmatics, gesture, play, language comprehension, and language expression. A criterion-reference assessment may be appropriate for diverse clients not represented in a standardization profile for standardized formal assessments.
Preschool Language Scales, 5th edition (**PLS-5**)	This language assessment is for birth to 7 years, 11 months and includes preverbal skills. Identifying expressive and receptive language skills is a critical component of assessment for ASD. This formal assessment is also available in Spanish.
Comprehensive Assessment of Spoken Language, 2nd edition (**CASL-2**)	This oral language assessment is for ages 3–21. There are a number of individual subtests that can be administered to assess skills in the following areas: lexical/semantic, pragmatic, syntactic, and supralinguistic.
Differential Ability Scales – II (**DAS-II**)	This test will assess processing and cognitive abilities to help identify learning disabilities and intellectual disability. It may be helpful to rule out other disorders or to diagnose a comorbid disorder such as autism with accompanying intellectual impairment. Translations in Spanish are available.
Mullen Scales of Early Learning	This assessment will evaluate expressive and receptive language skills, as well as motor skills (fine and gross motor).

INFORMAL ASSESSMENT

In addition to formal assessments with standardized scores and cut offs, informal assessments are a valuable tool that should not be excluded from the evaluation process (Table 2.3) formal assessments and informal assessments are. Although there are a number of different potential evaluation procedures, it is important to note that there should never be one single test or evaluation to diagnose for autism, especially since formal diagnosis is so heavily dependent upon parent and caregiver report and behavioral observations. Different tools and assessors should be used to confirm congruence in reports; simply put, behaviors should be identified across settings, contexts, informants, and evaluators.

TABLE 2.3   Informal evaluations.

Informal evaluation	Purpose
Language sample analysis (LSA)	Aside from formal assessment, evaluating the child's use of language in natural contexts is critical. LSA can be obtained via open-ended questions, picture books, and/or play as appropriate. The assessor should note the variety of language used, pragmatic skills, syntactic complexity, and mean length of utterance.
Play evaluation	Play skills should be evaluated as abilities in this area are often impacted in ASD. The assessor should note eye contact, use of gestures, play level, social overtures, appropriate toy play, responses to bids for joint attention, and initiation of play acts.
Parent interview	Parents are key components of assessment. They should provide information on developmental history as well as explain their concerns about their child's current functioning.
Natural environment observation	Observing a child in the natural environment may not always be feasible, but is a helpful component of a comprehensive evaluation. For young children, it may involve an observation at the child's home or other familiar environment. For older children, a school observation can indicate how the child is interacting with peers in the academic environment.
Review of records	This includes a review of prior assessments and reports. Ideally, reports should present similar findings and indicate social communication deficits and the presence of restricted and/or repetitive behaviors.

THE GENDER DISPARITY

Since ASD was first "discovered," there was a noted gender disparity in diagnostic rates. Researchers find the male to female ratio to be three to one, suggesting that the diagnostic criteria are closer than previously assumed and girls are at risk for not receiving targeted intervention because of gender bias (Looms et al., 2017).

As illustrated in Figure 2.4, current ASD diagnostic rates continue to identify more boys than girls with the disorder. Researchers continue to acknowledge girls may present with different ASD symptomology than boys and, in fact, be underdiagnosed because they fail to demonstrate more classic and overt characteristics (Dean et al., 2017). Further illustrating gender differences, boys with autism reported

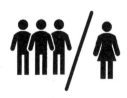

FIGURE 2.4   Note the gender disparity in ASD with more prevalence among boys than girls.

less social motivation for friendship than boys without autism and girls with and without autism (Sedgewick et al., 2016). Dworzynski et al. (2012) concluded that girls are less likely than boys to meet diagnostic criteria for ASD in the absence of accompanying behavioral or intellectual problems, suggesting a sex bias in diagnosis.

Evidence suggests that girls might be more adept at masking than boys and this use of camouflaging can contribute to reduced diagnosis (Mandy, 2019). School-age girls with autism may present with camouflaging behaviors like flitting, or moving swiftly, from task to task, rather than more clearly overt social isolation and solitary play observed in boys, in addition to linguistic camouflage features such as using fillers and pauses in conversation (Dean et al., 2017; Parish-Morris et al., 2017). As more evidence that girls with autism may be harder to distinguish from their neurotypical peers, findings indicate that girls with and without autism have similar friendships and social experiences, although girls with autism report more conflict and more difficulty in effectively resolving conflict (Sedgewick et al., 2019). Among toddlers, preschool girls diagnosed with autism tend to have more severe social communication deficits than preschool boys with autism (Ros-Demarize et al., 2020). In adolescence, girls with autism demonstrated more severe presentations on social responsiveness measures than boys with autism, while boys with autism demonstrated more severe restricted and repetitive scores than girls with autism on standardized measures (Katt et al., 2021). You should be aware of nuances specific to girls when noting potential symptoms of ASD and determining the need for referral.

KEY CONSIDERATIONS FOR EVALUATION OF ASD IN GIRLS

✓ *Discern between proximity and truly sustained social engagement.* Girls may "flit" from task to task, so they do not readily appear solitary; however, they lack sustained engagement in conversation or play with peers.

✓ *Note the appropriateness of conversation.* Girls may demonstrate highly verbal skills on age-appropriate topics, but lack typical flexibility and topic shifts in conversation.

✓ *Account for parent report.* Girls may be skilled in masking in socially demanding tasks like school, but then devolve in other contexts like at home with parents. This behavior may be dismissed as "moodiness" due to culturally dictated gender roles.

COMORBIDITY

While a client may have a primary diagnosis of autism, it is important to note that some clients may also present with symptoms of other disorders in addition to autism. The presence of **comorbid** diagnoses is not true in all cases, but ASD is noted to have increased instances of comorbidity with some additional diagnoses. For example, an additional diagnosis of *intellectual impairment* may be warranted in some cases and can serve to explain the significantly limited response to intervention in some clients. A number of comorbid conditions with autism have been identified including connections with:

- anxiety and depression
- attention defecit hyperactivty disorder (ADHD)
- obsessive compulsive disorder (OCD)
- sleep disorders
- gastrointestinal issues
- seizure disorders

Acknowledging comorbid conditions allows interventionists to determine how comorbidities may impact development, which might adversely impact progress toward speech and language goals (Chenausky et al., 2021). Research on the prevalence and significance of comorbid disorders are often evolving along with suggestions for assessment and intervention. For example, for children with autism and childhood apraxia of speech, specific evidenced-based interventions accounting for both diagnoses have shown mixed results and may require continuing evaluation to determine effectiveness (Beiting and Maas, 2021). As such, interventionists are strongly encouraged to keep up to date on the literature to best serve their clients.

The adage from Dr. Steven Shore, "If you've met one person with autism disorder, then you've met one person with autism disorder" becomes even more applicable, as ASD symptomology combined with the presence of comorbid conditions can contribute to significantly different presentations from case to case. In all cases, holistic, client-centered care is paramount. Prioritize parent concerns and child academic needs, while considering long-term implications. Refer to specialists when appropriate. Of critical importance when treating clients with autism and additional comorbid conditions, the interventionist must consider all diagnoses and treat conditions separately while considering the client's holistic needs. The most important concern should always be promoting optimal outcomes for our clients and supporting their diagnostic and intervention needs.

Active Learning Task

After reading the brief news magazine articles below, discuss how a child with autism and a comorbid diagnosis might present differently than a child with autism only.

Gastrointestinal symptoms more common in children with autism. *The ASHA Leader*, 2014, 19(7), 13. https://doi.org/10.1044/leader.RIB2.19072014.13.

Szarkowski, A. and Johnston, J. Dually diagnosed: autism and hearing loss. *The ASHA Leader*, 2018, 23(4), 20–21. https://doi.org/10.1044/leader.AEA.23042018.20.

CLINICAL APPLICATION

What might an ASD assessment look like in the real world? Here is a step-by-step approach of how we have approached ASD assessment in clinical settings when conducting a comprehensive evaluation.

So, your assessment starts when the client enters the clinic room, right? Not at all! Assessment starts before the client ever arrives. You should review the client's chart that might include prior assessments, teacher reports and education records, and client intake form. You want to get a picture of the client based on prior evaluations and look for consistency in reporting. Does the parent report the client has "a hard time saying what he wants," and his preschool teacher says, "he tantrums often?" This indicates congruence. You are essentially looking for behavioral characteristics across contexts that are areas of concern. Likewise, you might look for areas that are not consistent between reports. For example, you might see the parent report on the intake form that they "have no concerns, but the doctor wanted an evaluation." This also gives you critical information. You will want to explore the dichotomy of these two perspectives.

One of the most strikingly different reports we have ever received? A single mom of a four-year old boy reported no concerns. Why had she come for an assessment? She was with her son at Starbucks and another customer commented, "Oh, he talks so much for a boy with autism! Where does he go for speech?" ☺ Yep. That happened. After assessment, the child actually did meet criteria for an autism diagnosis, but the mother was never concerned about development because she thought autism was only "for kids who don't talk."

If the client has not sent pertinent case history prior to the appointment, we ask them to arrive early and we give the intake form paperwork to the parent to complete before they come in the room. The assessment starts the moment the family enters the door (sometimes in the parking lot if we see them walking up). We begin to listen for verbalizations, atypical vocal presentations, and how the client interacts with the family. We look at how they respond when greeted. We even leave the door open as they complete paperwork to overhear how they are interacting in the waiting room. All of that is key informal data.

As the client enters, we will typically start with informal assessment with clients irrespective of age. Generally, we think it is helpful to build rapport so the client and family are comfortable with you. As seasoned assessors, we can accomplish this relatively quickly. For newer clinicians, this may be more challenging. Generally, this is a skill that comes with repeated practice over time. Interpersonal skills are a critical foundation of intervention fields. Personally, we *love* this part of assessment. We get to put our personality on display to get people to let their guards down and feel at ease. In sessions, you can almost feel the difference in the room when clients do this. They let out a breath. They laugh. They ease into their chair. So how do you do this? Mostly, you focus on assuring them that you are warm and competent – we hope this is not a reach, so it should be easy! Smile and welcome them into your office space.

Make a bit of small talk. If nothing fails, an easy "Such a nice day outside!" or "I can't believe it's still snowing!" comment can do the trick. We often take note of clothing. Is the client's parent wearing a Laker jersey? Start to comment on last night's game. Is the child holding a superhero toy? Start talking about it! This approach sets the stage to building rapport and collect informal data. *So what kind of informal data do you want to collect?* Among other data, you may want to explore items similar to the checklist below.

Therapy Golden Nugget

Client Name: _____

Interventionist: _____

Area to assess	Y/N	Clinical notes
Behavioral observations for younger clients: • Does the child demonstrate **emotional regulation** skills? • Does the child transition into the clinic room? • Does the child attend to tasks or require frequent redirections? • Does the child engage in presented activities or require reinforcement and positive behavior support?		
Play observations for younger clients: • What level of play does the client demonstrate? • Does the child initiate play independently? If not, does the child respond to bids for play or imitate play? • During play, does the child make eye contact and demonstrate language skills?		
Receptive language: • Does the child follow directions? One step? Two-step? Multistep? • Does the child demonstrate understanding of simple what, where, who, questions? • Does the child respond spontaneously to posed questions or do they only respond when you also use gestures or give forced choices?		
Expressive language: • Does the child ask you any questions? • Does the child answer verbally? With gestures/signs? • With verbal responses, what is the mean length of utterance? • Does the child integrate eye gaze, facial expressions, and gestures with verbal output?		

The informal information above can be compared with the formal assessment results and caregiver report. Evidence shows natural language sampling can be more representative of language skills than skills demonstrated during standardized assessments like the ADOS-2 (Kover et al., 2014). As such, it is critical to value the information yielded from informal assessments procedures such as natural language samples and play observations independent of formal evaluations. Again, you are looking for consistency. Overall, we might allot 20–30 minutes or so for this portion depending on the child age, language level, and engagement, in addition to clinical constraints.

As lack of language is often an early concern that prompts parents to seek assessment, a formal language assessment should be completed. A child may only have a language delay and not autism. Likewise, a child without language delay may also have autism. Thus, it is critical to conduct a complete language assessment. We will select the type of assessment based on child age and initial impressions of language level. Typically, a younger child will do better on a play-based standardized assessment such as the Preschool Language Scales, fifth edition (PLS-5), while older children with more verbal abilities can exhibit their skills on assessments that call for more expressive output like the Comprehensive Assessment of Spoken Language, second edition (CASL-2), Clinical Evaluation of Language Fundamentals, fifth edition (*CELF-5*), or Oral and Written Language Scales, second edition (*OWLS-2*). Children with various types of verbal skills can benefit from standardized receptive and expressive vocabulary tests as well to help offer a complete picture of language abilities.

Caregiver Counseling

Following the assessment, it is critical to end your session with appropriate caregiver counseling, which can be challenging. Often, professionals do not receive adequate training on successfully delivering bad news, and the emotional burden this can take from the very start of one's professional career (Gold and Gold, 2018). Following an autism evaluation, your caregiver counseling should include your initial impressions as well as suggestions for things the parents can do at home to improve upon existing skills. Consider the importance of **soft skills** in your delivery, which includes what you say and how you say it. This critical juncture can often leave a lasting impression on parents and set the tone for their perception of healthcare professionals and clinical services. Interventionists should consider the emotions and grieving issues that can coincide with communication disorders and other disabilities including autism (Spillers, 2007).

Things to do include:

- Lead with positives: This can include things the child does well and/or affirming parents for seeking out an evaluation. For example, "He did pretty well on ___" or "I'm glad you all made the appointment to ask about your concerns. I know it can be hard to do that sometimes."
- Deliver "bad news" with care: "He is performing in the first percentile and is severely impaired" sounds grim and negative whereas, "He is not performing as well as his peers, so we want to get him the support he needs to improve" sounds much more positive and affirming.
- Offer active strategies that can be immediately employed at home: This may include direct and indirect language modeling, reading books, or more social time. Show parents how to do these things and then have them demonstrate them back to you so you can confirm that they understand. This might be particularly important as there may often times be a delay between diagnosis and treatment as families seek out services. While waiting to begin treatment, it is helpful to have strategies to use at home.
- End with hope: This can be something as simple as, "Early intervention has shown to be really helpful for getting kids to make improvements so I feel confident we can help." You might offer opportunities to connect with other parents and provide resources parents can review at home once they have more time to process evaluation findings.

Think about your body language, eye contact, and tone of voice as you deliver clinical results that might be confusing, unwelcome, and/or shocking to families. We strongly suggest using role playing tasks to help new professionals learn how to counsel families appropriately.

While there is no single "right way" to do it, we encourage professionals to lead with compassion, use language families can understand, make space for questions, and to clearly outline a path for clinical progress and client success. Importantly, we strongly encourage you not to avoid "bad news" because it can be uncomfortable. Avoidance does both the child and family a disservice. If you notice signs indicative of autism, it is important to share those concerns with parents appropriately so they can pursue assessment and appropriate intervention if necessary.

TIPS FOR AVOIDING PROFESSIONAL BURNOUT

- ✓ *Self-care*: It is important to take care of your own mental health needs so you can give the very best to your clients. Take time to rest and focus on things you enjoy so you can then do your job well.
- ✓ *Positivity*: Focus on the encouraging aspects of what you do. While it may be a challenge to disappoint families by alerting them of a disability, it is ultimately a positive thing to help them get the targeted care they need.
- ✓ *Reflect*: Consider the positive impact you have had on your clients' lives. For example, we keep a "Pick Me Up" folder on our phones. It has notes from parents, students, and clients that make us smile like the text shown here from a parent of a young child who was first misdiagnosed with apraxia before being diagnosed with autism. He was nonverbal at age three when he first began intervention. Two years later, he started in a general education kindergarten classroom because his speech and language skills were typical for his age. Being able to reference examples like that can be helpful during the difficult times in your profession. Intervention can be challenging, but it is all worth it in the end.

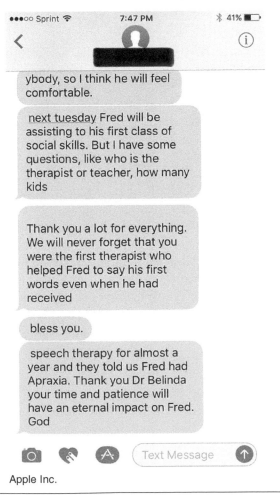

Apple Inc.

GOAL SETTING

Evaluations should naturally transition to setting targeted intervention goals to address observed deficits following a framework of expectations for age-appropriate typical development.

Active Learning Task

Goals should be written clearly enough to be discerned by others.

1. Consider the goals below. Do they pass the stranger test, so any person could clearly understand the targets?
   Goal 1: Student will produce regular past tense verbs.
   Goal 2: Student will understand commands.

2. After reading the section below, transform the goals above to be SMART.

What Is a SMART Goal?

A SMART goal is specific, measurable, attainable, relevant and time bound (Doran, 1981):

Specific	Goals should be clearly defined, which makes them easier to measure. For example, "Will use age-appropriate vocabulary" may be too general to objectively measurable. What is "age-appropriate?" How will we know when the goal is met? In contrast, "Will expressively identify 9 of 10 common farm animals" is much more specific and allows the interventionist to clearly document progress.
Measurable	Goals should be objective. It is important to create goals that are objective and quantifiable so progress can be clearly documented over time. Goals may include measures such as "X% accuracy," "X of X opportunities/trials," "X% consistency," etc. Additionally, they may include the amount of support such as "given minimal/moderate/maximum cues" or "given no more than one verbal prompt," etc.
Attainable	Goals should be able to be *reasonably attained*. That marker may look different for every child. For example, an unattainable goal for a nonverbal child might be "Will produce a 4+ word sentence in 9 of 10 trials." That goal might not be attainable because it is unlikely a nonverbal child will transition from using zero words to using complete sentences. A more attainable goal might be "Will label five common nouns in 5 of 10 trials given moderate cues." This goal might be more attainable given the child's baseline functioning.

Relevant   Goals should be relevant to the client's needs overall functioning. For example, a client preparing to graduate from high school may not be best served by targeting a goal on identifying farm animals. Rather, goals might be addressed that are more relevant such as targets that can be transferred into vocational skills.

Time Bound   Goals should have a projected date of completion. Some may write this as "In three months. . .," or "By month/year. . ." At the end of the time period, a note on progress can be documented and the goal can be classified as "met", "not met" or "in progress."

Active Learning Task

Now let's try to generate your own goals. Consider the baseline descriptions for a client of three-years and three-months with autism below. Based on the current level of functioning and age developmental norms, as well as your prior knowledge about typical speech and language acquisition, generate treatment goals for intervention. Goal 4 has been completed as an example.

After you create your goals, share with a peer for feedback.

Target area(s)	Goal #	Goal
Receptive language and auditory comprehension	1	[Your goal] Baseline: He currently demonstrates ability to follow one-step directions. Understanding of basic concepts size and colors were not observed per assessment report. Some prepositions such as in and on were reported to be understood receptively.
Expressive language/ expanding mean length of utterance	2	[Your goal] Baseline: He currently uses single words. He combines jargon, words, and gestures to communicate.
Vocabulary	3	[Your goal] Baseline: Does not demonstrate ability to name or point to at least 20 objects/pictures, but is able to name some objects, such as body parts.
Social language/ pragmatics	4	During structured and unstructured tasks, will use a 1–2 word utterance to demonstrate at least four pragmatic functions (i.e. initiate/respond to greetings, comment/ label, request, protest, respond to a question/request, turn take, and/or gain attention) with 80% accuracy given moderate (3–4) prompts/cues over three consecutive sessions as measured by data collection. Baseline: Currently combines gestures and sounds to request. When assistance is needed, he points or brings objects to caregivers. He does not seek out the attention of others or initiate interactions of shared enjoyment.

SUMMARY

Indications for an assessment for ASD include reduced social communication skills, language delays, the presence of restricted and repetitive behaviors, and poor play and/or conversation skills. In addition to ASD specific assessments, an evaluation for ASD should include a variety of formal and informal evaluation procedures including informal measures such as language sampling, play assessments, naming tasks, imitation tasks, and formal measures such as standardized assessments that explore receptive and expressive language, receptive and expressive vocabulary skills, and speech skills. Background information gathered from caregivers provides critical information to help ascertain the client's behavior across contexts such as the natural environment. Information gathered from caregivers should be collected using culturally responsive approaches that demonstrate cultural competence to meet the needs of diverse families. Common barriers to appropriate diagnosis of ASD in culturally, linguistically diverse families include differences in parent report, language barriers, and the inappropriate use of assessments that do not take cultural variation into account. Members of the assessment team can include all those who have expertise in ASD and/or the child. When generating treatment goals for students, they should be specific, measurable, appropriate, realistic, and timebound (SMART).

TEST QUESTIONS

1. The key difference between a diagnosis of autism spectrum disorder and a diagnosis of social pragmatic disorder is:
   A. The presence of communication challenges.
   B. The lack of intellectual impairment.
   C. The presence of restricted and/or repetitive behaviors.
   D. Difficulty with theory of mind.

2. Appropriate diagnosis of autism should include both formal and informal assessment measures.

3. Potential members of the diagnostic team may include:
   A. Parents
   B. Speech-language pathologist
   C. Applied behavior analyst
   D. All of the above

4. The M-CHAT-R/F is a formal, standardized assessment tool. True or false?

5. Any formal assessment for autism spectrum disorder should include a formal speech and language evaluation. True or false?

6. During assessment, a formal audiological evaluation should be conducted to rule out hearing impairment since symptoms may present similarly to autism spectrum disorder characteristics. True or false?

7. The ADOS-2 is an informal screening tool for autism. True or false?

8. Autism spectrum disorder may be diagnosed later in life even if there were never symptoms present in early childhood. True or false?

9. SMART goals are:
   A. Specific, measurable, altruistic, realistic, time bound
   B. Specific, measurable, attainable, realistic, time bound
   C. Singular, monitored, attainable, rational, time bound
   D. Specific, monitored, attainable, rational, time bound

10. A student goal revision from "Will use more expressive language" to "Will demonstrate a mean length of utterance of four" is an example of making a goal more:
    A. Measurable
    B. Specific
    C. Time bound
    D. A and B only

REFERENCES

Alsehemi, M., Abousaadah, M., Sairafi, R., and Jan, M. (2017). Public awareness of autism spectrum disorder. *Neurosciences (Riyadh)* 22 (3): 213–215.

Beiting, M. and Maas, E. (2021). Autism-centered therapy for childhood apraxia of speech (ACT4CAS): a single-case experimental design study. *American Journal of Speech-Language Pathology* 30 (3S): 1525–1541.

Beverly, B. and Matthews, L. (2021). Speech-language pathologist and parent perspectives on speech-language pathology services for children with autism spectrum disorders. *Focus on Autism and Other Developmental Disabilities* 36 (2): 121–132.

Broome, K., McCabe, P., Docking, K., and Doble, M. (2017). A systematic review of speech assessments for children with autism spectrum disorder: recommendations for best practice. *American Journal of Speech-Language Pathology* 26 (3): 1011–1029.

Camarata, S. (2013). Pediatric hearing impairment, autism, and autism spectrum disorder: implications for clinicians. *Perspectives on Hearing and Hearing Disorders in Childhood* 23 (1): 4–12.

Chenausky, K., Brignell, A., Morgan, A. et al. (2021). A modeling-guided case study of disordered speech in minimally verbal children with autism spectrum disorder. *American Journal of Speech-Language Pathology* 30 (3S): 1542–1557.

Cosentino, L., Vigli, D., Franchi, F. et al. (2019). Rett syndrome before regression: a time window of overlooked opportunities for diagnosis and intervention. *Neuroscience and Biobehavioral Reviews* 107: 115–135.

Crais, E. and Watson, L. (2013). Challenges and opportunities in early identification and intervention for children at-risk for autism spectrum disorders. *International Journal of Speech-Language Pathology* 16 (1): 23–29.

Dean, M., Harwood, R., and Kasari, C. (2017). The art of camouflage: gender differences in the social behavior of girls and boys with autism spectrum disorder. *Autism* 21 (6): 678–689.

Doran, G.T. (1981). There's a S.M.A.R.T. way to write management's goals and objectives. *Management Review (AMA FORUM)* 70 (11): 35–36.

Dworzynski, K., Ronald, A., Bolton, P., and Happe, F. (2012). How differenct are girls and boys above and below the diagnostic threshold for autism spectrum disorders? *Journal of the American Academy of Child and Adolescent Psychiatry* 51 (8): 788–797.

Gold, R. and Gold, A. (2018). Delivering bad news: attitudes, feelings, and practice characteristics among speech-language pathologists. *American Journal of Speech-Language Pathology* 6 (27): 108–122.

Hilton, C.L., Fitzgerald, R.T., Jackson, K.M. et al. (2010). Brief report: under-representation of African Americans in autism genetic research: a rationale for inclusion of subjects representing diverse family structures. *Journal of Autism and Developmental Disorders* 40 (5): 633–639.

Ijalba, E. (2016). Hispanic immigrant mothers of young children with autism spectrum disorders: how do they understand and cope with autism? *American Journal of Speech-Language Pathology* 25: 200–213.

Katt, A., Shui, A., Ghods, S. et al. (2021). Sex differences in scores on standardized measures of autism symptoms: a multi-site integrative data analysis. *Journal of Child Psychology and Psychiatry* 62 (1): 97–106.

Kayama, M. (2010). Parental experiences of children's disabilities and special education in the United States and Japan: implications for school social work. *Social Work* 55 (2): 117–125.

Keller-Bell, Y. (2017). Disparities in the identification and diagnosis of autism spectrum disorder in culturally and linguistically diverse populations. *Perspectives of the ASHA Special Interest Groups* 2 (Part 3): 68–81.

Kover, S., Davidson, M., Sindberg, H., and Weismer, S. (2014). Use of the ADOS for assessing spontaneous expressive language in young children with ASD: a comparison of sampling contexts. *Journal of Speech, Language, and Hearing Research* 57 (6): 2221–2233.

Looms, R., Hull, L., and Mandy, W. (2017). What is the male-to-female ratio in autism spectrum disorder? A systematic review and meta-analysis. *Journal of the American Academy of Child and Adolescent Psychiatry* 56 (6): 466–474.

Mandell, D., Ittenbach, R., Levy, S., and Pinto-Martin, J. (2010). Disparities in diagnoses received prior to a diagnosis of autism spectrum disorder. *Journal of Autism and Developmental Disorders* 37 (9): 1795–1802.

Mandy, W. (2019). Social camouflaging in autism: Is it time to lose the mask? *Autism* 23 (8): 1879–1881.

Moore, V. and Goodson, S. (2003). How well does early diagnosis of autism stand the test of time? *Autism* 7 (1): 47–63.

Nguyen, C.T., Krakowiak, P., Hansen, R. et al. (2016). Sociodemographic disparities in intervention service utilization in families of children with autism spectrum disorder. *Journal of Autism and Developmental Disorders* 46 (12): 3729–3738.

Norbury, C. and Sparks, A. (2013). Difference or disorder? Cultural issues in understanding neurodevelopmental disorders. *Developmental Psychology* 49 (1): 45–58.

Parish-Morris, J., Liberman, M., Cieri, C. et al. (2017). Linguistic camouflage in girls with autism spectrum disorder. *Molecular Autism* 8: 48.

Paul, R., Chawarska, K., and Volkmar, F. (2008). Differentiating ASD for DLD in toddlers. *Perspectives on Language Learning and Education* 15 (3): 101–111.

Petrocchi, S., Levante, A., and Lecciso, F. (2020). Systematic review of level 1 and level 2 screening tools for autism spectrum disorders in toddlers. *Brain Sciences* 10 (3): 180.

Pileggi, M., Brane, N., Bradshaw, J. et al. (2021). Early observation of red flags in 12-month old infant siblings later diagnosed with autism spectrum disorder. *American Journal of Speech-Language Pathology* 30 (4): 1846–1855.

Ravindran, N. and Myers, B. (2012). Cultural influences on perceptions of health, illness, and disability: a review and focus on autism. *Journal of Child and Family Studies* 21 (2): 311–319.

Robins, D.L., Casagrande, K., Barton, M. et al. (2014). Validation of the Modified Checklist for Autism in Toddlers, Revised with Follow-up (M-CHAT-R/F). *Pediatrics* 133 (1): 37–45.

Ros-Demarize, R., Bradley, C., Kanne, S. et al. (2020). ASD symptoms in toddlers and preschoolers: an examination of sex differences. *Autism Research* 13 (1): 157–166.

Sedgewick, F., Hill, V., Yates, R. et al. (2016). Gender differences in the social motivation and friendship experiences of autistic and non-autistic adolescents. *Journal of Autism and Developmental Disorders* 46: 1297–1306.

Sedgewick, F., Hill, V., and Pellicano, E. (2019). "It's different for girls:" gender differences in the friendships and conflict of autistic and neurotypical adolescents. *Autism* 23 (5): 1119–1132.

Seung, H. (2013). Cultural considerations in serving children with ASD and their families: Asian American perspective. *Perspectives on Language Learning and Education* 20 (1): 14–19.

Spillers, C. (2007). An existential framework for understanding the counseling needs of clients. *American Journal of Speech-Language Pathology* 16 (3): 191–197.

Swineford, L. (2017). Screening for ASD in toddlers: an update on recommendations and practices. *Perspectives of the ASHA Special Interest Groups* 2 (1): 5–10.

Wang, J., Hedley, D., Bury, S., and Barbaro, J. (2019). A systematic review of screening tools for the detection of autism spectrum disorder in mainland China and surrounding regions. *Autism* 24 (2): 285–296.

Westby, C., Burda, A., and Mehta, Z. (2003). Asking the right questions in the right ways: strategies for ethnographic interviewing. *The ASHA Leader* 8 (8): 4–17.

Wiley, A.D. (2016). Unlocking disparity of services for Latino children with autism spectrum disorder: Are mothers the answer? Doctoral dissertation, Claremont Graduate University. Emeryville, CA: ProQuest Dissertations. doi: 10143608.

Zuckerman, K., Sinche, B., Mejia, A. et al. (2014). Latino parents' perspectives on barriers to autism diagnosis. *Academic Pediatrics* 14 (3): 301–308.

Zwaigenbaum, L., Bauman, M., Stone, W. et al. (2015). Early identification of autism spectrum disorder: recommendations for practice and research. *Pediatrics* 136 (Supplement 1): S10–S40.

FURTHER READINGS

Jiang, X., Matson, J., Cervantes, P. et al. (2017). Gastrointestinal issues in infants and children with autism and developmental delays. *Journal of Developmental and Physical Disabilities* 29: 407–417.

Kanner, L. (1943). Autistic disturbances of affective contact. *The Nervous Child* 2: 217–250.

La Buissonnière-Ariza, V., Wood, J.J., Kendall, P.C. et al. (2018). Presentation and correlates of hoarding behaviors in children with autism spectrum disorders and comorbid anxiety or obsessive-compulsive symptoms. *Journal of Autism and Developmental Disorders* 48: 4167–4178.

Lord, C., Luyster, R.J., Gotham, K., and Guthrie, W. (2012a). *Autism Diagnostic Observation Schedule, Second Edition (ADOS-2) Manual (Part II): Toddler Module*. Torrance, CA: Western Psychological Services.

Lord, C., Rutter, M., DiLavore, P.C. et al. (2012b). *Autism Diagnostic Observation Schedule*, 2e. Torrance, CA: Western Psychological Services.

Sannar, E., Palka, T., Beresford, C. et al. (2018). Sleep problems and their relationship to maladaptive behavior severity in psychiatrically hospitalized children with autism spectrum disorder (ASD). *Journal of Autism and Developmental Disorders* 48: 3720–3726.

Sokolova, E., Oerlemans, A., Rommelse, N. et al. (2017). A casual and mediation analysis of the comorbidity between attention deficit hyperactivity disorder (ADHD) and autism spectrum disorder (ASD). *Journal of Autism and Developmental Disorders* 47: 1595–1604.

CHAPTER 3

Identifying Social Communication Challenges

Learning Objectives

By reading this chapter, interventionists will be able to:

1. List at least five different types of social communication challenges for individuals with autism spectrum disorder (ASD).
2. Explain the difference between conventional, instrumental, and descriptive gestures.
3. Define **theory of mind** and explain why it is an important social communication skill.
4. Explain the connection between gestures and language development.
5. Generate at least two different goals and treatment activities to target increasing social communication skills for individuals with autism.

It is critical to note that autism spectrum disorder is a condition with widely variable presentations across different individuals. While language skills vary from nonverbal to verbally fluent, social communication challenges are one of the most persistent difficulties in ASD. Challenges may be readily apparent or nearly unnoticeable to those untrained to identify them. Additionally, findings have noted differences in social challenges between girls and boys with autism, as girls with ASD appear to have distinct abilities to camouflage their social challenges and experience more stress and anxiety (Allely 2019).

Autism Spectrum Disorders from Theory to Practice: Assessment and Intervention Tools Across the Lifespan, First Edition. Edited by Belinda Daughrity and Ashley Wiley Johnson.
© 2023 John Wiley & Sons Ltd. Published 2023 by John Wiley & Sons Ltd.

Social communication challenges may also change over time and may present differently across contexts. As such, in assessment, evaluators may benefit from conducting assessment across contexts, such as in a formal clinic setting, and also in a natural setting like in the classroom or at recess. Such a comprehensive approach allows the evaluator to assess social communication challenges, where such challenges might be exacerbated, and how those challenges are adversely impacting functioning in the natural environment.

Before reviewing challenges, it is critical to understand typical development. Social communication, like language, play skills, and gross motor milestones, develops in a hierarchy in distinct stages. It is important to note that skills do not develop overnight. Rather, they develop and refine over time. In general, one should consider the child from a holistic approach. Consider the child's skills across contexts with a variety of partners, including familiar and unfamiliar adults and peers.

All children develop slightly differently and there is a wide presentation of typical development so individual differences should be considered. The absence of just one particular skill may not be clinically relevant. As such, remember to look for consistency by probing for the absence of key skills across a variety of settings to confirm a true delay. For example, common settings for children will be home, community, and school. You must communicate with parents and/or key stakeholders like teachers to inquire about skills across settings because the child may have a different presentation with you as a clinician in your therapy room than at home and/or school where the child spends significant time. In assessment, we always ask parents, "Is this typical of his/her usual behavior/skills?" It is important to remember that, a child who might be tired or sick will present very differently than when alert and active. It is critical to get the most accurate picture of the child, rather than reporting on only a single moment in time. Consider the chart in Table 3.1, with social milestones summarized by the American Speech–Language–Hearing Association (ASHA).

TABLE 3.1   Social milestones summarized by the American Speech–Language–Hearing Association.

Child age (in years)	Skills expected
0–1	✓ Prefers to look at faces and eyes ✓ Prefers the human voice to other sounds ✓ Smiles at people ✓ Follows a person's gaze ✓ Participates in vocal turn taking with an adult ✓ Vocalizes to gain attention ✓ Demonstrates joint attention skills ✓ Uses gestures to request and direct attention ✓ Plays simple social games such as peek-a-boo
1–2	✓ Brings objects to show for the purpose of sharing ✓ Points and vocalizes to make requests ✓ Demonstrates eye contact when others are talking ✓ Participates in limited verbal turn taking ✓ Integrates verbal output and gesture

TABLE 3.1 (Continued)

Child age (in years)	Skills expected
2–3	✓ Expresses basic emotions ✓ Introduces and changes topics ✓ Provides details to increase understanding
3–4	✓ Uses fillers to acknowledge others' comments (e.g. okay, yeah) ✓ Repairs conversation when not understood ✓ Adapts speech for different listeners (e.g. will demonstrate infant directed speech toward younger children)
4–5	✓ Demonstrates theory of mind (by age four) ✓ Uses more effective language to discuss feelings and emotions ✓ Demonstrates rapid topic shifts
5+ (school age years)	✓ Demonstrates conversational skills with increased conversational turns (includes topic maintenance and conversation repair) ✓ Demonstrates increased perspective taking (reads body language, facial expression, voice tone) ✓ Demonstrates social conventions such as politeness

Source: Adapted from ASHA and CDC guidelines as of 2020.

We encourage the use of checklists to help identify key social skill needs, especially since social interaction skills challenges shift over the course of development. Simmons et al. (2014) found measures like the Yale in vivo Pragmatic Protocol valid for helping to classify the specific pragmatic challenges of individuals with ASD. Social interaction challenges can be best captured by both observation and caregiver and/or client interview, as clients with autism may perform better in decontextualized environments such as standardized assessments, effectively communicating knowledge of what to do in theory, while they continue to demonstrate difficulty in practice as evidenced by poor execution when in social scenarios. Developed checklists such as the Communication and Symbolic Behavior Scales from Wetherby and Prizant (2002) can also be helpful.

Active Learning Task

In Search of Evidence-Based Practice

The American Speech–Language–Hearing Association (ASHA) defines evidence-based practice as an integration of clinical expertise acquired via training and professional experience, evidence gathered from scientific literature such as peer-reviewed journals and client observation, and client and caregiver perspectives.

1. Seek out scientific evidence you can apply to clinical intervention for a student with autism addressing social communication challenges in intervention. Exchange peer-reviewed journal articles with a classmate and share approaches.

(continued)

(continued)

2. Separate students into small groups and have each group search at least two journal articles to investigate a social communication challenge (eye contact, play, etc.). Have each group present on their findings to the class.

A NOTE ON CULTURAL VARIATION

Cultural differences also contribute to variation in client presentation. Clinicians should be intentional in considering cultural factors when evaluating social communication skills. Research highlights that cultural variables can impact ASD assessment because clinicians must be aware of how a child's social development is influenced by environmental factors (Huang 2016). Almehmadi et al. (2020) recognized the need to study social interaction conventions among adolescents with ASD in Saudi Arabia because there are noted cultural differences in Arab countries in comparison with English-speaking countries where ASD research is primarily conducted, putting forward key cultural differences in social acts like apologies and politeness. Research exploring cultural differences among Canadian and Vietnamese families with and without children with hearing loss found no significant difference relative to hearing status, but did find that Canadian families demonstrated more conversational turns than Vietnamese families, indicating that culture communication practices impact factors like language and social interaction (Ganek et al. 2018). Clinicians unaware of such cultural norms risk categorizing such differences as deficits, rather than appropriately recognizing them as cultural variations.

Also significant, research indicates neuro typical children who are adopted internationally demonstrate significantly different pragmatic communication performance than their non-adopted peers, further indicating the importance of cultural variance in regards to social interaction skills (Hwa-Froelich and Matsuo 2018). For example, in some cultures, making eye contact may be considered rude or engaging in conversation with unknown adults may be culturally inappropriate. To account for differences, interventionists should confirm a complete review of the client and their family's cultural background, research appropriate social norms for individuals of that culture, and interpret observed social behaviors through a cultural lens.

During assessment, we always ask if the child's behavior during the assessment is typical of their behavior at home in the typical environment. We also ask what is typical and expected in the home environment. While it is important for clinicians to consider cultural factors by investigating cultural norms, we strongly encourage clinicians to ask direct questions to individualize assessment, rather than making generalizations that may prove to be invalid for a particular client and family. You might try saying, "Typically, we expect children this age to ___. Does that sound right for what you might expect of children in your culture or community?" Overall, you must understand culture before making determinations about the child's presentation and/or challenges to be able to make culturally appropriate diagnostic decisions. This cultural awareness is critical across all allied health providers, as there are noted differences across cultures that impact children's attention, self-regulation skills, compliance, self-control, delay of gratification, and executive function skills (LeCuyer and Zhang 2015). For example, consider the differences between collectivist cultures like those in China, Japan, Korea, Indonesia, and Costa Rica compared with individualistic cultures like the United States, Canada, United Kingdom, Germany, and Australia. Key cultural differences include individualist perspectives that stress the importance of individual promotion without dependence on others, which contrasts a collective culture mindset of sharing responsibility among an entire group. Evidence suggests different cultures even perceive and use emotions expression in different ways (Table 3.2; Hareli et al. 2015).

Active Learning Task

Find at least one peer reviewed journal article illustrating social differences between cultures.

TABLE 3.2   Examples of social skills differences across cultures.

Comparison	Group studied		References
Girls and boys	Iranian kindergarteners	Teachers rated girls higher on social skills and boys higher on hyperactivity.	Abdi (2010)
Native American and White children	Preschool children	Parents identified different social skills as important to them. For example, Native American parents rated attends to your instructions and speaks in an appropriate tone of voice at home as one of their top 10 important items, while White parents did not.	Powless and Elliott (1993)
Black and Latino and White children	Elementary school-age children	Black, Latino, and White children told stories differently within the same structured task, suggesting cultural influences in narrative production.	Gorman et al. (2011)
American children and Chinese children	Adolescent and young adults	Chinese respondents viewed accepting credit for good deeds less favorably than their American peers (preferred lying for modesty).	Fu et al. (2011)

NONVERBAL SOCIAL COMMUNICATION CHALLENGES

Nonverbal social communication challenges include all the different ways we communicate messages without using words. As an indication of how important these skills are, consider the effectiveness of miming. Movies with Charlie Chaplin and other actors told entire stories without words by using body language and facial expressions, and these stories were clearly understood by massive audiences.

Active Learning Task

Watch a movie or TV clip with the sound muted. We generally use scenes from a soap opera or telenovela because they are particularly expressive. Can you determine the characters' feelings and what the scene is about? After making your predictions, watch the clip again, this time with sound. Were your predictions accurate?

Joint Attention

Joint attention begins early in childhood as an infant learns to look at objects and back at the caregiver in the first year of life (Owens 2020). Joint attention has long been recognized as a key milestone in preverbal communication skills because it positively predicts later language outcomes (Bruinsma et al. 2004; Nowell et al. 2020). Evidence suggests specific interventions targeting joint attention can influence both immediate skills like pointing to share interest and later skills like language development (Gulsrud et al. 2014).

GOAL SPOTLIGHT

- During structured play tasks, client will respond to bids for joint attention by making eye contact in four of five opportunities.
- During play tasks, client will initiate bids for joint attention to share in three of five opportunities following a model.

Therapy Golden Nugget

To target increasing joint attention among children with low engagement, consider the importance of affect. Try to increase joint attention and engagement by increasing your own use of gestures (particularly index finger pointing), directed facial expressions, eye gaze, and vocal inflection. Before trying this with a client, practice with a partner in class by demonstrating high affect with a common object like a pencil or paper clip.

Note: If high affect alone is not effective with a client, try to prompt joint attention by adding physical touch like tickling.

Eye Contact

Eye contact remains one of the key social communication challenges for individuals with autism. Research has shown that eye gaze remains significantly reduced for children with ASD, even in comparison to peers with other intellectual and developmental disabilities (Hahn et al. 2019). To understand eye contact deficits, one must understand the role of eye gaze in communication and its development among typically developing children. Neurotypical children demonstrate a preference for faces. Infants at increased risk of developing autism demonstrate less preference for faces, which might preface deficits in social communication and language development (Droucker et al. 2013). So why does eye gaze matter? As infants attend to faces, they learn about the world around them, including critical social and emotional information gathered from facial attenuation. Later, eye gaze indicates what someone is thinking as a nonverbal communication cue.

🔦 GOAL SPOTLIGHT

Read the goal examples and then practice making your own.
- Client will demonstrate eye contact in response to having their name called in 7 of 10 opportunities given no more than two verbal presses.
- During conversation tasks, client will appropriately integrate eye gaze with verbal output with 80% consistency given minimal cues, as reported by teacher, caregivers, and/or clinical data.
- Client will _____

In young children, this domain can be assessed along with response to name, as most children respond to their name being called by looking at an adult after one to two presses, even if they are engaged in a task like playing with toys. Conversely, children with autism may not respond to their name being called or might appear to turn to the caller without establishing eye contact. Other children with autism might not seem to respond to their name at all, even when an adult gets closer, attempts to break their visual field, or insinuates touching.

Abnormal eye gaze is an early indicator of an autism diagnosis. Evidence suggests that toddlers with autism display gaze indifference as opposed to gaze aversion, indicating a lack of connection between the importance of eye gaze and social stimuli (Moriuchi et al. 2017). Adults respond to infants' gazes by continuing or terminating interactions, using eye gaze as cues to determine their actions. Direct eye gaze influences a bidirectional interaction between adults and infants, resulting in infants demonstrating more vocalizations and more neural connectivity (Leong et al. 2017). Difficulties with eye gaze can persist over time. While this is a common target in early intervention population, some teens and adults with ASD report feeling sensory overload when compelled to make eye contact (Trevisan et al. 2017). Interventionists should consider the child's total programming needs, together with client and family preferences, to determine whether eye gaze is an appropriate target for intervention.

Therapy Golden Nugget
"The Eyes Have It" To illustrate to clients that people often assume that what you are looking at is what you are thinking about, present at least five trials of eye gaze where the client has to predict your current thought.

CLINICAL APPLICATION

In assessment, clinicians should assess client eye gaze. This can be done during play or during conversation. Does the client initiate eye gaze? Do they integrate eye gaze during conversation and play interactions? Is their eye gaze coordinated with vocalizations? It takes the ability to build clinical rapport to clearly distinguish atypical eye contact from typically developing children who may present as shy or reticent to engage with novel people. If a child is shy, make sure to allow time for the child to warm to you by supporting natural interactions. Once sufficient rapport is established, you can correctly evaluate eye gaze. When typical, it should be clearly present, appropriate, and used across contexts.

Gestures

Clearly defining gestures is a critical area for interventionists who want to target this domain (Ellawadi and Weismer 2014). Evidence suggests that differences in gestures are readily apparent among infants as early as 8–14 months of age at high risk for ASD (West et al. 2020). Gestures encompass an array of different types. Consider the types of gestures below as specified in the Autism Diagnostic Observation Schedule, second edition (ADOS-2):

- *Conventional gestures* include actions like clapping or waving.
- *Instrumental or informational gestures* include actions like pointing, nodding or shaking your head, or shrugging.
- *Descriptive gestures* represent an object or event. An example is gesturing to drive a car or brush your teeth.

In addition to types of gestures, children with autism are often limited in the intention of their gestures, often using gesture with the intention of requesting, while demonstrating limited instances of gesture use for more social means such as pointing or giving for the purpose of showing or sharing. In treatment, this might look like a client pointing to a toy out of reach to get you to give it to them, while not giving or showing the toy to you to engage socially. When exploring a client's use of gestures, you should consider types, frequency, and function. Importantly, gestures should be used simultaneously with verbal output as a method of supplementing the communicative message (Owens 2020). Findings indicate that specific gesture imitation training may help facilitate verbal imitation skills as use of gestures is a critical component in language development (Ingersoll and Lalonde 2010; Ham and Bartolo 2012). Use of gestures appears correlated to use of verbal language output in young children. This trend appears to continue over time with gesture use in teens, with ASD appearing to underly strengths and weaknesses in speech and language development (Braddock et al. 2016).

GOAL SPOTLIGHT

Read the goal examples then practice making your own.
- Client will imitate conventional gestures during semi-structured play tasks given minimal cues in 8 of 10 opportunities.
- Client will request a distal object via gesture (e.g. index finger point) in 7 of 10 trials given a model.
- Client will _____.

Active Learning Task

Individually or in small groups, generate an intervention activity for each of the clients below to address the noted goals. What kind of tasks would you use and why? What evidenced-based practices influenced your choices? Think, pair, share, to exchange ideas.

Quick client snapshot: Two years old. Nonverbal. Cries and tantrums to request objects.

Goal: Client will demonstrate an index finger point to indicate a request for objects in 8 of 10 opportunities without cues across two consecutive sessions.

Quick client snapshot: Three years old. Points and gives items to request only.

Goal: Client will show objects during play-based tasks in 7 of 10 opportunities given moderate cues across three consecutive sessions.

Quick client snapshot: Eight years old. Verbally fluent. Poor use of nonverbal communicative acts integrated into speech.

Goal: Client will demonstrate use of at least two descriptive gestures while relating a narrative in 8 of 10 opportunities given minimal cues across three consecutive sessions.

Facial Expressions and Body Language

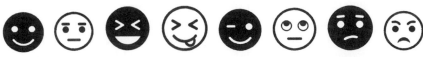

These areas can be challenging for individuals with autism, particularly as it pertains to appropriately matching conversation and/or interpreting body language in others. They can have difficulty both reading facial expressions in others and demonstrating appropriate facial expressions themselves. A very common intervention task is using emotions cards to get children with autism to infer emotions using nonverbal cues like facial expressions. Such tasks can be challenging for children with autism, particularly if they continue to have difficulty looking at faces, which is a critical foundation to being able to identify and discriminate facial expressions. Even for children who are highly verbal, evidence indicates potential difficulty with appropriately allocating visual attention as children with ASD tend to fixate on the mouth when looking at faces, which differs from the behavior of their typical peers (Neumann et al. 2006). This focus can contribute to inaccurate interpretations of facial expressions, especially considering how much social information is derived from the eyes and the face as a whole when inferencing emotions. Challenges recognizing emotion appear related to **theory of mind** deficits and can have continuing implications for children as they enter school, when such challenges can manifest during narrative comprehension tasks like understanding the internal states of characters or assuming their perspectives (Prelock 2015).

Therapy Golden Nugget
<ul><li>For younger children, consider beginning by contrasting two opposite emotions like *happy* vs. *sad*.</li><li>For older children, consider incorporating this target in age relevant tasks like interpreting the meaning of emojis or noting how the inclusion of an emoji might change the meaning of a text message.</li></ul>

CLINICAL APPLICATION

In informal assessment, you might consider showing pictures of different emotions and asking children to identify them. For example, in a visual field of three (or more or less as appropriate), you might ask, "Show me happy/sad/excited/scared/etc." You might then present an emotion and ask the child to identify how the person is feeling. This task explores the child's ability to receptively and expressively identify emotions given nonverbal cues (facial expressions).

A NOTE ON THEORY OF MIND

What is **theory of mind**? Theory of mind is a child's ability to discern other's mental states and understand how those states might differ from their own. This skill is generally achieved around age four in typically developing children. Assessment of this skill is achieved via false-belief tasks, which indicate that children with autism have more difficulty ascribing beliefs to others in comparison with peers (Baron-Cohen et al. 1985). Many standardized formal language assessments for children will include a false-belief task to assess this skill, but you can also assess this informally by setting up a false-belief task of your own. One of the most common is the Sally-Ann task developed by Baron-Cohen et al. (1985).

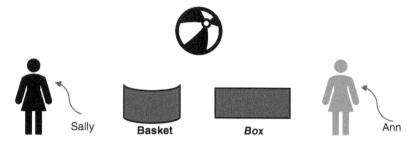

Show the child the dolls and items and, as you act out the actions, say: *Sally has a ball. She puts her ball in a basket and goes out to play. Then Ann comes in. Ann takes Sally's ball and puts it in the box. Sally comes back.* Ask the child: *Where will Sally look for her ball?*

This task called, The Sally Ann Task, is a way to see whether children can infer the states of others and differentiate their own beliefs from the beliefs of others. This skill of perspective taking is the foundation for understanding that people can have different internal states and mental representations. You could also assess this skill with your own version of a false-belief task. For example, you can put carrots into an empty bag of Skittles and ask a child what is inside. The child would likely answer "Candy". Next, show the child the contents of the bag so the child can learn that their belief is wrong. Then you might say, "Let's go to my friend in the next room. What will my friend think is in the bag?" If the child has developed theory of mind, the child will still answer "Candy," knowing that this new person is now operating under the same prior false belief that the child held. However, a child who has not developed theory of mind will answer "Carrots" because the child is assuming that all people know what they know – they have yet to discern that people hold different states of knowledge and beliefs.

VERBAL SOCIAL COMMUNICATION CHALLENGES

Verbal social communication challenges include the quality and use of expressive language skills in the varied nuanced ways we shift our styles and approaches depending on context to communicate our intended meanings.

Tone and Suprasegmental Speech

Individuals with autism may present with difficulty demonstrating appropriate vocal inflection and tone. **Suprasegmental** aspects of speech include intonation, timing, and stress of words, phrases, and sentences (Small 2020). These suprasegmental aspects carry meaning. Without them, our speech can sound robotic or monotone, lacking feeling and emotion. Individuals with autism may present with difficulty in demonstrating appropriate vocal inflection and tone. Evidence suggests children with autism do demonstrate pitch range and variability, but they demonstrate shallower spectra and less harmonic structure than their typical peers (Bonneh et al. 2011). Evidence suggests that these challenges with tone and suprasegmental aspects of speech among individuals with autism require direct intervention to target improvement (Holbrook and Israelsen 2020).

GOAL SPOTLIGHT

Read the goal example. Then practice making your own goal.
- Client will use vocal tone to connote emotion given minimal cues in four of five opportunities.
- Client will _____.

Try saying the sentence "I really want to go" in at least three different ways. Using different tone and stress, the sentence can have different meanings even though the content (words) is the same (Table 3.3).

Conversation and Topic Maintenance

Often, children with autism, even those who are highly verbal, can struggle with initiating and maintaining conversation appropriately with others. Evidence is

TABLE 3.3   A sentence can have different meanings with different tone and stress.

Sentence with stress	Inferred meaning
I really want to go.	Stress on "I" indicates emphasis. Maybe the person speaking really wants to go when the other people do not.
I really want to go.	Stress on "really" indicates an emphasis on wanting to go as if asking for permission or pleading.
I really want to go.	Stress on "want" indicates maybe the person wants to go but is not able to.

consistent across direct observation, data from parents, and firsthand accounts that social skills challenges such as conversation skills are delayed in ASD, which adversely impacts friendship development (Daughrity 2019; Brinton et al. 2004). Deficits may include making contingent comments and reciprocating social communication questions to extend a communicative exchange with a partner.

In assessment, this area may be included on some standardized assessments, but it is best assessed informally. Some individuals with autism may respond appropriately on a formal test, indicating they know what to do; however, their skills in execution of the skill may be limited. Here is an example of a sample script you might use in assessment.

To client: Hey there! So what did you do this weekend?
Client response.
To client: "Oh that sounds fun." Followed by a distinct pause to see if the client spontaneously asks about your weekend. If not, continue by saying, "Oh I had a GREAT weekend and did something super fun. . ."

This is followed by another distinct pause to see if the client then responds to this dangler to ask a related question. If the client continues not to ask a question, offer one more opportunity by saying, "Do you want to know what I did this weekend?"

Here are examples of how you might report your findings in a diagnostic report.

- The client spontaneously reciprocated social communication questions to demonstrate an appropriate to-and-fro.
- The client responded appropriately to danglers in conversation to ask questions and extend a conversation.
- The client did not ask questions in conversation contributing to a stilted exchange that lacked reciprocity.

You also want to note whether the client makes contingent comments on your responses. During an informal language sample, try to make at least two different positive or negative statements in an attempt to yield a related comment and prompt related questions (Table 3.4). Importantly, you want to note in your assessment if the client's skills are consistent across contexts:

- Did the client demonstrate conversation skills with you?
- Did the client initiate conversation or only respond?
- Were skills consistent with parent report?
- If you are able to observe the client in the natural environment with peers, does the child demonstrate appropriate conversation skills with age-matched peers?
- If you are unable to observe the child with peers directly, what do the child's teachers or caregivers report on their peer conversation?

TABLE 3.4   Positive and negative statements.

Sample scripted statement	Sample appropriate comments/questions
Example negative statement	
Oh man I spilled my coffee everywhere this morning. I had to change my shirt!	Oh no! That sucks. Bummer.
Example positive statement	
I'm going to Disneyland tomorrow! I'm so excited.	Cool! Sounds fun! Who is going with you?

In addition to parents and teachers, if you are able, you want to provide other key stakeholders with opportunities to provide feedback on the client's typical performance. You might ask other adults with knowledge of the child like a therapist, paraprofessional, social skills teacher, or other reliable informant of the child's usual behavior.

> ### GOAL SPOTLIGHT
>
> Read the goal example then practice making your own goal and generating an intervention idea to target the goal.
> - Client will maintain a topic of conversation for a minimum of four conversational turns given minimal cues in 8 of 10 opportunities.
> - Client will extend a topic of conversation by asking a contingent question or making a contingent comment in three of five opportunities given moderate cues.
> - Client will _____.
> Intervention idea: _____.

> ### Therapy Golden Nugget
>
> In this task, the client can select a Memoji sticker and be prompted to either initiate or maintain a conversation for as many conversational turns as appropriate for your client. This can be done as an oral activity or a written activity such as simulating a text message exchange.
>
> *or*
>
> The client can infer the character's emotion based on the facial expression. Prompt the client to expressively identify the emotion. To extend the task, you can ask the client to make an inference and generate a plausible social scenario by asking "Why do you think he/she feels that way?" "What happened?"

> *or*
>
> You can create social scenarios and provide the stickers below. Ask the client to match the sticker to the scenario as appropriate.
>
> *or*
>
> You can provide the client with a target emotion and prompt your client to create a Memoji sticker to match that emotion.

EXECUTIVE FUNCTION

Executive Functioning Skills often presents as a concerning area for highly verbal children with autism from school age to adult years. According to the information processing model, executive function includes the steps of attention, discrimination, organization, and memory (Owens 2020). Deficits in this area can present as a client being absent-minded or lazy, which are frequently ascribed negative assumptions when educators fail to note these aspects as distinct challenges associated with autism spectrum disorder. Remember that, despite a child's academic abilities, social skills deficits can continue throughout their lifespan and may present in various ways throughout their school-age years and beyond. For example, we once evaluated a teenager who had recently changed high schools. His records showed a diagnosis of autism, but his parents opted not to disclose his diagnosis to his new school so he could "have a fresh start." In reviewing his midterm grades, nearly every teacher commented on the same challenges. *John misses deadlines. John does not submit assignments. John understands the material, but he doesn't do the work. John does not seem focused.* One teacher who reported allowing John to submit all of his late assignments without penalty said that he was doing excellent. These reports indicate how easy it can be for a student like John to slip through the cracks, especially in the context of educating dozens of other students. John was not behavioral. His teachers mostly described him as "quiet." He was a C to D student, largely because he failed to submit work. During his evaluation, he scored within the typical range on his speech and language assessments, but he demonstrated deficits in pragmatics (language use) and executive functioning. When asked, he said he often did assignments, but just forget to turn them in. He also reported feeling overwhelmed in classes because of all the different expectations and demands. In John's case, intervention targeting increasing his ability to multitask and developing organizational strategies that he could employ independently might make a significant difference in his ability to appropriately access his academic curriculum and demonstrate his understanding of class concepts.

In assessment, this area might be assessed via looking at reports from the natural environment. How does the child do in school? How do they manage responsibilities at home? Such reports might help to begin determining if this higher-level skill is an area of concern. If so, it is certainly a target for intervention.

Practical solutions may include working on generating schedules, graphic organizers, checklists, and visual supports (Zenko 2014). Clinicians may target skills like time management, in addition to supporting common daily tasks like setting an alarm to wake up for school/work, completing home tasks like making the bed or cleaning up, and/or relaying important messages to persons of authority.

Why are these skills important? We once had a female teen client with ASD who was highly verbal and in a special education setting. She was repeatedly having toileting issues even though she was able to use the restroom independently. When I probed her about this, she reported, "Well I asked my teacher, but she was helping John (another student) and told me to wait until she was done, but she took too long." She went on to say that she didn't want to leave class without asking because she didn't want to get in trouble. In this case, we worked on role-playing to reframe "Can I go to the bathroom?" to "Ms. X, I'll be right back from the restroom." The toileting accidents immediately stopped, as did the teasing from classroom peers. As illustrated in the above example, deficits in executive functioning are often highly problematic in independent settings such as older grade levels and higher education or work when an individual is largely expected to self-organize, prepare, and solicit help as needed.

SOCIAL RECIPROCITY AND RAPPORT

Social reciprocity and rapport are social communication skills that are often considered highly variable and qualitative; however, standardized assessments now often include quantitative scores of these domains. In the ADOS-2, items such as "shared enjoyment in interaction," "amount of social overtures," "quality of social overtures," "quality of social response," "level of engagement," and "overall quality of rapport" are quantitatively scored. To illustrate this point to students, we often give the following example of typical social reciprocity and rapport. Imagine you are waiting at your airport gate, and you look up and lock eyes with a toddler. Naturally, you smile. Most children will also smile back. If you keep looking at them and make a silly face because that comes naturally to you, then you better be ready to go because you have just made a friend who will expect reciprocated engagement for the near future. This example reflects the clear feeling of experiencing an engaged and socially reciprocal child. Even children who are shy to strangers clearly demonstrate these skills among familiar adults like parents, grandparents, and babysitters. The interaction is warm. It compels even the most hardened person to crack a smile.

In assessment, we do not encourage clinicians to attempt a specific task to evaluate this domain. Rather, we encourage them to consider the interaction in full and then document the impressions in the diagnostic report. This ensures that the clinician is not only considering one task, especially one that the child might have been particularly interested in; rather, it compels the evaluator to consider the full scope of the interaction and then summarize the exchange. In intervention, such items typically demonstrate improvement via targets on increasing play and use of gestures, among other social communication skill areas.

Active Learning Task

Attempt this engagement task with a child at your next available opportunity – maybe a family ahead of you in the grocery store line or on the bus or as you pass a child in a stroller out for a walk with a caregiver. How does the child react to your smile and wave?

OBTAINING FIRSTHAND REPORTS

During the course of your assessment, do not neglect to also include **self-reports** on functioning from clients themselves. For school-age clients, consider asking them questions such as "Do you have friends?" or "Do you have a hard time with playing with other kids sometimes?" Such self-reports can be included in your evaluation as another point of evidence to explore consistency. The self-report may also indicate that clients are aware of their own challenges. As such, in the diagnostic report, we may write, *The client reported not having friends, which is consistent with parent report.*

For example, we often ask clients, "Tell me about your friends." Often, clients unaware of their challenges or the nuances of friendship will respond by listing all of the kids in their classroom. This indicates the client is unable to name true friends. We will typically follow up by asking "What do you and your friend(s) do together and when do you see each other?" This question gives an opportunity to note whether the client can identify mutual interests with a peer and whether the client interacts with the peer in different contexts such as school and on weekends.

The inclusion of self-reports is increasingly important as clients get older, when peer interaction naturally becomes more self-supported, rather than facilitated by parents. As clients mature, allowing them to provide firsthand accounts encourages client buy-in and also honors their personal opinions and beliefs, which become increasingly important as the ultimate goal to support client success is to promote self-evaluation and critique to facilitate independence.

Another area to probe for firsthand report is an understanding of relationships. As clients get older, you want to evaluate their understanding of romantic relationships and how they might differ from friendships. A client's response indicates an understanding of different types of relationships with varying degrees of intimacy.

CLINICAL RELEVANCE

Social communication challenges contribute to difficulty in developing and maintaining friendships. Preschool-age children with better social communication skills such as joint attention report higher quality friendship development during school-age years (Freeman et al. 2015). Evidence suggests highly verbal children with ASD in mainstream education settings report poorer quality friendships than their neurotypical peers and have more challenges with peer relationships in school (Kasari et al. 2011). While there is evidence that school-age children with autism do have friendships and are not socially isolated, it is noted that adults play an active role in supporting friendships for children with ASD (Calder et al. 2013). Friendships serve critical roles of facilitating emotional intimacy as well as serving as a protective factor against bullying for school-age children.

In schools, clinicians often must connect deficits to their adverse impact on the child's ability to access their academic curriculum. Among inclusive preschool programs integrating children with autism with their neurotypical peers, findings revealed use of gestures and language skills largely predicted program invitation (Siller et al. 2020). This finding suggests social communication skills can be used to determine success in inclusive educational settings. In later academic years, consider the need to interact appropriately with peers for group projects and presentations. Social communication challenges would adversely impact children with autism who might struggle during such tasks, thus adversely impacting their ability to fully access their academic curriculum, despite being highly verbal and presenting with typical speech and language skills.

Highly verbal children with ASD may also struggle with academic tasks like reading comprehension activities that call for taking the perspective of a character or making inferences. Such skills require the ability to deduce emotions and demonstrate theory of mind to take on the point of view of others. These skills may be challenging for children with autism, which would adversely impact their ability to appropriately participate in such academic tasks.

The relevance of social communication skills is evident across the lifespan. In younger years, such skills are critical in supporting language development and academic success. As individuals get older, such skills are critical to relationship development and successful navigation of higher education and vocational settings. As such, social communication skills are critical across the lifespan as challenges will have adverse impacts on functioning across contexts.

Reporting on Social Communication Challenges in your Diagnostic Report

You will want to provide clear descriptions of what you observed about the client's social communication skills during your assessment. The challenge for new professionals can be summarizing this information and writing clinically, rather than creating a long descriptive narrative about every behavior you observed. In addition to properly summarizing your observations, report writing requires professional and clinical writing skills. Ways to shift to clinical writing are described in Table 3.5, and examples of clinical language include those in Table 3.6.

Including Social Communication Strengths

In addition to reporting deficits, do not neglect to include strengths. This information is critical to beginning intervention as the clinician will want to target new goals while

TABLE 3.5 Ways to shift to clinical writing.

Informal language	Clinical language
The client had a big problem with . . .	*The client had significant difficulty . . .*
The client did __ over and over again.	*The client repeatedly ___.*
The client didn't do a good job playing.	*The client demonstrated difficulty during play.*
The client really had bad eye contact.	*The client demonstrated significant difficulty with appropriate eye gaze.*

TABLE 3.6 Examples of clinical language.

What you saw	What to write
Client didn't start conversation.	The client demonstrated infrequent initiations and responses to bids for conversation.
Client gestured sometimes and talked, but didn't do this at the same time.	The client demonstrated poor coupling of gestures with verbal output.
Client rarely had eye gaze.	The client demonstrated fleeting eye gaze throughout the assessment.
You called the client's name several times and the client never acknowledged you.	The client demonstrated poor response to name despite multiple presses.
When you called the client's name, the client turned to look at you. The client did not make eye contact during other opportunities.	The client demonstrated eye contact when called, but demonstrated poor use of eye gaze integrated with verbal output.
Client kept changing topics during conversation.	The client demonstrated poor topic maintenance in conversation.
Client gestured to be picked up and to get a toy. Client did not gesture for other reasons.	The client's use of gestures was restricted to pointing for the purpose of requesting.
Parent said client behavior in the evaluation was the same as home.	The client's social communication challenges were consistent across standardized assessment, clinical observation, and parent and client report.
Client has typical speech and language. Client doesn't use language to interact.	In spite of age-appropriate speech and language skills, the client demonstrates significant social communication challenges that adversely impact conversation and social interaction skills.
Client has the most trouble when with peers.	The client demonstrates limitations in social communication skills that are manifested in unstructured social contexts such as recess with peers.

(continued)

TABLE 3.6   (Continued)

What you saw	What to write
Client said work is hard because of unwritten social rules.	The client reports social communication difficulties that create challenges in their work settings.
Client had social challenges during assessment. Parent confirmed social challenges. Client reported no challenges.	While social communication challenges are evident in clinical observation and consistent with parent report, the client demonstrates poor awareness of their errors in social interaction.
Client has trouble with relationships and/or workplace interactions.	When asked about their social communication challenges, the client's responses indicate difficulties are significantly adversely impacting their social interaction skills.
Client understands nuances of friendships and romantic relationships. Client has trouble with these connections in daily life.	The client demonstrates awareness of friendships and intimate relationships, but reports difficulty applying social communication skills to successfully maintain peer relationships.

building on existing strengths. Generally, we like to report the strengths first and then discuss areas for improvement.

With each statement, you might provide a clear example or two of how you reached that conclusion. Remember, your report will serve as the document to support the client in obtaining intervention services. Other professionals may read your document to look for consistency, wanting to confirm that the client performed similarly across contexts in different settings with different professionals. Examples may look like:

- The client did respond when his name was called and responded to bids for joint attention. For example, the client responded to the clinician calling his name by establishing eye contact. The client did not initiate bids for joint attention.

For the interventionist, this provides valuable information that the client can respond to name and does respond to bids for joint attention. Those strengths can be used as a foundation to build new skills like increasing initiation of joint attention during play.

- During spontaneous conversation, the client appropriately integrated gesture with verbal output and gave contingent responses to questions posed by the clinician. The client did not respond to danglers to spontaneously reciprocate social communication questions to extend a conversation. For example, the client answered questions in conversation to identify favorite foods and sports. However, the client did not ask question of the clinician, which contributed to a stilted conversation that lacked a natural to-and-fro.

In intervention, a clinician would know the client is responsive in conversation. Goals would appropriately target reciprocating questions to begin. For example, a clinician might target this skill by getting the client to first answer the question and then ask it back, which targets conversational turn taking skills. A clinician may describe conversation as a game of volleyball or hot potato so the client can visualize the importance of keeping the conversation going, rather than only answering and letting the conversation end. Documenting strengths gives a clinician an idea of where to begin in intervention by using the skills a client does have to target those skills in need of support. In considering a strengths-based approach, one also wants to document those things a client does well or relatively well, rather than only consider areas of growth.

Active Learning Task

Read the lesson plan example below. Using the goals you generated for this three-year-old client with autism in Chapter 2, create your own lesson plan with tasks to support the goals. Make sure to include evidence-based practice and clear descriptions. Include visuals as appropriate so others can clearly interpret your session plan. Once complete, exchange plans for peer review and feedback.

Sample Intervention Plan

Student Name: Nohlan   **Primary Diagnosis:** Autism

Chronological Age (CA): 3;3

BEHAVIORAL SUPPORTS: Environmental arrangement, visual schedule, positive reinforcement, sensory breaks.

Evidenced-Based Practice

Banda, D. and Grimmett, E. (2008). Enhancing social and transition behaviors of persons with autism through activity schedules: a review. *Education and Training in Developmental Disabilities, 43*(3), 324–333.

Koegel, L., Matos-Freden, R., Lang, R., Koegel, R. (2012). Interventions for children with autism spectrum disorders in inclusive school settings. *Cognitive and Behavioral Practice, 19*(3), 401–412.

Ledford, J.R., King, S., Harbin, E.R., Zimmerman, K.N. (2018). Antecedent social skills interventions for individuals with ASD: what works, for whom, and under what conditions? *Focus on Autism and Other Developmental Disabilities, 33*(1), 3–13.

Matson, J., and Boisjoli, J. (2009). The token economy for children with intellectual disability and/or autism: a review. *Research in Developmental Disabilities, 30*(2), 240–248.

Piller, A., and Barimo, J. (2019). Strategies to calm and engage children with ASD: challenges with sensory processing are a hallmark of autism spectrum disorder. Occupational therapists share suggestions for addressing a child's off-task behavior. *ASHA Leader, 24*(4), 56–63.

Therapy Plan

(+) Correct without prompting; (−) Incorrect with prompting or no response; (P) Prompted | (%)

(continued)

(continued)

Activity name (goals targeted)	Instructions (goals)
Preparation prior to session	Prepare materials: Brown Bear book with manipulatives: prepare board book with laminated copies of animals and Velcro to adhere during book share Brown Bear coloring worksheet Sensory box Token economy board Transparent prize box "I want" sentence strip. Ensure the space is set up appropriately: environmental arrangement.
Introduction of therapy rules and visual schedule (3, 4)	Show the token board and go over the following speech rules, which are posted on the wall: (a) listen to teacher, (b) calm body, (c) eyes looking and (d) always try my best! For each rule, display good and bad examples and ask if that's what it means. For example, with eyes looking to the floor in a silly position, ask "is this eyes on teacher?" Record yes/no answers (goal 4). After going over each one, explain that if we follow these rules we will get tokens on our board. Explain that the board can be exchanged once it is full for a prize in the prize box. Briefly grab the prize box for show and put it back out of reach and sight. Keep the token board on the table as a visual reminder of the need for good behavior. May refer to this if behavior needs to be redirected. Next, using the visual schedule, explain how it works by demonstrating that once tasks are complete, we move it to "finish" to signify that we are done, and we are moving to the next task. Have Nohlan practice "put on/off" the visuals and model/hand-over-hand this part if necessary. If Mom is in the room, ask to observe if this may at all help with transitions at home, and a visual schedule can be created for home use as well.
Read Brown Bear book with prepared Velcro manipulatives	Explain that we will now read a book. Read the book to him with a very engaging voice. Each page is an opportunity to elicit language. You might read and say "let's see who is next!" and respond with enthusiasm when he labels. When labeling the animals, get Nohlan to first label what the animal is. For example, "who is that?" (3). If he responds with "bear," expand the utterance to two words such as "brown bear" or a carrier phrase "I see bear." Note whether he imitates this. Also note what he is successfully able to label out of all the animals in the book.

If he cannot label the animals, then flip through the pages and ask "Can you help me find yellow duck? Find duck. Yellow duck." See if he points to the right manipulative and let him place it onto the page (3). Note whether this is successful. Note if he does any of the following: (a) label, (b) request, (c) request to gain attention, etc. Overall, note the pragmatic functions of his behavior during the task (4).

Sensory break	Explain that he's earned a break. Use a visual timer.

Allow for autonomy in selecting toys and exploring provided sensory items. Note items he prefers that could be used as reinforcers.
When he has a minute left, offer a verbal warning and a visual cue by showing the timer. Set the visual schedule close-by. Announce the end of the break verbally ("All done break" and sign *all done*) and by showing the visual timer. Signify its end by moving the break icon to finished, and ask him to help clean up. If he demonstrates with difficulties, remind him of our token board and review behavior expectations (class rules).

Brown Bear coloring worksheet
(2, 4)

After showing the book, explain that now we get to color all our friends with a coloring worksheet. Bring out the worksheet and crayons, with the crayons away from him on your side. Using the "I Want" sentence strip, the goal of this activity is to: (a) expand utterances to two words, (b) facilitate verbal requests with word or two words (i.e. want red). He has to ask for the crayons. Start by asking him what he wants to color first.
If he points, ask him what he is pointing to. If no response, give phonemic cue or if appropriate, a gestural cue. If there is still no response, provide answer and ask him to imitate. Note responses.
If he responds with what correctly, praise him, and ask him what color he'd like.
If he points, ask him what he is pointing to. If no response, give phonemic cue or if appropriate, a gestural cue. If there is still no response, provide answer by using sentence strip and model "Want _____. Now you say!" You may supplement *want* with the sign for want. (2, 4)
If he responds with the right color, expand with the help of the sentence strip and model "Want ____. Now you say!" (2, 4)
If he responds verbally but incorrectly, prompt him to the right answer with a phonemic cue or a gestural cue. Note responses.
While coloring, ask him "What is that?" Prompt expansion of the utterance with attributes such as "That's a brown bear! What is it?" "That's a big bear!" (2, 4) Note any imitations and spontaneous productions of two-word utterances.

In clinical practice, interventionists often find that many social communication areas can overlap and intersect with one another. In targeting social communication deficits across all age levels, interventionists should consider the exact nature of the deficit(s) to generate targeted, measurable goals and related treatment activities. Otten and Tuttle (2010) specify the social skills challenges shown in Figure 3.1 to help interventionists readily identify the area of need.

Skill deficits indicate that the student does not know how to perform the skill or has difficulty discriminating which skill to use in which situation. Clients with autism have to discern the appropriate social rule for the situation and recognize that a specific social behavior can be appropriate in one context and inappropriate in another. Intervention might target breaking skills into concrete steps, directly instructing each component, and then practicing each step via targeted activities.

Active Learning Task

Imagine you have a high school student with autism who demonstrates difficulty making introductions to meet classmates. Develop social skill steps for "making introductions" by breaking down the skill into at least four smaller, measurable steps that would allow you to teach each skill distinctly.

Performance deficits can occur when clients with autism know how to do the skill but have challenges executing it at an appropriate level. Alternatively, the student might have mastered knowledge of the skills, but have challenges discriminating which skills to use based on the context.

Therapy Golden Nugget

Interventionists might use role-playing tasks to practice performing the targeted skill. Consider videorecording the interaction and then using the video to provide direct feedback and have the client identify areas of strength and growth; for example, "What did you do well?" and "What area(s) should we continue to work on?"

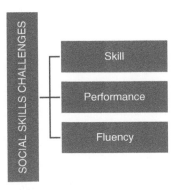

FIGURE 3.1   Social skills challenges.

Fluency-based challenges might mean your client does the skill appropriately in one setting, but fails to do it in another. This is particularly true among clients who successfully demonstrate skills within the therapy setting, but stakeholders such as teachers or parents continue to report challenges in unstructured settings. For example, we once had a high-school client with autism successfully meet goals targeting increased independence such as ordering food for herself. However, while she mastered the skill and performance in the clinic room, she demonstrated difficulty across settings. For example, she often struggled in crowded and busy spaces. In observation in the school lunch line, upon being asked what she wanted to eat by the cafeteria worker, the client did not respond quickly enough or use skills to communicate her need for more time to respond. The cafeteria worker quickly asked her to step aside until she was ready and served other students. With the unexpected change, the student never successfully got her lunch. In this example, an interventionist might consider a two-pronged approach. One target might be to teach community members to allot more time for students to communicate successfully, while another target might be to direct the client to increase self-advocacy skills.

Therapy Golden Nugget

Community integration tasks might be used to help the client practice the skill in more natural settings. For example, a client targeting repairing communication breakdowns might demonstrate the skill well in the clinic room where there are limited distractions and demands. However, the client might respond differently if attempting to demonstrate the skill in practice such as going to a coffee shop and ordering correctly in the midst of increased noise, a busy barista, and a line of waiting customers. Among all the deficit areas, attainment can be challenging because social rules are complex and vary based on context. Interventionists should address the social communication targets most useful and appropriate for client functioning, while considering reported and observed challenges.

SUMMARY

A variety of social communication challenges may present in individuals with autism. These challenges can vary across contexts, can present with different levels of severity, and can change over time. Some, but not all, impacted areas of social communication can include joint attention, play skills, eye gaze, body language, use of gestures, response to name, use of tone and suprasegmental aspects of speech, initiations, topic maintenance, and executive functioning. There are different types of gestures that include *conventional, instrumental or informational*, and *descriptive* gestures. Use of gestures is correlated with language development, with children who use communicative gestures demonstrating more expressive language learning skills. Theory of mind is the recognition that others can have different mental states. This skill is typically achieved by age four, but can be limited in children with autism, which can contribute to adverse social and academic impacts. Providers working with clients with ASD must be able to effectively describe social communication challenges and should look for consistency among raters to confirm areas of deficit.

REFLECTIONS ALONG THE PATH

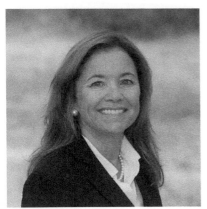

Lynn Kern Koegel, Ph.D.

It is a pleasure to write about my experiences working in the area of autism. The longer I'm in the field, the more I realize that there is still so much that we need to do to support autistic individuals and their families. During my early career years, autism was considered "low incidence," with about 1 in 2500 children receiving the diagnosis. At that time, institutionalization was common, even for very young children. Fortunately, interventions were beginning to move away from a parental causation theory, wherein parents were separated from their children. Newer procedures, based on learning theory, with parents included as an integral and important part of the process, were showing that children could indeed learn. Albeit effective, the children exhibited a fair number of interfering behaviors during these early drill-type adult-driven interventions. Thus, our team of speech–language pathologists and psychologists began researching ways to help improve the children's "motivation," and found that areas such as choice, task variation, interspersing maintenance tasks, rewarding attempts, and providing natural rewards were helpful. Eventually we combined them as a package, which focused on improving expressive communication (Koegel et al. 1987). This was initially described as the "natural language paradigm," but later we found that when key core areas are targeted, positive collateral improvements are seen in untargeted areas, and thus the intervention was renamed "pivotal response treatment" or "*PRT*." These naturalistic procedures are now widely used and can be measured via correct responding, improved rate of responding, decreased latency times, and improved affect. These techniques have resulted in considerably more autistic children using expressive verbal communication and can also be applied to other areas, such as play, language, academics, social conversation, and pragmatics.Lynn Kern Koegel, Ph.D.,

I was also fortunate to be able to work with a team of researchers, including Horner, Dunlap, R. Koegel, Carr, Anderson, Sailor, and Albin, to help develop the field of positive behavior support. There are many positive procedures to address interfering behaviors without the need for punishment. Although the motivational procedures are important for engagement, particularly as an antecedent intervention, the more evidence-based interventions we have in our repertoires, the better. Techniques such as priming, replacement behaviors, self-management, predictability, and desensitization can be helpful when developing a comprehensive program that is coordinated across environments. I have also found that, despite a huge increase in autism research, there are still many areas that remain under-researched, such as mechanisms responsible for improving first words (and intelligibility), social communication and friendships, employment, and leisure activities. Issues related to parental stress also continue to be a concern. We as a society need to learn how to give families the support they need to reduce their stress. However, we do know that carefully choosing the right pivotal areas, such as motivation, initiations and question asking, empathy, responding to multiple cues, and self-management, while incorporating motivational procedures into the intervention can make a huge difference in both targeted and global improvements.

In our busy lives, it is sometimes easy to forget to keep up with the research but using evidenced-based interventions is important. Going to conferences provides an opportunity to find out the latest effective techniques before publication. Collaborative efforts are also essential. Everyone working with an individual with ASD can contribute important information. We don't have all the answers yet, and everyone responds uniquely to interventions, so keeping the lines of communication open and cooperative will greatly benefit all involved. Lastly, focusing on the strengths of the individuals you work with during assessment and intervention helps us all appreciate the many abilities of individuals with ASD, while also attributing to better outcomes.

Lynn Kern Koegel, Ph.D., CCC-SLP
Clinical Professor, Stanford School of Medicine

TEST QUESTIONS

1. A child clapping is an example of a:
   A. Descriptive gesture
   B. Conventional gesture
   C. Instrumental gesture
   D. Informational gesture

2. Gestures that represent an event like surfing are:
   A. Descriptive
   B. Conventional
   C. Instrumental
   D. Informational

3. True or false? Eye contact is a challenge that typically resolves by age three in children with autism.

4. True or false? The Sally-Ann task is a type of false-belief task used to assess theory of mind.

5. Which of the following is not an example of evidenced based practice?
   A. Evidence from a peer-reviewed scientific journal
   B. Professional textbooks
   C. Facebook group
   D. Clinical expertise

6. Typical children develop theory of mind by age:
   A. Two years
   B. Three years
   C. Four years
   D. Six years

7. Which of the following may be included in diagnostic reports (select all that apply)?
   A. Clinical observation
   B. Parent report
   C. Client report
   D. Teacher report

8. Short answer question: Discuss four different social communication challenges that individuals with autism might exhibit.

9. True or false? In evaluating social communication challenges, individuals may exhibit different strengths and weaknesses in different contexts.

10. True or false? "The client did bad with staying on topic when talking" can be transformed using clinical language to "The client demonstrated difficulty maintaining a topic during conversation."

REFERENCES

Abdi, B. (2010). Gender differences in social skills, problem behaviors and academic competence of Iranian kindergarten children based on their parent and teacher ratings. *Procedia – Social and Behavioral Sciences* 5: 1175–1179.

Allely, C. (2019). Understanding and recognising the female phenotype of autism spectrum disorder and the "camouflage" hypothesis: a systematic PRIMSA review. *Advances in Autism* 5 (1): 14–37.

Almehmadi, W., Tenbrink, T., and Sanoudaki, E. (2020). Pragmatic and conversational features of Arabic-speaking adolescents with autism spectrum disorder: examining performance and caregivers' perceptions. *Journal of Speech, Language, and Hearing Research* 63: 2308–2321.

Baron-Cohen, S., Leslie, A., and Frith, U. (1985). Does the autistic child have a "theory of mind"? *Cognition* 21: 37–46.

Bonneh, Y.S., Levanon, Y., Dean-Pardo, O. et al. (2011). Abnormal speech spectrum and increased speech variability in young autistic children. *Frontiers in Human Neuroscience* 4: 237. https://doi.org/10.3389/fnhum.2010.00237.

Braddock, B., Gabany, C., Shah, M. et al. (2016). Patterns of gesture use in adolescents with autism spectrum disorder. *American Journal of Speech-Language Pathology* 25 (3): 408–415.

Brinton, B., Robinson, L., and Fujikii, M. (2004). Description of a program for social language intervention. *Language, Speech, and Hearing Services in Schools* 35 (3): 283–290.

Bruinsma, Y., Koegel, R., and Koegel, L. (2004). Joint attention and children with autism: a review of the literature. *Mental Retardation and Developmental Disabilities Research Reviews* 10 (3): 169–175.

Calder, L., Hill, V., and Pellicano, E. (2013). 'Sometimes I want to play by myself': understanding what friendship means to children with autism in mainstream primary schools. *Autism* 17 (3): 296–316.

Daughrity, B. (2019). Parent perceptions of barriers to friendship development for children with autism Spectrum disorders. *Communication Disorders Quarterly* 40 (3): 142–151.

Droucker, D., Curtin, S., and Vouloumanos, A. (2013). Linking infant-directed speech and face preferences to language outcomes in infants at risk for autism Spectrum disorder. *Journal of Speech, Language, and Hearing Research* 56: 567–576.

Ellawadi, A.B. and Weismer, S.E. (2014). Assessing gestures in young children with autism spectrum disorder. *Journal of Speech, Language, and Hearing Research* 57: 524–531.

Freeman, S., Gulsrud, A., and Kasari, C. (2015). Brief report: linking early joint attention and play abilities to later reports of friendships for children with ASD. *Journal of Autism and Developmental Disorders* 45 (7): 2259–2266.

Fu, G., Heyman, G., and Lee, K. (2011). Reasoning about modesty among adolescents and adults in China and the U.S. *Journal of Adolescence* 34 (4): 599–608.

Ganek, H., Smyth, R., Nixon, S., and Eriks-Brophy, A. (2018). Using the language environment analysis (LENA) system to investigate cultural differences in conversational turn count. *Journal of Speech, Language, and Hearing Research* 61: 2246–2258.

Gorman, B.K., Fiestas, C.E., Peña, E.D., and Clark, M.R. (2011). Creative and stylistic devices employed by children during a storybook narrative task: a cross-cultural study. *Language, Speech, and Hearing Services in Schools* 42 (2): 167–181.

Gulsrud, A., Hellemann, G., Freeman, S., and Kasari, C. (2014). Two to ten years: developmental trajectories of joint attention in children with ASD who received targeted social communication interventions. *Autism Research* 7 (2): 207–215.

Hahn, L., Brady, N., and Versaci, T. (2019). Communicative use of triadic eye gaze in children with down syndrome, autism Spectrum disorder, and other intellectual and developmental disabilities. *American Journal of Speech–Language Pathology* 28: 1509–1522.

Ham, H.S. and Bartolo, A. (2012). Exploring the relationship between gesture and language in ASD. *Perspectives on Language Learning and Education* 19 (2): 56–65.

Hareli, S., Kafetsios, K., and Hess, U. (2015). A cross-cultural study on emotion expression and the learning of social norms. *Frontiers in Psychology* 6: 1501. https://doi.org/10.3389/fpsyg.2015.0150.

Holbrook, S. and Israelsen, M. (2020). Speech prosody interventions for persons with autism spectrum disorders: a systematic review. *American Journal of Speech–Language Pathology* 29: 2189–2205.

Huang, S. (2016). Cultural competence in bilingual social communication assessment: a case study. *Perspectives of the ASHA Special Interest Groups* 1 (14): 29–41.

Hwa-Froelich, D. and Matsuo, H. (2018). Pragmatic language performance of children adopted internationally. *American Journal of Speech–Language Pathology* 28 (2): 501–514.

Ingersoll, B. and Lalonde, K. (2010). The impact of object and gesture imitation training on language use in children with autism spectrum disorder. *Journal of Speech, Language, and Hearing Research* 53 (4): 1040–1051.

Kasari, C., Locke, J., Gulsrud, A., and Rotheram-Fuller, E. (2011). Social networks and friendships at school: comparing children with and without ASD. *Journal of Autism and Developmental Disorders* 41 (5): 533–544.

Koegel, R.L., O'Dell, M.C., and Koegel, L.K. (1987). A natural language teaching paradigm for nonverbal autistic children. *Journal of Autism and Developmental Disorders 17* (2): 187–200.

LeCuyer, E. and Zhang, Y. (2015). An integrative review of ethnic and cultural variation in socialization and children's self-regulation. *Journal of Advanced Nursing* 71 (4): 735–750.

Leong, V., Byrne, E., Clackson, K. et al. (2017). Speaker gaze increases infant-adult connectivity. *Proceedings of the National Academy of Sciences* 114 (50): 13290–13295.

Moriuchi, J., Klin, A., and Jones, W. (2017). Mechanisms of diminished attention to eyes in autism. *American Journal of Psychiatry* 174 (1): 26–35.

Neumann, D., Spezio, M., Piven, J., and Adolphs, R. (2006). Looking you in the mouth: abnormal gaze in autism resulting from impaired top-down modulation of visual attention. *Social Cognitive and Affective Neuroscience* 1 (3): 194–202.

Nowell, S., Watson, L., Crais, E. et al. (2020). Joint attention and sensory-regulatory features at 13 and 22 months as predictors of preschool language and social-communication outcomes. *Journal of Speech, Language, and Hearing Research* 63 (9): 3100–3116.

Otten, K. and Tuttle, J. (2010). *How to Reach and Teach Children with Challenging Behavior (k-8): Practical, ready-to-use interventions that work.* San Francisco, CA: Jossey-Bass.

Owens, R.E. (2020). *Language Development: An Introduction*, 10e. New York, NY: Pearson.

Powless, D. and Elliott, S. (1993). Assessment of social skills of native American preschoolers: teachers' and parents' ratings. *Journal of School Psychology* 31: 293–307.

Prelock, P. (2015). DSM-5 changes: understanding the social challenges in children with ASD. *Perspectives on Language Learning and Education* 22 (1): 5–12.

Siller, M., Morgan, L., and Fuhrmeister, S. (2020). Social communication predictors of successful inclusion experiences for students with autism in an early childhood lab school. *Perspectives of the ASHA Special Interest Groups* 5 (3): 611–621.

Simmons, E., Paul, R., and Volkmar, F. (2014). Assessing pragmatic language in autism spectrum disorder: the Yale *in vivo* pragmatic protocol. *Journal of Speech, Language, and Hearing Research* 57 (6): 2162–2173.

Small, L.H. (2020). *Fundamentals of Phonetics: A Practical Guide for Students*, 5e. Pearson.

Trevisan, D., Roberts, N., Lin, C., and Birmingham, E. (2017). How do adults and teens with self declared autism spectrum disorder experience eye contact? A qualitative analysis of first-hand accounts. *PloS One* 12 (11): e0188446.

Wetherby, A.M. and Prizant, B.M. (2002). *CSBS DP™ Infant-Toddler Checklist*. Baltimore, MD: Paul H. Brookes Publishing Co.

West, K., Roemer, E., Northrup, J., and Iverson, J. (2020). Profiles of early actions and gestures in infants with an older sibling with autism spectrum disorder. *Journal of Speech, Language, and Hearing Research* 63 (4): 1195–1211.

Zenko, C. (2014). Practical solutions for executive function challenges created by the unique learning styles of students with autism spectrum disorder (ASD). *Perspectives on School-Based Issues* 15 (4): 141–150.

FURTHER READINGS

Lock, J., Shih, W., Kretzmann, M., and Kasari, C. (2015). Examining playground engagement between elementary school children with and without autism spectrum disorder. *Autism* 20 (6): 653–662.

Wong, C. and Kasari, C. (2012). Play and joint attention of children with autism in the preschool special education classroom. *Journal of Autism and Developmental Disorders* 42 (10): 2152–2161.

CHAPTER 4

Early Intervention and Autism

Learning Objectives

By reading this chapter, students will be able to:

1. Describe speech and language developmental milestones for neurotypical preschool age children.
2. Contrast neurotypical speech and language development with common characteristics and deviations for individuals with an early autism diagnosis.
3. Define and describe key aspects of joint attention and the marked deficits in joint attention present in individuals with an early autism diagnosis.
4. Define and compare levels of play and describe common deficits and areas of need for individuals with an early autism diagnosis.
5. Describe methods of collaboration with other professionals involved in the therapeutic process for a young child with autism.
6. Plan for a therapy session with a young child with an autism diagnosis considering timing, presentation of material, and organization of material.

A little boy is carried into your office. He barely looks at you, making noises with glottal stops and hums upset that he is being put down, he starts screaming, throws his body to the floor, and then attempts to find the door. His parents look stressed and are holding on to him for dear life. Dad says "sorry, we don't want him to start throwing things around your office." Day one of therapy has just begun.

Autism Spectrum Disorders from Theory to Practice: Assessment and Intervention Tools Across the Lifespan, First Edition. Edited by Belinda Daughrity and Ashley Wiley Johnson.

UNDERSTANDING NEUROTYPICAL DEVELOPMENT

For young neurotypical clients, research shows that the **critical learning period**, often referred to as the first six years of life (Snow 1987), represents the opportunity for repair and development of new skills. During this time, a child can best be described therapeutically as a sponge, ready to soak up all information that is given to them. Similar to a sponge, the liquid, or therapy absorbed, will be retained. Some may fall off, but most will stay in place and ultimately dries into the sponge, creating an imprint that will last throughout the sponge's lifetime. Therapeutically, that imprint can be considered to be *mastery and generalization* (Brignell et al. 2018).

For a student with an early autism diagnosis, the sponge analogy may or may not hold true. In fact, the *variability in performance* is what makes it a challenge for interventionists to predict outcomes for language skills, social pragmatic skills, and overall level of functioning for a young client who has an autism diagnosis. Some clients with autism may present with neurotypical language skills, or even advanced language skills. However, many may present with severe delays in expressive and receptive language early on. With the newest *Diagnostic and Statistical Manual of Mental Disorders, fifth edition* (DSM-V) criteria, the key qualification in diagnosis of autism is the presence of social communication delays along with restrictive repetitive patterns of behavior (American Psychiatric Association 2013).

Therapy Golden Nugget
Analyzing the DSM-5 criteria through a clinical lens indicates that clients with autism encountered in the therapy room may all look different.

Active Learning Activity

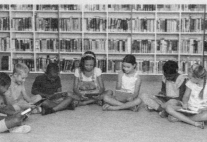

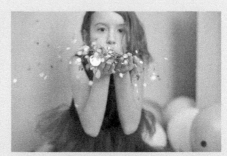

WavebreakMediaMicro/Adobe Stock   Credit: bondarillia/Adobe Stock

Clinical Profile #1
• Has a few words and phrases
• Parents say that he can read chapter books
• No conversation skills
• Limited meaningful language

Clinical Profile #2
• Extreme restricted behaviors; flaps hands often
• Fleeting eye contact
• Could not sit for a formal evaluation
• Does not sit independently

Consider the two clinical profiles listed above. Identify three possible obstacles with executing therapy and potential solutions to overcome the obstacle. Compare and contrast with a peer.

CONSIDERING NEUROTYPICAL DEVELOPMENT

When planning to do therapy with a young child who has autism, it is critical to understand and plan using typical language milestones (American Speech and Hearing Association 2022). This will assist the interventionist to qualify the child based on current performance and to develop realistic and meaningful, developmentally appropriate goals. The standard should be to support the child to use and understand language at or above their age level. However, the complex world of a child with autism can be challenging to understand and it may be easy to lose sight of what you need to be working on first and knowing what is next. Table 4.1, adapted from the American Speech and Hearing Association, depicts normal speech and language milestones along with accompanying therapeutic tasks.

Although there is variation in presentation of language skills, when you compare speech and language development for a child with autism to typical milestone limits, you may see variation. In fact, studies show that many children with an autism diagnosis will be delayed in development of many speech and language milestones, mostly reported as delayed onset of the first word and first phrase. In comparison with clients with other similar delays, including atypical development and pervasive developmental disorder – not otherwise specified, a client with autism is the most delayed in language and gross motor developmental milestone limits of all of these groups in comparison with their neurotypical peers (Matson et al. 2010).

In therapy, one challenge present for a client with autism and language development is *variance in communication trajectories*. This is best described as a building block effect. Normally, blocks will build upon each other getting higher as more blocks are added to the full structure. This should describe the natural flow of therapy with a neurotypical client. On the contrary, many clients with autism develop in different, irregular patterns. One of our adults clients, whom we've seen from early intervention age to now, refers to his different way of learning as his "unique wiring."

You may experience **regression**, described as sudden loss of skills that were previously mastered, or a **plateau**, where you have reached a peak and skills remain the same. When you experience this in therapy, it is important to not feel defeated or frustrated; rather, switch your therapy to help engage the client in a different manner. On the contrary, you may even experience abnormal acceleration, where skills are very quickly acquired, even more so than you expected (Luyster et al. 2005; Rogers et al. 2004; Pearson et al. 2018; Brignell et al. 2018; Matson et al. 2010; Figure 4.1). Of course, acceleration is a wonderful thing to experience during therapy sessions!

Variances in development of skills will also depend on environmental factors such as parent participation, socioeconomic status, and child factors, such as nonverbal IQ, comorbidities, autism spectrum disorder (ASD) symptoms, play skills, and gender. All these variables can be contributing factors to progress in addition to interventionist factors such as use of effective evidence-based practices and clinical flexibility, which may be heavily influenced by years of prior formal and informal experience and expertise.

To better understand external factors, it is best to thoroughly read the case history and to obtain background information from the parent through parent interviews when possible. For example, nonverbal IQ is often assessed and discussed in the

TABLE 4.1 Early language developmental milestones and therapeutic activities.

Typical age of development	Receptive language skillset	Expressive language skillset	Therapeutic activity
 Prostock-studio/Adobe Stock 7 months – 1 year	Localizes to sounds with head turn and eye gaze. Coordinates eye gaze to look at what someone is pointing to.	Babbles long syllable strings.	Noise toys hidden behind therapists, under objects, or around therapy room.
	Responds to name with a head turn and established eye contact.	Uses sounds (ooh, ahh, oh, huh, boo) and gestures (points, signals, pulls hand) to get and keep attention.	Segmenting objects in a book, using them for identifying common objects (seen in story for context) and for develop the clients matching pointing, and showing target pictures.
	Understands words for common items and people (i.e. cup, car, mommy).	Points to objects with one finger and will show others.	No David! Book series to develop early gestures such as a head shaking and indicating yes/no.
	Responds to common phrases to get attention like "stop!" "come here!" "no!"	Uses gestures and facial expressions for social purposes (shaking head "no" reaches for "up," smiles and laughs, waves).	
	Plays simple routine games (peek-a-boo, high fives) Listens for one to two minutes.	Says a few simple words which may not be clear.	
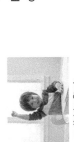 Tierney/Adobe Stock 1–2 years	Points to body parts when asked.	Consistently develops toward and past first 50 words.	Freeze dance! Using a manual stop sign, help the child to regulate their body and follow simple commands.

2–3 years		
Follows simple one step directions	Names pictures in books.	"Simon says" + body parts. Give simple directions incorporating touching or pointing to various body parts.
Responds to simple wh-questions (who, what, where).	Practices words they like.	Mr. Potato Head for identification and labeling.
Points to pictures in a book when you name them.	Asks simple questions (who, what, where?).	Carrier phrase development I + See + Object using sign and verbalizations to develop increased utterance length.
Listens to stores songs and rhymes for up to four minutes.	Puts two to three words together or more.	Use wordless picture books to stimulate language production and also increase labeling.
Understands opposites.	Has a word for almost everything.	Red light, green light game!
Follows two-step related directions.	Talks about objects events or occurrences not in immediate real.	Large box, object, and child to practice preposition expression and understanding.
Understands new words quickly.	Understands basic prepositions.	Expressive recall of past activities with parent participation.
Understands basic prepositions.	Uses simple sentences.	Silly Sentences activity set to encourage sentence construction and use.
	Understood by familiar listeners.	
	Asks "why" questions.	

Source: American Speech–Language–Hearing Association (2020).

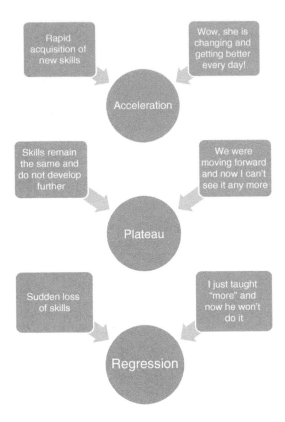

FIGURE 4.1   Clinical manifestations.

diagnostic report. Through reading the diagnostic report, there have been times that we have found nonverbal children who have an IQ of 110 (above average range). These clients may present as severely delayed. However, with repetition and practice, we have seen them demonstrate abnormal acceleration in the therapy sessions and ultimately present as children with gifted savant-like abilities. Without reading diagnostic information, we would have been unaware of the potential of the client.

FAMILY INVOLVEMENT

Family involvement is an additional critical component for success in therapy sessions with young children with autism (Shamash and Hinman 2022). Remember, as the interventionist, you spend a total of a few hours a week with a child in the best-case scenario. Families, however, make up the remainder of that time when a child is not in the early intervention setting. Empowering and sharing knowledge about their child's abilities and knowledge about autism is critical especially for parents of early-intervention-age children with a recent diagnosis (Wiley et al. 2016; Shamash and Hinman 2022).

While a parents knowledge about autism may vary based on a variety of factors, taking time to assess and develop a parent's or caregiver's knowledge in this area can lead to increased parent self-efficacy and lower parent stress levels (Shamash and Hinman 2022, Wiley et al. 2016; McConachie and Diggle 2007). One example in practice is to provide the parents with examples of how the child's behaviors relate to specific characteristics of autism (Figure 4.2).

Many interventionists suggest including the parent in the session when possible, to teach strategies and to assist. In fact, **parent-mediated interventions** are a proven treatment method which increases joint engagement and play skills, while generalizing across natural environments (Kasari et al. 2010, 2015). This could be positive for some clients and not the best idea for others. Discretion is key. At the bare minimum, it is best to share what has gone on in therapy via a progress note, home packets, or dedicating the last few minutes of the therapy session to the parent to share successes, challenges, and key strategies.

Strategies to Promote Parent Engagement

- ✓ Engage in regular check-ins on client progress.
- ✓ Do not overwhelm parents with information – provide a concise summary.
- ✓ Use the contact method most convenient to both you and the parent (email, text message, smartphone apps, face to face, handwritten notes, etc.).
- ✓ Communicate in the parent's primary language (this might be different than the child's primary language) via an interpreter if needed – remember to also use documents in the parent's primary language.
- ✓ Showing what to do might be more helpful than telling what to do.
- ✓ Encourage questions and transparency – invite parents to observe and participate as they feel comfortable.

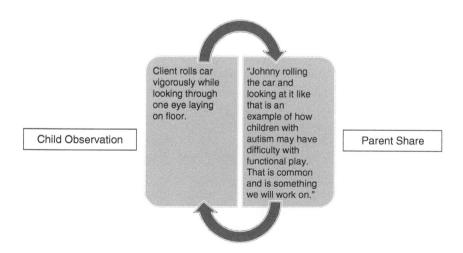

FIGURE 4.2 Providing parents with examples of how the child's behaviors relate to specific characteristics of autism.

Active Learning Task

Using the example above, complete the examples below to practice providing parents with examples of how the child's behaviors relate to specific characteristics of autism. For added practice, after completing the table, practice role playing to consider your direct implementation in your future practice.

Child observation	Parent share: What can you say to the parent observing?
Child retreats to corner to play with toys alone.	
Child reaches for toy instead of asking for it.	

EVIDENCE-BASED APPROACHES

Interventionists working with early-intervention-age children on the autism spectrum must use practices that are based on scientific evidence. These practices have been tried and true and are a specific requirement when working with children who have autism and their families. In an age where the internet, social media, and other media outlets are prevalent, it is very easy to find approaches that claim to be "effective" or shift the lives and wellbeing of a child with autism (Siri et al. 2014). However, given the **critical learning period,** increased prevalence of the disorder, and parents desire to see change with their child, it is critical to rely heavily on methods that have been cited and proven as effective and grounded in empirical research.

Many textbooks will teach a student the information needed to pass a test and have knowledge about a subject and related terminology. However, this does not translate to being prepared and ready to execute when you are placed in a room with a young child with a recent autism diagnosis who is presenting with all of the characteristics you have read about (Sam et al. 2019). We can tell a parent in a debriefing session that you will use evidence-based practices, but without the practice component, are you really prepared to be able to commit and do it? For many novice interventionists, the honest response undoubtedly is "no." Being aware of the practices that are considered evidence based is not enough to lead an interventionist to physical practice. This common challenge has paved the way for the claim that scientific data, which can often present as sterile, must be translated for interventionists to feel comfortable to be able to use with their client and the clients families. Evidence-based practice must be individualized and adapted to child and family needs to be most effective; interventionists working with young children with autism must use their clinical judgment to determine best approaches.

One effective approach for assisting interventionists working with children with autism and their families is to use evidence-based practices, the Autism Focused Intervention Resources and Modules (AFIRM) project developed at the Frank Porter Graham Child Development Institute at the University of North Carolina at Chapel Hill. This online learning project has worked to use information compiled by the

National Professional Development Center on Autism Spectrum Disorders and reviewed by the National Clearinghouse for Autism Evidence and Practice, which has analyzed and organized evidenced-based practices for use with people with autism and also brought light to methods that are not proven to be effective or evidence based. The purpose of the AFIRM method is to train interventionist and parents to describe, practice, and monitor progress using the most common evidence-based approaches that have proven to be effective in working with children and youth with autism (Sam et al. 2019). The video modules, which are estimated to take two to three hours each, are organized as shown in Figure 4.3.

In the communicative disorders and sciences field, the American Speech and Hearing Association website is another great resource for evidence-based practice approaches with guidance for practitioners to be able to use the approach, learn about required training, and compare various methodologies for use with people with autism. For the purposes of working with young children with autism, below is a list of related evidence-based approaches to use. For more information, access the 2020 NCAEP Evidence-Based Practice Report (`http://NCAEP.fph.unc.edu`), AFIRM project (`http://afirm.fpg.unc.edu`), and ASHA Practice Portal Autism Database (`www.asha.org`).

- Antecedent-based interventions:
  Arrangement of events or circumstances that precede an activity or demand in order to increase the occurrence of a behavior or lead to the reduction of the challenging/interfering behaviors.
- Denver Early Start Model:
  The Denver Model is a child-led, play-based treatment approach that focuses on the development of social communication skills through intensive one-on-one therapy, peer interactions in the school setting, and home-based teaching created

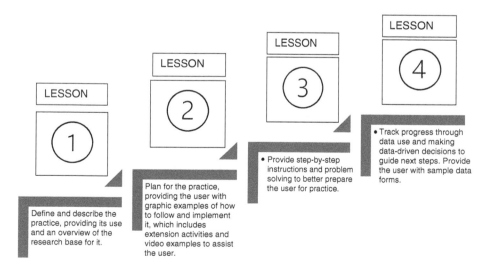

FIGURE 4.3 The autism focused intervention resources and modules.

by Rogers and Dawson in 2009. The Early Start Denver Model (created in 2010) for toddlers is an extension of the Denver Model; it combines developmental approaches with behavioral teaching strategies and can be delivered in a variety of settings (e.g. by the therapist and/or parents in group or individual sessions in the clinic or at home).

- **DIR®/DIRFloortime®:**
  A model that promotes development by encouraging children to interact with parents and others through play. The model focuses on following the child's lead; challenging the child to be creative and spontaneous; and involving the child's senses, motor skills, and emotions (Greenspan and Wieder 2007).

- **Exercise and movement:**
  Interventions that use physical exertion, specific motor skills/techniques, or mindful movement to target a variety of skills and behaviors.

- **Extinction:**
  The removal of reinforcing consequences of a challenging behavior to reduce the future occurrence of that behavior.

- **Joint attention symbolic play engagement regulation or JASPER:**
  A treatment approach that combines developmental and behavioral principles. This approach targets the foundations of social communication (joint attention, imitation, play) and uses naturalistic strategies to increase the rate and complexity of social communication. The approach incorporates parents and teachers into implementation of intervention to promote generalization across settings and activities and to ensure maintenance over time (Kasari et al. 2010, 2015).

- **Modeling:**
  Demonstration of a desired target behavior that results in use of the behavior by the learner and that leads to the acquisition of the target behavior.

- **Music-mediated intervention:**
  Intervention that incorporates songs, melodic intonation, and/or rhythm to support learning or performance of skills/behaviors. It includes music therapy, as well as other interventions that incorporate music to address target skills.

- **Naturalistic intervention:**
  A collection of techniques and strategies that are embedded in typical activities and/or routines in which the learner participates to naturally promote, support, and encourage target skills/behaviors.

- **Parent-implemented intervention:**
  Parent delivery of an intervention to their child that promotes their social communication or other skills or decreases their challenging behavior.

- **Pivotal response treatment (PRT):**
  Play-based, child-initiated behavioral treatment. Formerly referred to as "natural language paradigm," PRT's goals are: (i) to teach speech sounds, first words, and language; (ii) to decrease disruptive behaviors; and (iii) to increase social, communication, and academic skills. Rather than target specific behaviors, PRT

targets pivotal areas of development (response to multiple cues, motivation, self-regulation, initiation of social interactions, and empathy) that are central to a wide range of skills (Koegel and Koegel 2019). PRT emphasizes natural reinforcement (e.g. the child is rewarded with an item when they make a meaningful attempt to request that item).

- **Prompting:**
  Verbal, gestural, or physical assistance given to learners to support them in acquiring or engaging in a targeted behavior or skill.
- **Reinforcement:**
  The application of a consequence following a learner's use of a response or skills that increases the likelihood that the learner will use the response/skills in the future.
- **Social skills training:**
  Group or individual instruction designed to teach learners ways to appropriately and successfully participate in their interactions with others.
- **Video modeling:**
  A video-recorded demonstration of the targeted behavior or skill shown to the learner to assist learning in or engaging in a desired behavior or skill.
- **Visual supports:**
  A visual display that supports the learner engaging in a desired behavior or skills independent of additional prompts.

Active Learning Task

Access the AFIRM database (`http://afirm.fpg.unc.edu`) and identify one module of interest. Complete the module ending with the quiz. Send proof of accessing database and completing modules by printing the module certificate of completion.

IMPORTANCE OF CONNECTION

Establishing a natural connection is an important factor to be developed early on in therapy (Figure 4.4). As adults, one easy way to look at this would be to consider yourself in a therapy session with a psychologist. What would make you feel comfortable to talk with a therapist? What would make you feel uncomfortable and cause you to shut down or stop engaging with them? For many adults, the answer would be an ability to connect with the person you are talking to and also an ability to follow along with what they say when they are talking to you. This type of connection is exactly what is needed for a successful speech therapy session. However, most of our young clients, especially with autism, are unable to express that need and also may have challenges due to their difficulties establishing meaningful relationships or connection with others. This is a hallmark diagnostic feature for many children with autism and is included in the DSM-5 diagnostic criteria for a child to receive an autism diagnosis (American Psychological Association 2013).

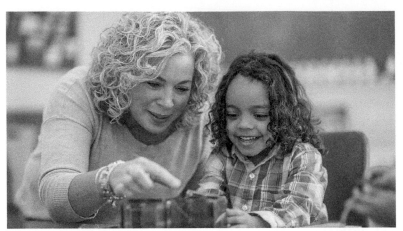

FatCamera/E+/Getty Images

FIGURE 4.4   Establishing a natural connection. Interventionist and client sharing in the same moment.

Therapy Golden Nugget

Objective: Client will respond to interventionist posed common social question; "what is your name?" Client will engage in joint attention by imitating large body movements as posed by clinician.

Materials: Client chairs in semicircle, interventionist chair in center of semicircle forearm length away.

Song lyrics:

> *Name, Name!*
> *What's in a name?*
> *I have a name*
> *AND*
> *YOU have a name*
> *What's YOUR name?*

Procedures: Interventionist will:
- Lead song with accompanying motor movements (i.e. hand clapping, pointing for I and YOU).
- Encourage student participation and copying of motor movements associated with song.
- Point to client to signal turn while posing final question.
- Say "What's your name?" once more.
- Lead client through production of the following phrase through sign or verbalization.

  My + Name + Is + _____.

- Encourage peers watching to exchange social nicety like a wave, "hi," or high five.

> **GOAL SPOTLIGHT**
>
> - Student will produce their name when prompted with a question posed by the clinician in four of five opportunities given minimal assistance.
> - Student will follow gross motor body movements as modeled by interventionist in four of five opportunities given moderate prompting.

One key characteristic of young children with autism is deficits in **joint attention skills** (Mundy et al. 1994). Joint attention is commonly defined as when two or more people sustain attention and focus on the same person, action, object, and are aware of the other's interests. A critical component of early development, joint attention is the way that a child learns the world. There are several factors that can be developed in a therapy session to repair or establish effective joint attention skills.

> **GOAL SPOTLIGHT**
>
> Client will demonstrate joint attention (turn taking, reciprocal play, sustained engagement) to complete a five-minute task with another in four out of five opportunities given minimal assistance.

The first and most crucial aspect needed for a successful therapy session is establishing eye contact with your client. There is a popular saying dating back as early as 58 BCE, found in the Bible, loosely translated as, "the eyes are the windows to the soul." For the purposes of this therapy manual, we share this statement to impart the importance of capturing your client's eyes as much as possible throughout the therapy session refer to Figure 4.4.

> **THERAPY VIEWPOINT**
>
> Establishing and sustaining eye gaze with a child will lead to understanding what the client is seeing, feeling, or thinking.

For a young client with autism, establishing and modulating eye-gaze behavior may seem like an impossible feat. In fact, atypical eye gaze is a hallmark diagnostic feature of autism. This lack of appropriate eye gaze behavior often occurs with adults who are not the child's caregiver or parent and more often in moments where there is an absence of toys or other objects for the client to interact with socially. In therapy settings, this may look like a client who refuses to look at you even for longer than a second but a parent who does not report any concerns with eye contact in the home setting. Parent report often is solely based on the level and type of personal interactions they have had with their child. The following are tips for establishing and encouraging sustained eye contact:

1. Draw attention to your eyes: Many SLPs suggest using a sticker featuring something the client likes on your forehead to motivate the client to orient

their gaze toward your face and eyes. Once you have them there, with the appropriate therapy strategies and activities, they may just stay there!

2. Pause preferred activities and demand eye contact: Moving an object toward your eyes to encourage looking is a dynamic way to increase ability to establish and sustain eye contact. Pair this move with a request (i.e. "Do you want more cars?").

3. Stay at your client's level: When engaging in therapeutic tasks, stay at the level of the child. It is easiest to encourage eye contact

Other key components of joint attention include reciprocal engagement, tracking, and imitation. These equally important aspects of joint attention can best be described as a child's ability to modulate eye contact and attention to follow along with someone to complete something or to look at various focal points (Cañigueral and Hamilton 2019). Sharing this experience, the child is expected to imitate what is seen. This is the way that a child learns and can build upon skills.

Active Learning Task

We know that establishing eye contact may not be an easy task to teach for a client who has atypical social communication. What can you do to help develop these critical skills? Given the above definition and examples, create three therapy activities that encourage the following aspects of joint attention?

- Reciprocal engagement
- Eye gaze and tracking
- Imitation

IMPORTANCE OF PLAYFULNESS

Mr. Rogers, world famous activist and child entertainer once said, "Play gives children a chance to practice what they are learning."

In a therapeutic setting as an interventionist facilitating change in a young client with an autism diagnosis, this quote could not be any truer. In fact, play-based methods are considered an evidenced-based approach proven to be an effective tool when working with a young child in the therapeutic setting (Sam et al. 2019). Clients with autism may present with delays in social communication, restricted interests, and limited engagement. In fact, when compared with neurotypical children and those with intellectual disabilities, children with autism present with less pretend play, decreased quality of play, and have increased difficulty spontaneously generating play (Lin et al. 2017). Therefore, incorporating play in the therapy room will work to engage parts of the brain that may need to be strengthened, taps into key areas of development, and of course encourages early social communication, which is a hallmark deficit for any child with an autism diagnosis.

Like language development, play also develops in a systematic fashion, which has often been organized and described chronologically by many authors. Review the following levels of play flowchart highlighted in Figure 4.5.

Early on, a child should be able to engage in **functional play**. In practical terms, this is a time where a child can pick up a play object and use it for its specific use. More specifically, a brush will be a brush being used to comb the hair, a car will be rolled on its wheels and may be accompanied by a "vroom" or "beep beep," and so on. This is a critical period, which indicates early play abilities. Around this time, we could expect a child to engage in **solitary play**, where a child plays alone and may not have an interest in engaging with other children.

As children mature chronologically and developmentally, you began to see onlooker behavior. This can best be described as your child being a spectator at the game. They watch other children and take an interest observing their play but are not quite ready to jump in and play along. Around this same time of onlooker behavior development, a child begins to develop symbolic play skills. This is where children will use objects, actions, or ideas, to represent other objects, actions, or ideas. For example, a set of blocks may magically represent a long train.

As these skills develop by two years old, a child is now ready to begin to engage with other children. The first step to this is parallel play, where a child will use the same objects and participate in the same activity beside another child, but not directly with that child. This is a critical period where children will learn how to play and will develop confidence to engage with another. Once this has developed, by around three years of age, a child is ready to engage in associative play, where the child interacts minimally with another child engaging in the same task. A great example of this may be where children are all playing on a piece of playground equipment but are using different pieces.

The final level of play, which develops typically around four years of age, is collaborative play. This looks just how it sounds; children playing together with a shared interest or goal. This is where games with rules come into play, playground chants, and organized activities or craft play starts to develop.

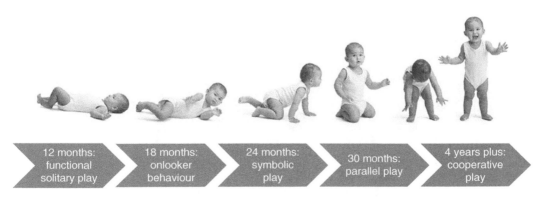

| 12 months: functional solitary play | 18 months: onlooker behaviour | 24 months: symbolic play | 30 months: parallel play | 4 years plus: cooperative play |

FIGURE 4.5 Levels of play flow chart. Source: Adapted from Centers for Disease Control and Prevention (2021), Parten (1932), Pathways.org (2022), Zero to Three (2022).

Active Learning Task

Watch the video clip:

Take a look at the video modeling, which is teaching symbolic play skills. Take time to consider the following questions with a peer.

- How many objects do you see in this video, what does each object represent?
- Describe the therapeutic space in the video. What about this will capture a young clients eye?
- How do you best describe the level of playfulness depicted in the video? How may this or may this not assist a client to feel encouraged to copy and engage?

Informally assessing where a child may be in terms of play skills and beginning to engage the child to increase the quality and diversity of play interactions will prove to be beneficial in the development and therapeutic process when working with a young child with autism (Lin et al. 2017). Figure 4.6 shows a list of play items that may prove beneficial for interventionists to have in their "tool box" when working with a young child with autism;

As tempting as it might be, especially for a new interventionist, we encourage you not to overpack your bag and include all these items! More does not mean better. Having too many play options can be overwhelming for both you and the child, and can contribute to disorganization, with a session lacking clear structure. Instead, select a few items and then determine how you can maximize their use to deliver age-appropriate, targeted intervention within play-based tasks using evidence-based approaches.

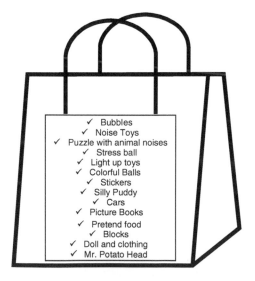

FIGURE 4.6   Play items for the interventionist's "tool box."

ORGANIZATION IN THERAPY

For young children with autism, there may be several challenges, which have been discussed throughout this chapter, like a shortened attention span, limited experience in the therapy and classroom settings, the presence of challenging behaviors, and limited joint attention. When given the task of being one of the child's first interventionists, it can be intimidating and may feel like an impossible feat. While no one can promise what may be the "golden ticket" to get a young child to engage, we can assist early interventionists to be well prepared to be "dressed for success."

In years of private practice and mentoring clinical fellows in our profession, we find one common challenge is language use. As a rule of thumb, we suggest limiting prompts and responses presented to young children with language delays to three to four words. Research shows that wording should be direct and concise when giving prompts to people with language delays. In theory, if you have challenges in understanding or expressing language, it can be conceived that it would be challenging to listen, comprehend, and then respond to prompts that are language rich. Complexity in language can increase as a child develops skills and abilities. However, less verbiage leaves room for less interpretation and more action on the part of the client.

Active Learning Task

Consider the following directives. Produce a phrase that follows the three- to four-word parameters shared in the Organization of the Therapy section of this chapter.

- You want your client to sit down and complete your activity; you will reward him with car play when he finishes.
- You want your client to point to the pictures of the bear, elephant, giraffe and monkey among all these other common objects.

Another component to consider when planning and presenting therapy is the frequency and duration of tasks presented in a therapy session. We suggest high frequency and short duration as a framework when planning therapy. More specifically, fill your session with a high number of activities. There, of course is a happy medium between enough and too much. For a session that lasts 50 minutes, we recommend that novice interventionists to prepare four tasks. The activities should last 13 minutes, which is short enough for a child to reduce boredom, but long enough for a client to have opportunities to produce the expected behavior.

ENVIRONMENTAL ARRANGEMENT

For a young child with autism, environmental arrangement is an evidence-based practice that has proven to be successful when implemented by interventionists in tandem with other strategies such a prompting and appropriate therapeutic approach. The idea of keeping a'child's therapeutic environment "clean" seems counterintuitive. In fact, one may believe it is simply the absence of materials, a neat space, somewhere where a child can sit down and, in essence, get to work. However, this type of environment can be considered "sterile," resulting in the lack of engagement, positive interactions, and motivation to respond to an intervent'onist's prompts. *Environmental arrangement* means using various strategies to manipulate the contexts to improve the likelihood that a specific behavior occurs (Ledford et al. 2017). This can include organizing physical materials and social arrangements.

For the purposes of this manual, *an appropriately arranged therapeutic space* when working with a young child with autism must be considered inviting and organized, with materials hidden from the clients' grasp. It is also helpful to include tangibles within viewpoint, but with limited access to the client. When successfully organized, consistently implemented, and paired with appropriate prompts using evidenced-based therapeutic approaches, therapists will see increased engagement and more positive interventionist–client interactions with young clients with autism (Ledford et al. 2017).

Therapy Golden Nugget			

How "Arranged" Is My Therapy Space?

Take a moment and ensure that you are ready for a successful therapy session for an early-intervention client. Complete the first and last column of the chart below each time you prepare to begin therapy with a new client.

Completed (✓)	What do I need to achieve for my client?	What does that look like?	What could I do with my existing space and materials?
	My space should be INVITING.	A child should feel comfortable to play and engage in your space. Regardless of size!	
	My space should be ORGANIZED.	Too many items can promote sensory overload which will distract or discourage a client with autism.	
	My space should be free of any MATERIALS not intended for my client to grab.	Strategically place materials out of their reach!	
	Have tangibles in my view and reach point.	Keep a few items that will shape a clients behavior in a safe place nearby or on your body.	

Sources: Adapted from Canavan (2015).

Active Learning Task

Deconstruct therapy spaces 1–5 and answer the following questions.

- How is the space organized?
- Does this space avoid possible client distractions?
- How do you think this space would make a client feel if they had to sit and engage in it?
- What are the positive and negative aspects of the therapy space in these images?
- Look at the room that you are in right now. How can it be best organized to serve a young client with autism?

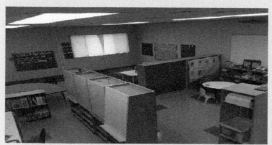

Therapy Space #1

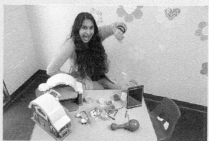

Therapy Space #2

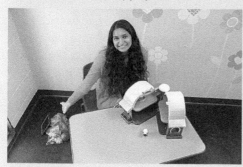

Therapy Space #3

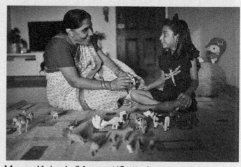

Mayur Kakade/Moment/Getty Images

Therapy Space #4

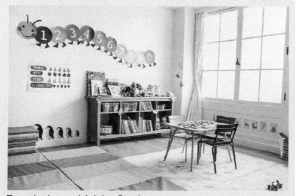

Rawpixel.com / Adobe Stock

Therapy Space #5

THE IMPORTANCE OF INTERPROFESSIONAL COLLABORATION

Traditionally, early intervention services for children with ASD have been provided by individual interventionists, such as SLPs, occupational therapists, applied behavior analysis specialists, and educational specialists such as the classroom special education teachers and resource specialists. For SLPs and related interventionists, therapy is often referred to as being "in a bubble" where services are pulled out and addressed in a group setting. One problem with this method is that providing pullout therapy can often show progress in an isolated environment and not as it relates to more complex settings like the classroom. Collaborative teamwork has been documented as one of the most critical components of instructional practice and, consequently, student outcomes (Goddard et al. 2007; Moolenaar et al. 2012). Progress is typically reported individually, and shared among team members at annual meetings, often referred to as individual educational plans or individual family service plans. Alternatively, collaboration between providers often facilitates more progress for the young child with autism and clearer communication among interventionists across various disciplines (Barnett and O'Shaughnessy 2015).

It can be hypothesized that it is counterintuitive for a service provider to work singularly when providing early intervention services for a student who presents with a variety of deficits that correlate directly with overall functioning. As current research findings suggest, working in isolation and convening annually is not the most productive or efficient during the critical period. Despite the current trend in service delivery, for decades, research has shown that the most crucial component of intervention for ASD is providing comprehensive services across all disability categories. This means that all services should have an emphasis on targeting adaptive behaviors, communication, cognitive ability, and social interaction to decrease the severity of the ASD (Cunningham 2012). Often, for a variety of reasons, this type of best practice does not occur. When thinking of the idea of progress and the ability to deliver services to children with ASD, it is important to consider how can we best meet the needs of our students in an efficient, but also realistic manner?

Recently, there has been a paradigm shift in evidence-based practice in speech and language pathology and psychology/psychiatry, which shows that using a collaborative model in providing services is more effective and efficient in working with young children with ASD (Friend et al. 2010; Brookman-Frazee et al. 2012). Current literature mentions the critical need for interventionists to work collaboratively and explore the effects of working directly alongside other services (Wilson et al. 2011) on overall levels of functioning. Specifically, Brookman-Frazee et al. (2012) reports that blended methods with an emphasis on behavior adaptation, communication skills, and developmental teaching has proven effective in working with young populations. With service providers collaborating to provide services, providers will have a more comprehensive understanding of the student's current level of functioning and strengths and weaknesses across domains.

SUMMARY

Autism is a complex neurodevelopmental disorder that does not present itself in a homogeneous fashion. There are a range of evidence-based practices and intervention approaches in early intervention that should be modified and individualized to meet the unique needs of each client and family. Early intervention will not be the same for each client; every client with autism might respond differently to intervention and you have to use your clinical judgment to determine best practices. Interventionists are responsible for using evidence-based approaches with clients with autism. To do so, you much follow a clear framework that considers typical milestones and remain abreast of evolving clinical research findings. Additionally, collaborating with key stakeholders is critical for intervention success to promote optimal outcomes.

REFLECTIONS ALONG THE PATH

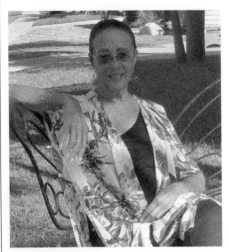

Diane Bernstein MA CCC-SLP

Congratulations on choosing one of the premier careers in the fields of allied health sciences and education. You will have the opportunity to work with infants, children and adults in intervention centers, schools, universities, clinics, hospitals, skilled care nursing/rehabilitation facilities and private practices separately or at the same ti'e. It's your choice! I did it at the same time and loved it.

Communication is the primary modality humans use to interact and connect with each other. They talk about their thoughts, hopes, dreams, joys and emotions. When the development is delayed in young children because of premature birth, genetic disorders, cerebral palsy, autism and other diagnoses, parents are deprived of the joy of hearing their child make their first communicative attempts using signs, words, or sentences in the right order with clear articulation. Each language has its own set of sounds and grammatical rules for developing speech. Since we can't explain those rules to infants and toddlers, they have the daunting task of figuring them out on their own, just by listening to us talk. This textbook will provide you with the therapeutic knowledge for helping them acquire those skills.

You will feel compassion for the teen with autism who has learned to stay on topic during a conversation with peers, or recognize the meaning of prohibitive facial expressions from peers when they are about to make an inappropriate remark that should not be heard by the group; the dysfluent client who has learned the technique for starting words or dropping secondary characteristics; the senior adult whose speech has been restored after a stroke or is now able to swallow food and enjoy a meal with family. These are just a few of the ways your therapy skills will enable clients to improve their quality of life at home, school, work and in functional and social settings.

While paperwork is the "bane of our existence," you may as well embrace it. Develop techniques for balancing it with the rest of your life. Reports must be done to prove our depth of knowledge, efficacy of therapy, and for agencies to provide funding. Research provides the empirical evidence by which we learn, grow and enhance our skills. New areas are frequently being considered to add to the field of communicative disorders. The latest include treatment of the "long hauler effects" on COVID 19 survivors, and teaching stroke patients how to re-engage in "pillow talk" to enhance interpersonal relationship communication. How lucky we are to have a career which is constantly being reinvented! You will never get bored or "burn out." There is always something new and interesting to learn.

And finally . . . therapy. Your goal is to improve the quality of your c'ients' lives when developing treatment plans. Critical areas to include for new skills to generalize are the 'lient's cognitive skills, areas of interest and life experiences. Ask yourself, does the client understand how to respond? Does the client understand the vocabulary I am using? Do I need to simplify the instructions? Equally important as a therapist, always listen carefully to your 'lient's response. You must be able to determine *when and where the 'lient's breakdown occurs during the activity, based on their level of understanding, and how to restructure the task to improve it.* You will have challenging clients from whom you will learn the most about therapy and human behavior. Once you have had the experience of evaluating and providing therapy across a wide variation of diagnoses, you will develop confidence, intuition and your own unique therapy style.

You have made your choice. Go for it.

Diane Bernstein MA CCC-SLP
Program Coordinator/Clinical Supervisor, 40 years

TEST QUESTIONS

1. A client with autism may demonstrate difficulty with sustaining eye gaze.

2. Teaching a clients parents about autism is offensive.

3. When looking to work with a young client with an autism diagnosis, it is critical to consider neurotypical language developmental milestones.

4. While language develops in a hierarchal fashion in typical development, play skills develop more idiosyncratically and unpredictably across young children.

5. Making a sound associated with an animal like "moo" may confuse the child. Its best to just use the real name.

6. Symbolic play is a higher level of play than functional play.

7. In intervention with young children with autism, only one evidence-based practice should be employed in therapy.

8. A sudden loss of language or skills that were previously mastered is known as:
   A. Language delay
   B. Aphasia
   C. Regression
   D. Articulation disorder

9. In JASPER, the "SP" stands for:
   A. Speech and language
   B. Symbolic play
   C. Special education
   D. Specified paradigm

10. _____ is an engagement state where the child is watching other people playing.
   A. Solitary play
   B. Onlooking
   C. Collaborative play
   D. Parallel play

REFERENCES

American Psychiatric Association (2013). *Diagnostic and StatistiIanual of Mental Disorders*, 5e. Arlington, VA: American Psychiatric Publishing.

American Speech-Language-Hearing Association. (2022). Autism spectrum disorder: Overview. Available from www.asha.org/Practice-Portal/Clinical-Topics/Autism (accessed 30 January 2022).

Barnett, J. and O'Shaughnessy, K. (2015). Enhancing collaboration between occupational therapists and early childhood educators working with children on the autism spectrum. *Early Childhood Education Journal* 43: 467–472.

Brignell, A., Williams, K., Jachno, K. et al. (2018). Patterns and predictors of language development from 4 to 7 years in verbal children with and without autism spectrum disorder. *Journal of Autism and Developmental Disorders* 48 (10): 3282–3295.

Brookman-Frazee, L., Stahmer, A.C., Lewis, K. et al. (2012). Building a research-community collaborative to improve community care for infants and toddlers at-risk for autism spectrum disorders. *Journal of Community Psychology* 40 (6): 715–734.

Cañigueral, R. and Hamilton, A.F. (2019). The role of eye gaze during natural social interactions in typical and autistic people. *Frontiers in Psychology* 10: https://doi.org/10.3389/fpsyg.2019.0056.

Canavan, C. (2015). Sensory overload: creating an autism-friendly environment. In: *Supporting Pupils on the Autism Spectrum in Primary Schools*, 56–78. London: Routledge.

Centers for Disease Control and Prevention. (2021). CDC's developmental milestones. Available from https://www.cdc.gov/ncbddd/actearly/milestones/index.html (accessed 30 January 2022).

Cunningham, A.B. (2012). Measuring change in social interaction skills of young children with autism. *Journal of Autism and Developmental Disorders* 42: 593–605.

Friend, M., Cook, L., Hurley-Chamberlain, D.A., and Shamberger, C. (2010). Co-teaching: an illustration of the complexity of collaboration in special education. *Journal of Educational and Psychological Consultation* 20 (1): 9–27.

Goddard, Y.L., Goddard, R.D., and Tschannen-Moran, M. (2007). A theoretical and empirical investigation of teacher collaboration for school improvement and student achievement in public elementary schools. *Teachers College Record* 109 (4): 877–896.

Greenspan, S.I. and Wieder, S. (2007). The developmental individual-difference, relationship-based (DIR/Floortime) model approach to autism spectrum disorders. In:

Clinical Manual for the Treatment of Autism (ed. E. Hollander and E. Anagnostou), 179–209. Washington, DC: American Psychiatric Publishing.

Kasari, C., Gulsrud, A., Wong, C. et al. (2010). Randomized controlled caregiver mediated joint engagement intervention for toddlers with autism. *Journal of Autism and Developmental Disorders* 40 (9): 1045–1056.

Kasari, C., Gulsrud, A., Paparella, T. et al. (2015). Randomized comparative efficacy study of parent-mediated interventions for toddlers with autism. *Journal of Consulting and Clinical Psychology* 83 (3): 554–563.

Koegel, R.L. and Koegel, L.K. (2019). *Pivotal Response Treatment for Autism Spectrum Disorders*, 2e. Baltimore, MD: Paul H. Brookes Publishing Co.

Ledford, J.R., Zimmerman, K.N., Chazin, K.T. et al. (2017). Coaching paraprofessionals to promote engagement and social interactions during small group activities. *Journal of Behavioral Education* 26 (4): 410–432.

Lin, S., Tsai, C., Li, H. et al. (2017). Theory of mind predominantly associated with the quality, not quantity, of pretend play in children with autism spectrum disorder. *European Child & Adolescent Psychiatry* 26 (10): 1187–1196.

Luyster, R., Richler, J., Risi, S. et al. (2005). Early regression in social communication in autism spectrum disorders: a CPEA study. *Developmental Neuropsychology* 27 (3): 311–336.

McConachie, H. and Diggle, T. (2007). Parent implemented early intervention for young children with autism spectrum disorder: a systematic review. *Journal of Evaluation in Clinical Practice* 13 (1): 120–129.

Matson, J.L., Mahan, S., Kozlowski, A.M., and Shoemaker, M. (2010). Developmental milestones in toddlers with autistic disorder, pervasive developmental disorder – not otherwise specified and atypical development. *Developmental Neurorehabilitation* 13 (4): 239–247.

Moolenaar, N.M., Sleegers, P.J., and Daly, A.J. (2012). Teaming up: linking collaboration networks, collective efficacy, and student achievement. *Teaching and Teacher Education* 28 (2): 251–262.

Mundy, P., Sigman, M., and Kasari, C. (1994). Joint attention, developmental level, and symptom presentation in autism. *Development and Psychopathology* 6 (3): 389–401.

Parten, M.B. (1932). Social participation among preschool children. *Journal of Abnormal and Social Psychology* 27 (3): 243–269.

Pathways.org. (2022). How kids learn to play: 6 stages of how play development. Available from `https://pathways.org/kids-learn-play-6-stages-play-development` (accessed 30 January 2022).

Pearson, N., Charman, T., Happé, F. et al. (2018). Regression in autism spectrum disorder: reconciling findings from retrospective and prospective research. *Autism Research* 11 (12): 1602–1620.

Rogers, L.J., Zucca, P., and Vallortigara, G. (2004). Advantages of having a lateralized brain. *Proceedings of the Royal Society of London B: Biological Sciences* 271 (Suppl_6): S420–S422.

Sam, A.M., Cox, A.W., Savage, M.N. et al. (2019). Disseminating information on evidence-based practices for children and youth with autism spectrum disorder: AFIRM. *Journal of Autism and Developmental Disorders* 50 (6): 1931–1940.

Shamash, E.R. and Hinman, J.A. (2022). Assessing caregiver stress and coping at time of autism spectrum disorder diagnosis. *Early Childhood Education Journal* 50: 97–106.

Siri, K., Lyons, T., Bradstreet, J.J., and Arranga, T. (2014). *Cutting-Edge Therapies for Autism*, 4e. New York, NY: Skyhorse Publishing.

Snow, C.E. (1987). Relevance of the notion of a critical period to language acquisition. In: *Sensitive Periods in Development: An interdisciplinary perspective* (ed. M. Bernstein), 183–209. Hillsdale, NJ: Erlbaum.

Wiley, P., Gentry, B.F., and Torres-Feliciano, J. (2016). *Autism: Attacking Social Interaction Problems, a Therapy Manual Targeting Social Skills in Children 4–9*. San Diego, CA: Plural Publishing.

Wilson, K.P., Dykstra, J.R., Watson, L.R. et al. (2011). Coaching in early education classrooms serving children with autism: a pilot study. *Early Childhood Education Journal* 40 (2): 97–105. https://doi.org/10.1007/s10643-011-0493-6.

Zero To Three. (2022). The development of play skills from birth to 3. Available from https://www.zerotothree.org/resources/series/the-development-of-play-skills-from-birth-to-3 (accessed 30 January 2022).

FURTHER READINGS

VandenBos, G.R. (2015). *APA Dictionary of Psychology*. Washington, DC: American Psychological Association.

Wiley, A.D. (2014). Collaboration Rotation and Technology: Innovative service delivery models for preschoolers with autism. Lecture presented at American Speech and Hearing Association National Convention in Orange County Convention Center, Orlando Florida, November 2014.

CHAPTER 5

School-Age Children Part One: Early Years

Learning Objectives

By reading this chapter, interventionists will be able to:

1. Explain frequent questions families of students with autism have when transitioning to school.
2. List common challenges for students with autism during elementary school years.
3. Identify at least two different positive behavior support strategies that can help clients with autism in the school setting.
4. Create intervention plans that address goals for students with autism in the school setting.

Entering school can be an exciting time for most families. For families of children with autism, the transition into elementary school can be full of questions and anxiety for both students and parents (Nuske et al. 2019). Will their child make friends? Will the teacher support the child's needs? For interventionists, our role becomes one of helping children with autism best access their academic curriculum and better address social skills deficits to promote successful peer engagement. For families, our role becomes one of promoting and teaching advocacy, as well as providing appropriate counseling during critical transition periods such as kindergarten, middle school,

Autism Spectrum Disorders from Theory to Practice: Assessment and Intervention Tools Across the Lifespan,
First Edition. Edited by Belinda Daughrity and Ashley Wiley Johnson.

high school, and post-high school. The purpose of this chapter is to help interventionists understand common challenges for students with autism and their families during early school-age years to develop strategies to promote skills that support school success.

TRANSITION TO SCHOOL

Pre Diagnosis

Despite all we know about early diagnosis and intervention, as evidenced by the average age of diagnosis of autism spectrum disorder (ASD) being older than four, there are still a number of children who are not diagnosed during this critical early childhood period of early intervention years from birth to three (Ozonoff et al. 2018). Some children not diagnosed in preschool years may be more readily identified in school, as expectations for social interactions increase and symptomology becomes more apparent in context around age-matched peers (Lord 2018). For these children, a diagnosis is often obtained during their first few years in school, especially as their social communication deficits adversely impact their academic achievement and school participation. Some families may have never suspected a developmental or speech delay, especially without peers for comparison if the child did not have siblings or attend preschool. In fact, children whose parents report low symptom severity of ASD are often diagnosed years after their counterparts with more severe symptomology, resulting in a minority of cases being diagnosed before age three (Sheldrick et al. 2017). Some families may have noticed areas of concern, but decided to "wait and see" if issues resolved on their own. Some families may have received early intervention services for speech and language and/or other delays, but never received an official diagnosis of autism.

Challenges are typically first noticed by the classroom teacher who, with training on typical child development and many typical peer references for comparison, might report concerns to parents. Initially, a classroom teacher might report concerns to an interventionist like a speech–language pathologist (SLP) or school psychologist to inquire about needs for a formal evaluation. For these families, the transition to school can be particularly challenging as they are simultaneously learning how to accept an autism diagnosis *and* how to navigate special education services to meet their child's needs.

Obtaining a Diagnosis

The first step to receiving intervention services in schools is receiving a formal evaluation and diagnosis. Typically, school districts will conduct their own assessments even if the child has an existing diagnosis or received services in early intervention. Appropriate assessment should include the same elements as reviewed in Chapters 2 and 3. Assessment in the school district includes members of the individual education plan (*IEP*) team, which differs from the individualized family service plan (*IFSP*) team in early intervention (Figure 5.1).

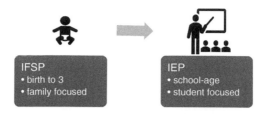

FIGURE 5.1 Transition from home to school: from individualized family service plan (IFSP) to individual education plan (IEP).

Individualized Family Service Plan

The IFSP team is composed of members of the early intervention team including service providers like the SLP, occupational therapist, physical therapist, and psychologist, as well as case managers and parents. The IFSP is centered around the family. Some services may be offered in the home as well as in clinics. Because this plan is in early intervention, the family is at the center of care. Goals might include elements of caregiver education so parents can stimulate speech and language development in the natural environment – the home. The idea is that the child's challenges impact the family as a whole and progress for young children is strongly correlated to family support.

Individual Education Plan (IEP)

The IEP team also includes service providers like the SLP, occupational therapist, physical therapist, and psychologist, as well as parents. It will also include additional members from the school like the general education classroom teacher, the special education classroom teacher, the resource teacher, and the adapted physical education teacher. Unlike the IFSP, the focus of the IEP is the student and the impact of the student's disability on accessing the education curriculum. Goals center on supporting the student's academic success under the guidelines of every child being able to access a free and appropriate public education, (FAPE).

An IEP is a legal document that dictates a child's educational plan and support services in the United States. IEPs are typically reviewed annually for progress and then extensively reviewed at least every three years. The review process typically involves all parties responsible for the child's care in the school with an emphasis on collaborative input to support the child's educational needs. This kind of documentation and process is similar outside of the United States; for example, in the United Kingdom and Ireland, the term is "special education needs" often referred to as SEN. This review process serves the same function as the IEP to provide additional provisions to support children with disabilities like autism in school. Scotland uses the term "additional support needs" to represent the same type of support.

While terminology differs across countries, terms also differ between states in the United States. For example, in California, case managers in early intervention can support families with autism across the lifespan and assist with helping families navigate the transition of services. As an interventionist, it is critical to find out about the key stakeholders and terminology in your state so that you can be knowledgeable about parents' experiences and also be able to provide additional support and education about the process as a whole. Transition planning generally begins a few months prior to the child's third birthday.

Children with ASD who transition into the school district and qualify for an IEP may not qualify for all support services, such as speech and language intervention, if they exceed eligibility criteria. Different school districts may have different eligibility criteria for services. For example, one school district may specify children need to score below a certain percentile rank or standard deviations from the mean of a formal assessment in order to qualify. This eligibility process can be frustrating for families as they navigate different systems to make sure their children have the appropriate support services to promote school success. Parent perspectives on IEP development indicate challenges working with schools to access appropriate for their children; however, increased satisfaction is connected to teacher satisfaction and relationships with school stakeholders (Kurth et al. 2020).

DETERMINING AN APPROPRIATE EDUCATION SETTING

The findings of the assessment report and review of records should contribute to the determination of an appropriate education setting for the child. Options can vary widely depending on school district and even schools themselves. Parents and the IEP team should collaborate to determine the best setting for the child to achieve academic success. The goal should be for the child to be academically successful. Placing a child in an inappropriate environment results in a child being inadequately academically challenged or being taught in a manner that prevents learning and appropriate access to the academic curriculum. Inappropriate academic classroom placement can lead to maladaptive behaviors and less positive attitudes toward learning and the academic environment as a whole (Figure 5.2).

Special education or self-contained classrooms can be appropriate for some children with autism with moderate to severe delays. These children require significant adaptations to best access their academic curriculum. They benefit from smaller class sizes with additional adult support. The traditional curriculum is adapted to be more functional to meet the students' unique learning needs.

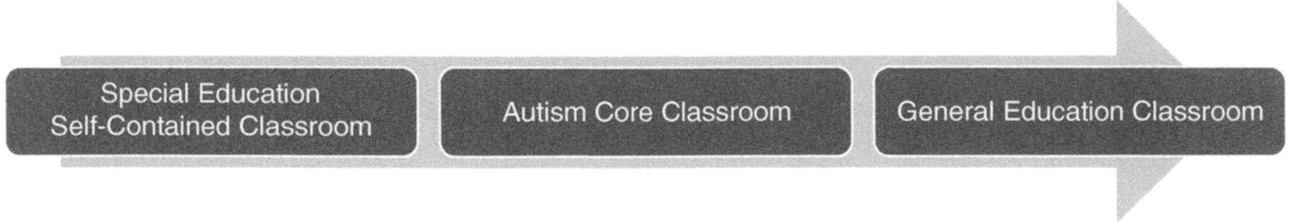

Special Education Self-Contained Classroom → Autism Core Classroom → General Education Classroom

FIGURE 5.2   Most to least restrictive educational environments.

Autism core classrooms may be offered by some schools. These settings offer the standard academic curriculum, while offering adjustments specifically to support students with autism. Modifications may include smaller class sizes, additional adult supports, teachers with training in autism, and positive behavior support strategies like visual schedules and token economies.

General education or mainstream settings to be appropriate for some students with autism with less symptomology, especially if they have typical or minimal delays in language skills and cognition. Some students may need appropriate supports can help them access the general education curriculum of their typically developing peers. At times, highly verbal children with autism are placed in general education settings with the idea of typical peer models being critical to social success. However, proximity to neurotypical peers does not automatically facilitate social success. In fact, children with autism in general education settings are often at higher risk of being socially isolated and lacking fully developed peer social networks (Rotheram-Fuller et al. 2010). In such cases, clinicians may consider support services like targeted interventions for social skills development to make friends. For example, studies have shown that brief interventions for playground staff improve peer interactions among children with autism in general education in elementary school settings, and are beneficial and contribute to increased peer engagement (Kretzmann et al. 2015). Despite evidence of their success, such interventions targeting key stakeholders like playground personnel have often proven unsustainable over time because of competing school demands and other barriers (Locke et al. 2015). Additionally, clinicians may consider strategies for educating typical peers on how children might exhibit differences and how to be more inclusive during unstructured social interaction times like lunch and recess. Such proactive approaches may support inclusive classrooms, reduce bullying, and promote the acceptance of neurodiversity among young children.

Therapy Golden Nugget

If you work in a school setting, consider opportunities to broaden your impact. Offer to make brief presentations to students to help them understand autism and how it might make a peer act differently. Ask students what they might do if they saw a peer being bullied. Prompt younger students to think about how they might get all students involved in playing games at recess. Think about starting a weekly lunch club where students with autism and their neurotypical peers can build relationships during semi-structured tasks like engaging in activities that might be related to the student with autism's interests. Get creative! Taking the therapy out of the clinic room when possible is a golden opportunity to promote generalization and to make your intervention matter in context.

GOAL SETTING

It is important to note that many school-age children with autism will have intervention goals in the areas of expressive and receptive language. Thus, goals may be similar to those of children with other disorders targeting increasing expressive and receptive language skills. While the goals may be similar, the child with autism may have specific accompanying behavioral differences from their peers. As such, consider your training in providing direct and indirect language stimulation, while making accommodations for the specific needs of children with ASD.

Given that children with autism are a unique population, clinicians should consider evidenced-based practices and determine appropriate tasks to support client engagement and progress in intervention. For example, evidence suggests children with autism can learn new grammatical forms given intervention approaches that include both explicit and implicit instruction methods (Bangert et al. 2019). Evidence also suggests school-age children with autism can improve in narrative production to create more complex, structured stories with more age-appropriate language given targeted intervention (Gilliam et al. 2015).

Your goals should be directly informed by your formal and informal assessment results. Some students with autism may be highly verbal and present with challenges that adversely impact their academic performance. Other students with autism may be less verbal and require supports to effectively communicate their wants and needs within their school setting. Your goal selection should be determined by a combination of:

- *Area(s) of need*: What are areas of delay according to formal and informal assessment?
- *Greatest functionality*: What are areas that will make the most significant impact for the student academically and socially?
- *Domain scope*: Which areas may serve to support one another? Consider selecting goals in different domains as appropriate: receptive, expressive, pragmatic speech.

Consider areas in which you might collaborate with other key professionals to support the student's goals. You might want to see which areas are also being targeted in other contexts.

BEHAVIORAL SUPPORTS FOR CHILDREN WITH AUTISM IN THE CLASSROOM

While behavior support is the primary expertise of behavior interventionists and applied behavior analysis professionals, all professionals, such as SLPs and other professionals supporting students with disabilities like autism, benefit from employing positive behavior support strategies to promote successful intervention (Bopp et al. 2004). All the following strategies are aspects of positive behavior support approaches to support students with autism in the classroom and other structured settings. It should be noted that such strategies can often be employed effectively for other children without autism. We often teach students that the use of such strategies provides additional support and do not adversely impact any students. As such, it is typically beneficial to use such approaches in a proactive manner as behavior is best managed in the absence of maladaptive behaviors, rather than only in the presence of problems (Otten and Tuttle 2011). Beyond clinicians working with children with autism, all adults working with children benefit from employing positive behavior support approaches in classrooms to promote positive and engaging classroom environments. All of the following examples are real life examples of supports we have used clinically and/or observed in the classroom environment. These accommodations can be helpful across contexts for any professionals working with students with autism.

Classroom Accommodations

Environmental arrangement is a proactive method of setting a student up for success by arranging the space in advance for the student to be successful. In group environments like classrooms or small intervention groups, this might mean sitting the student closer to the front of the room within easy access to the teacher. It might mean selecting particular students to sit with each other based upon behavioral needs.

THERAPY VIEWPOINT

No matter how large or small your space is, use the corners especially for **elopers**! Setting the child on the floor or in a chair in the corner with you directly in front helps to cut large spaces into much smaller and manageable work zones.

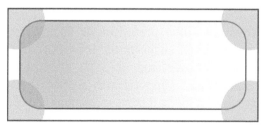

While considering the physical space set up of your work, also consider the visual space. Try to reduce visual clutter by putting away unnecessary items. Be mindful of posters or items on your walls to make sure your space is not too visually distracting for your clients with autism. Other accommodations may mean using different seating options like cube chairs, which provide more physical assistance for children with limited trunk support (Figure 5.3). This type of suggestion may come from an occupational therapist. However, we believe all interventionists should be aware of different options that can facilitate success for students with autism in the classroom who may have sensory integration challenges, which can negatively impact self-regulation

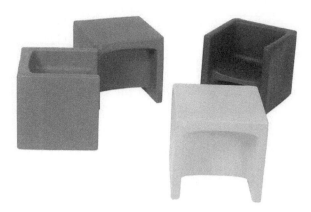

FIGURE 5.3   Cube chairs.

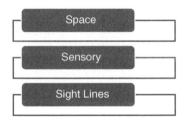

FIGURE 5.4   Different options that can facilitate success for students with autism in the classroom.

skills without targeted intervention (Case-Smith et al. 2014). Interventions should consider the teachers' input surrounding different options that can facilitate success for the students with autism in the classroom (Figure 5.4).

Collaborating with other allied professionals such as occupational therapists might help to employ a variety of suggestions to support students in the classroom such as pencil grips that may help students with writing tasks. While this seems minimal, identifying the correct supports will reduce the stress associated with common classroom activities. Other supports may include items such as weighted lap bands, fidget spinners, or stress squeeze balls.

Behavioral Shaping Supports

The example in Figure 5.5 was used for a child with autism who exhibited frequent hand flapping. His behavior was distracting for his peers and also prevented him from actively attending to classroom instruction. The visual cue card served as a specific reference to address the behavior. Note the instruction is framed positively. It tells the student *what to do*, rather than what not to do. This approach helps to replace the unwanted behavior with a new behavior, as it is impossible to do both at the same time. The cue card was placed on the student's desk and served as a visual reminder for him without the need for frequent adult verbal reminders.

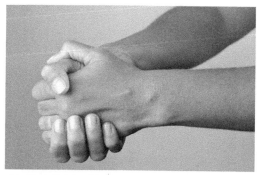

Jopstock/Adobe Stock

FIGURE 5.5   Visual cue card.

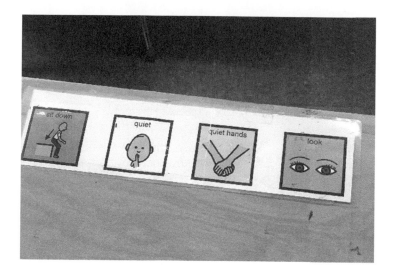

FIGURE 5.6   Visual behavior reminders: "Sit down," "Quiet", "Quiet hands," and "Look."

The primary purpose of behavioral shaping tools is to promote positive behavior support to elicit desired behaviors. Students with autism, as well as many other students, benefit from frontloading, which empowers students to know from the very beginning what is expected of them. By using positive behavior support, you can shape behavior into desired expectations and address potential behavioral issues before they occur and become problematic. Any interventionist can use these approaches in any setting.

The example in Figure 5.6 is another visual behavior reminder that provides simple classroom "rules" and allows the student to reference the behavior expectations as needed. The expectations are simple: sit down, quiet hands, and look. Note the instructions provide visual support with pictures and simple text support. When offering cue cards like this example, items displayed should match the child's language and cognition level.

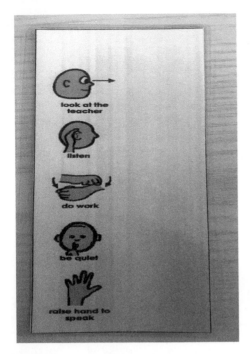

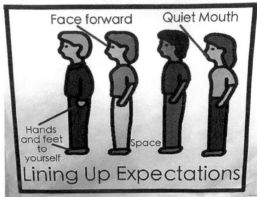

FIGURE 5.7   Examples of physical behavioral expectations charts.

The next example (Figure 5.7) shows another behavior support, but includes more icons and text. Clinicians may decide the best supports to use, based upon the student's language and cognition. Using a cue card with too many instructions or too much text can be ineffective because the child will not understand it. Typically, we find it helpful to start simple and then gradually increase the level of difficulty as needed and if appropriate:

- larger pictures
- less text
- limited directions.

We always directly refer to the cue card first. We will point at each picture to read the text and review the expectations for the child. Depending on needs, we may review the card intermittently throughout the session. We are also intentional about wanting to "catch the child being good." We want to praise the child frequently when they are doing the behaviors on the card. For example, "I love how you are sitting down." "Great job looking!" "John has quiet hands" (while giving a thumbs up 👍). This serves the purpose of giving the child positive attention and recognizing their efforts of emotional regulation skills to demonstrate expected skills. Recognizing positive behaviors is critical, as some school environments only attend to maladaptive behaviors. We have seen lots of classrooms, social skills groups, and small group therapy sessions with lots of *No! Stop that! Get down!* Such environments are negative with lots of what-not-to-do statements and can single out children with autism who might have difficulty understanding directions or demonstrating self-regulation skills. Instead, adults should try to reframe statements and focus on positive behavior support by praising good behaviors, rather than chastising negative behaviors. We often set a standard of wanting to have at least a two to one ratio: We praise positive behaviors twice as much as we reject negative behaviors. This practice helps to create a positive environment for students in intervention and can contribute to a positive classroom experience.

- *Overall*, consider the following formula to support your intervention:

  Gesture + Voice + Acknowledge = Good behavior shaping practices

- *Gesture*: Point to the visual display (cue card, visual schedule, behavior expectations, etc.). The visual should be clearly displayed in the environment.
- *Voice*: Clearly verbalize the expectations in language commensurate with the child's level. Be firm without raising your voice. Clear, simple language is best.
- *Acknowledge*: Offer verbal praise or redirection in response to student behavior. We are adamant about offering behavior specific praise. Our pet peeve is when we hear clinicians saying, "Good job!" "Great!" and so on, because the child is not definitively clear on what is being praised. Rather, try saying "Great job sitting" or "Good job answering. I like how hard you're working." These statements are now both positive and specific. Now the child knows exactly what behaviors are earning positive praise and the child can increase those behaviors as they seek more positive reinforcement. It is also critical to offer your praise using high affect, as your tone of voice can help to communicate your message, especially for children with autism who have receptive language deficits.

Remember, the goal is to capably manage behaviors so you can successfully conduct your intervention. You will not be an effective clinician, no matter how talented you are, if you cannot manage behaviors. Thus, your approach to behavior should be just as planned and organized as your approach to your intervention.

In addition to individual supports, whole group supports may also assist children with autism to be successful. Often, adults may give instructions to students without specifying how to do such tasks because we often operate under the assumption that children should know what to do. For children with autism, explicit instruction and visual support is often helpful (Banda and Grimmett 2008). Displaying visual support does not adversely harm any student, and it may serve as a helpful reminder for students with autism and some of their peers, so they can be successful in completing common tasks during the school day.

For elementary school-age children with autism, visual schedules should contain pictures to help with comprehension. A schedule can consist of pictures alone or be accompanied by some text commensurate with the student's language level. Schedules should represent general schedules for the day to help the child know what to expect. Adults should explicitly review visual schedules prior to the start of activities and then frequently throughout the day. It is less important to have perfect pictures than it is to consistently and clearly explain the visual schedule to the student. Do not underestimate how important this is, even for minimally verbal students with ASD. Again, use of a schedule provides routine, which provides structure for all students, but especially for students with autism. A good visual schedule and routine helps to set the tone and manage a student's behavioral expectations Table 5.1.

Active Learning Task

Review the example visual schedule, John's Schedule. With a classmate or on your own, create a visual schedule specific to your discipline for a potential student using text and visuals as appropriate for the student age and language level. List the activities for your therapy session so your client with autism will know what to expect.

John's Schedule	
Get Dressed	
Go to School	
Take Bus Home	
Snack Time	
Homework Time	

Token boards or *token economy systems* can be used in positive behavior support. With this system, tokens are given in response to a child demonstrating a desired behavior. Later, those tokens are exchanged for a reward. There are a few points to keep in mind to make this system successful:

- The expectations to earn a token need to be clear. It may be that the child is earning tokens for behaviors and/or for attempts during intervention.
- The reward must be motivating. Every child might be motivated by different objects or activities, so you might ask parents for ideas or observe what toys the child tends to gravitate to.

TABLE 5.1 Common terms used in the individual education plan.

What is it?	Also known as	Need to know
Accommodations		Allow students to complete the same tasks as their neurotypical peers with some variations or adjustments.
Addendum		May be included at any point to indicate a change in originally planned services and/or supports.
Free and appropriate public education	FAPE	This concept also helps to guide intervention services. Students are often granted services to address deficits that will help them to appropriately access their academic curriculum.
Frequency	Quantity	IEP documents will typically include details on the amount of services. Standards vary, but some school districts may write this as "X hours per month" or "X minutes per week."
Individualized family service plan	IFSP	Commonly used in early intervention services when intervention plans include the child and the entire family as key members of the plan. This focus on the family in addition to the child presupposes that, for young children, caregiver education and caregiver mediated intervention are critical to child success and achieving optimal outcomes.
Individualized education plan	IEP	This is a legally binding document used in schools to dictate intervention services. Unlike the IFSP, the focus is clearly shifted to the child as opposed to the family. Further, the IEP is guided by interventions to directly promote the child's educational achievement. Diagnosis alone does not determine access to services. Rather, inability to access the curriculum becomes the marker for receiving intervention.
Least restrictive environment	LRE	This term often guides schools in providing the most inclusive environment for students with disabilities as possible. This guide can be interpreted widely based upon a student's needs, but ultimately seeks to include students with autism and other disabilities with their typically developing peers as much as possible.
Objectives	Intervention targets	Objectives in IEPs are typically marked by short- and long-term goals. Short-term goals can be intended to span a few months, while long-term goals may represent the target for the full academic year.

(*continued*)

TABLE 5.1 (Continued)

What is it?	Also known as	Need to know
Primary disability		An IEP will specify the primary disability, a formal diagnosis that serves as the catalyst to make a child eligible for intervention services. There can be a secondary diagnosis documented as appropriate.
Service delivery		There are a number of options for service delivery in schools. They can include **pull-out services** that take the child out of the classroom, **push-in services** where interventionists enter the classroom and work with the student during class, or consultative services where the interventionists will work directly with the classroom teacher, rather than the student, to suggest strategies that can be employed throughout the school day. Additionally, services can be offered individually or in a small group (or a combination of both). Services may also be delivered via traditional face-to-face intervention or via telepractice with the assistance of a paraprofessional.
Signature page		All parties must sign the IEP document to indicate they have read the plan and agree to the items specified for the given time period.

- The reward should be withheld unless earned. With that in mind, the reward needs to be appropriate to the setting.
- The system should be consistent. This builds trust and the client knows that the system is reliable.
- Token chart complexity should be commensurate with the student's current level of behavior, attention to tasks, and overall needs. As such, the chart may be connected to immediate or delayed reinforcement. Immediate reinforcement is often used when first introducing a token economy system. In such cases, the child may perform a task and then instantly receive a preferred item or activity as the child is learning to link task performance to reward. Later, the child may be able to tolerate more delayed reinforcement that offers rewards only intermittently in a less predictable manner, which would help to increase the child's flexibility during tasks. This differential schedule of reinforcement is a critical component of behavior management.

Figure 5.8 shows a general token board. The Velcro pieces are situated so the chart can be used for 5 or 10 tokens at a time, depending on the child's needs. A child who can tolerate longer tasks can work for 10 tokens at a time. Additionally, the child might earn

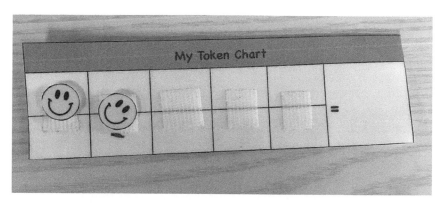

FIGURE 5.8   Token economy system.

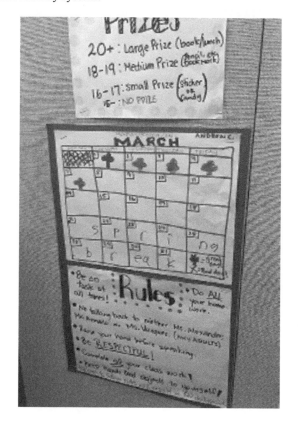

FIGURE 5.9   Delayed reinforcement system.

a token for every two or three attempts instead of a token after every trial. It is also not specified what the child is working for. You might discuss the break verbally with the child in advance or they may even earn the tokens first, then ask the child for their preferred activity. Alternatively, you could add an image to represent the reinforcer.

The calendar token system (Figure 5.9) is an example of a delayed reinforcement schedule, as the student is working for a reward each month.

Timers can be helpful to transition between activities for clients. Often, temporal concepts like "five more minutes" really are not salient enough for a child with autism to understand. Using timers on your phone, visual timers via many free apps, or other methods like sand timers, which are very inexpensive, can be effective. These methods offer a visual representation of time that allows the child to better anticipate the end of one task and the start of another. This practice is often more appropriate than an abrupt "Time's up!" that may be anxiety producing or prompt maladaptive behaviors in protest.

Using engaging activities with appropriate difficulty is important as a method of positive behavior support. Often, children may demonstrate maladaptive behaviors when tasks are too challenging and also when tasks are not challenging enough. This is also true of children with autism. For this reason, it is important to know about both strengths *and* weaknesses. You want to target challenging skills that build upon existing strengths so that students are not overwhelmed by tasks they perceive as too taxing to be achieved.

All the items described above may be used in both individual and group contexts. In small group contexts, **interdependent group-oriented contingencies** may be useful where success of the group depends on the success of each individual. These approaches tend to mirror adult systems such as the success of a company being dependent upon every worker's individual contributions. Such approaches may be helpful to employ peer support in helping students follow clear behavioral expectations, although individual supports may continue to be needed with some students as appropriate.

In summary, while your primary role may not be targeting behavior, any person working with children with autism must support behavior needs effectively to be effective in targeting the specific skills in their own domain. Thus, employing evidenced-based practices for supporting behavior needs is a core skill for all interventionists supporting students. At times, some behavior needs may require more specific and advanced support. Such instances may prompt you to collaborate with other disciplines to appropriately address concerns that preclude the student from fully benefiting from your expertise. However, all interventionists should be equipped with basic skills in managing and supporting behavior needs as a foundation to engaging with clients appropriately in a positive way.

 THERAPY VIEWPOINT

Quick Look at Behavior Supports
To support my student(s) with autism and behavior needs, I will use:
- visual schedules
- checklists
- behavior cue cards
- appropriate environmental arrangement
- sensory supports
- token charts
- behavior specific verbal praise
- motivating rewards
- (visual) timer.

Lesson Plans

All professionals, especially pre-professionals and those at the early career stage, should prepare lesson plans to effectively design intervention. For pre-professionals, this process is particularly helpful as it serves to help you think through your concrete plans for activities to target goals. As you select activities, you may also consider your plan for instruction: How do you plan to teach the targeted skill? Often, we see students may plan activities but fail to plan how to respond when clients do not produce the intended target. Students should anticipate clients not responding correctly. If clients could demonstrate the correct response, the target most likely would not have been selected as a goal for intervention. As such, we encourage students to think about how they will teach the goal and then assess for increased client production and generalization across contexts with fading support.

An important question to ask yourself while planning is "But *why*?" Your clinical approach should be informed by evidenced-based practices, which should reflect your knowledge of prevailing intervention practices evidenced by research and your understanding of your client as you predict which practices will be best suited to that client and family. This individualization of clinical practice should continue to evolve as you monitor your client's response to therapy. Ask the questions: Is my client making progress? Is this approach working? Is there another approach that might work better? Keep in mind that evidenced-based intervention is only successful if it is in fact working for your client. You need to consider individual differences, family preferences, service delivery setting, and behavior needs when selecting approaches to target plan goals.

Importantly, other than just being prepared for your sessions, clients with autism can benefit from frontloading information so they know what to expect from their time with you. As such, clear planning benefits both the client and the interventionist.

Active Learning Task

Part I
The following exchange was submitted by a former graduate student during her clinical placement. Identify areas of the lesson plan that are unclear. How might you better specify your plans so that it could pass the stranger test and nearly anyone could implement it?

Lesson Plan

Client: Michael M. (ASD dx)
Chronological Age: five years, two months
Grade level: Kindergarten
Goal: Michael will use words expressing quality (size, color, etc.) to describe a noun in 7 of 10 trials with mild prompting.

Activity #1
Materials: Book.

(*continued*)

Steps:

1. Clinician will read book to client and will ask questions along the way to set up opportunities for him to use adjectives.
2. Clinician will guide client with questions if he has difficulty expressing himself.
3. Verbal praise will be awarded for successful and non-successful attempts.

Activity #2
Materials: Colorful objects set up all around the room.
Steps:

1. Clinician and client will play a game of "I spy" with the various colors used in the book.
2. Clinician will start off by saying "I spy something red. . ." and ask if the client sees anything in the room that is red.
3. If client has difficulty, I will ask him yes/no questions to guide him.
4. Verbal praise will be awarded for successful and non-successful attempts.

Goal: To improve his receptive skills, Michael will follow 1-step directions with 70% accuracy with mild prompting.

Activity #3
Materials: Following directions worksheet, crayons.
Steps:

1. Clinician will read directions on the worksheet out loud and will use mild prompting if he does not understand the directions.

Part II
Redesign the above lesson plan to make it clear, so that it will pass the "stranger test" – anyone could implement the activities. Specify the prompts that will be provided and the exact questions and/or directives to be used during each task.

Now consider the lesson plan in Table 5.2 of another school-age client with a primary diagnosis of ASD. Compare and contrast the plan in Part I and the following plan. Are the activities clear? Is clear evidenced-based practice included? How would you address the goals by:

- including relevant evidenced-based practices
- including positive behavior-support strategies
- including age-appropriate activities that target the stated goals
- including at least one carryover task for families to implement at home.

To Do
Share the lesson plan with a professional. Solicit feedback. What constructive criticism did the person provide?

TABLE 5.2 Sample lesson plan.

Client initial: E

Age: 6 years 3 months

Goal	Procedure	Rationale
Identify the intervention goal	This needs to be specific. **Exactly what** do you plan to do to address the goals? Is the activity age appropriate? Include **specific tasks, language structures, words, word combinations, gestures, cues, behavior strategies, etc.**	Why did you target this goal? The goal is already set so the rationale needs to be based upon **typical developmental norms.**
Given a reading selection, the client will make inferences, with 80% accuracy, given minimal to no prompting.	**Activity 1** The clinician will spend a few minutes greeting the client and explain what they will be targeting throughout the session. Materials: *There Was an Old Lady Who Swallowed a Fly* (book) • Fish activity with pictures • Mr. and Mrs. Potato Head • Tic-Tac-Toe worksheet • Roll-N-Go worksheet • Visual schedule with options Procedure: The clinician will introduce the book *There Was an Old Lady Who Swallowed a Fly.* They will read the book to the client and ask her the following questions as they read the book: • Why do you think she would swallow a fly? • Why would she swallow a spider? • Why would she swallow a bird? • Where do you think she is at? • Do you think she was hungry? • Do you think she will keep eating? • Why would she swallow a cat? • Why do you think she swallowed the goat? • Do you think she is full after eating all those animals? • What do you think is going to happen next?	These goals were targeted for this session because the client should be making appropriate inferences from a reading passage or pictures, understand the use of pronouns, and articulate the /l/ phoneme correctly for his age.

(continued)

TABLE 5.2 (Continued)

Client initial: E

Age: 6 years 3 months

Goal	Procedure	Rationale
To increase language skills, the client will understand the use of pronouns (he, she, they, his, her, them) with 80% accuracy, with minimal to no prompting.	**Activity 2** The clinician will give the client the option to either work on describing the pictures on the fishes or playing with Mr. and Mrs. Potato Head. Fishes option: The clinician will introduce the fish activity to the client. The fish will have a magnet and pictures on them displaying either a male or female engaging in an activity. The client will describe 10 pictures using the proper nouns (he, she, they, his, her, them). After describing 10 fish, the fish will be displayed upside down on the table and the client and clinician will take turns in fishing them one by one and describing what they see. The clinician will provide a prompt, cue, or model when necessary (i.e., is that a boy or a girl? So is that a he or a she?) Mr. and Mrs. Potato Head option: The clinician will begin the activity by demonstrating Mr. and Mrs. Potato Head. They will bring out the body parts from each box one at a time by asking the client to label them. For example, the clinician will bring out Mr. Potato Head's body out and ask the client, "Whose body is this?" The client is expected to answer appropriately for each body part such as "Its his body." If the client answers incorrectly, such as "It's him body," the clinician will correct the client by asking him "Is it him body, or his body?" The clinician will continue the activity by bringing out one body part at a time and ask the client "Whose body part is this" If the client does not respond, the clinician will elaborate by saying "Is it his or hers?" (while pointing to each Potato Head). Whenever the client does not know whose body part it is, the clinician will advise her to look for clues. For example, when deciding whose ears belong to who, the clinician will say "These have earrings, does Mr. Potato Head wear earrings?" and the answer is "Nooooo, he's a boy, boys don't wear earrings, so these ears are for her," providing visual cues by pointing to Mrs. Potato Head. The clinician will also show her earrings to the client to further explain the concept of earrings. The clinician will also encourage the client to ask for help when she cannot attach a body part to a body. The clinician will provide the client with behavior specific praise such as "I like the way you are thinking", "You used the correct word!". By the end of the activity, the client will help to clean up the toys.	

To increase intelligibility, the client will produce the phoneme /l/ in the initial position of words, given minimal to no prompting.	**Activity 3** The client will be given the option to work on the Roll-N-Go game or the Tic-Tac-Toe worksheet. The clinician will begin the activity be describing how to play the game. The clinician will say "We have to decide who wants to be the "X" and the "O." We must get three of our target object (X or O) in a row. Wherever we decide to put our target object, we must produce the target word that begins with the /l/ sound in the initial position. Whoever wins two of three games gets to get something from the treasure box. The client will be asked to articulate the names of objects that contain the phoneme /l/ in the initial position from the Roll-N-Go game. The clinician will provide a prompt, cue, or model when necessary such as "Make sure you put your tongue up."

Behavior: Sensory related breaks will be given when necessary. Verbal praise will be given throughout the session.

Home carryover activity: The family will be encouraged to target familiar objects around the house that have the /l/ sound in the initial position such as *lemon, lime, lemonade, leaf*, etc., and will work with their child in producing those names appropriately. Whenever the child does not produce the /l/ appropriately, she can be reminded to put her tongue up.

Active Learning Task

Example of Goals for an Elementary School-Age Student with Autism
Let's explore the goals below created by an SLP graduate student intern in a clinic rotation with students with ASD.
Short-Term Goals for Edward C.
Client chronological age: 7 years 10 months

1. Will discriminate between correct and incorrect productions of /t/ in the initial position of words, given minimal cues, with 80% accuracy, across two consecutive sessions.
2. Will discriminate between correct and incorrect production /d/ in the initial position of words, given minimal cues, with 80% accuracy, across two consecutive sessions.
3. Will reduce the phonological process of backing in the initial position of words, given minimal prompting, with 80% accuracy, across two consecutive sessions.
4. Will identify common objects when named, given minimal cues, with 80% accuracy, across two consecutive sessions.
5. Will demonstrate understanding and use of pronouns (he, she they, his, her, theirs), given minimal cues, with 80% accuracy, across two consecutive sessions.

How would you change any of the above goals and why? Are they all SMART (specific, measurable, attainable, relevant and time bound) goals? Based on the client's age, include rationales for why these goals are being targeted by identifying typical age of acquisition of the targeted skills.
Go further: Using the goals above, create your own lesson plan to address the intervention targets.

COMMON SCHOOL DAY CHALLENGES

Recess

Even for those who thrive inside the classroom, recess can be one of the most challenging school scenarios for children with autism during early school years; they typically benefit from targeted support to increase social initiations and engagement (Vincent et al. 2018). Unlike the classroom, the playground is even less predictable and deficits in social interaction skills can become readily apparent. Further, playground time is often less regulated and facilitated by adults, leaving children with interaction difficulties largely on their own to navigate the rules of peer engagement. Helping children with autism have success on the playground is essential to help build peer friendships, which also reduces chances of peer bullying (Cappadocia et al. 2012). Collaboration is critical to ensure success, as clinicians and classroom teachers may not be readily present during unstructured social interaction times like lunch or recess; rather, involving paraprofessionals, classroom aides, and playground personnel may be key to success for children with ASD (Kretzmann et al. 2015).

How Can Interventionists Support Children with ASD During Recess?

1. *Incorporate traditional playground games into your sessions:* Use **social skill steps** to explain the importance of games with rules, good turn taking skills, and being a good sport. If you see children with autism in a small group setting, use playground games in your sessions to give the child with autism a chance to practice games in a low-risk setting before getting to the playground.

2. *Enlist peers:* Many evidenced-based approaches to address social skills for children with autism in inclusive settings in schools enlist the support of typical peers to some degree (Dean and Chang 2021). You can help to teach neurotypical peers to demonstrate more tolerance and acceptance of their classmates by teaching about neurodiversity and differences. You can enlist support from more empathetic classmates to help serve as advocates and peer buddies. In schools, consider starting a peer buddy group specifically for recess time to help prevent social isolation on the playground. This can work by prompting socially strong and empathetic peers to find children alone at recess and inviting them to play. Creating roles for these typical peers such as a "playground ambassador" can help to enlist peers to make sure all classmates, including those with autism, are involved at recess and reduce bullying of children who are isolated during unstructured interaction time.

3. *Set up for success:* It is helpful to structure peer interactions. Often, children are dismissed for recess as in "Go play!" and they are expected to form their own groups and games. This can be better facilitated for children with autism by creating some structure before recess begins. For example, when preparing to transition to recess, create pairs or playgroups with specific activities. Ask children before they go to the playground, "*Who* are you going to play with?" and "*What* are you going to play?" This prompts students with autism to consider these points before they get on the playground and play alone. If they have difficulty answering the questions, you can suggest play partners and activity ideas based on their interests. For example, you can assign six students to soccer and four students to basketball. At times, students with autism struggle with sports games due to difficulty comprehending rules and/or challenges with motor coordination. We often suggest setting up social table-top activities such as puzzles or chalk stations to offer less physical activities as options.

Potential Goals and Interventions

Great goals to target in this area include targets related to play skills and peer interaction.

GOAL SPOTLIGHT

Student will demonstrate joint engagement in play with peers during recess for a minimum of 10 consecutive minutes given minimal adult facilitation/support as measured by clinical data and/or paraprofessional staff report.

What Might This Look Like in Clinical Practice?

An interventionist can consider collaborating with paraprofessional staff like playground personnel to improve peer play during recess (Kretzmann et al. 2015). A clinician can consider modeling appropriate peer play, such as shadowing the child during recess and playing kickball or soccer with the target child and peers. First, the clinician might prime for this activity with the child in individual therapy by asking, "How do we play kickball with our friends?" The clinician might help the child develop concrete skill steps for the process of joining a game, asking to play, following rules appropriately, demonstrating good sportsmanship, etc. (Wiley et al. 2016). The clinician might use **video modeling** to prompt the child to identify appropriate and inappropriate behaviors related to the task. Once the child has been exposed to what to do, the clinician should shift to engaging in the natural context during recess to assess the child's execution of the task and fluency of skills. Lastly, the clinician may provide live coaching and modeling to the student as needed before fading out of the activity as appropriate.

Transitions

Transitions between tasks can be challenging for children with ASD, especially transitioning between preferred to non-preferred tasks. Often, children with autism thrive on structure and routines. Sudden disruptions can lead to challenging behaviors.

How Can Interventionists Support Children with ASD?

Establish routines for transitions. Start with a visual schedule that outlines the plan of the day using pictures and/or language that matches the child's language level. Visual schedules can increase or decrease in complexity as appropriate to fit the child's needs. Even children with autism who are highly verbal can benefit from a visual schedule. We strongly suggest implementing them in classrooms. In fact, many high-quality classrooms will already contain a visual schedule usually in the front of the classroom. This practice is effective for all children, including students who are typically developing, but especially for children with autism to help manage transitions (Banda et al. 2009). Generally, children thrive on structure and consistency, and using a visual schedule helps them to know what to expect next. Upper elementary grades may have a written schedule on the board.

Some classes might include a visual like the images of clock hands to help children learn how to tell time. If not already in place, this type of schedule can be very helpful for children with autism to show them the activities of the day.

While most elementary school classrooms do include some kind of visual schedule, many classrooms do not automatically include a structure specifically for transitions. Often, kids are expected to transition abruptly and without warning. This expectation can be particularly challenging for children with autism. Employing a structure for transitions can help reduce challenging behaviors and increase effectiveness in classroom settings (Iadarola et al. 2018). Consider the following Schedules, Tools, and Activities for Transitions in the Daily Routine (*STAT*) Program approach developed by Iadarola et al. (2018) Table 5.3.

This type of transition reinforcement is helpful for all children, but can be particularly useful for children with autism. The focus is on preparing students for the upcoming transition (rather than changing abruptly), clearly communicating what you expect and how you expect it to be done, and using positive reinforcement to prompt compliance. In many cases, step 7 may not be needed if all students are following instructions.

Students often respond to positive reinforcement directed at peers and will adjust their behavior so they can be the recipient of verbal praise. This is also true of children with ASD, as this positive behavior support strategy can help to prevent problem behaviors and reduce their prevalence (Neitzel 2010). We stress the importance of highlighting positive behaviors, rather than negative behaviors. For example, in our classes, we might be doing a transition and 6 of 10 kids are doing the right thing. Rather than focusing on the four, we use high positive affect and verbal praise to highlight the six such as smiling and saying, "Wow! We love how (student name) is lining up quietly!" "Look at how (student name) is following directions! Great job!" This practice both acknowledges the children who are following directions and prompts the children not following directions to correct their behavior in hopes of also receiving positive praise.

TABLE 5.3   Steps to prepare for successful transitions.

#	Step	What to say
1	Warning for the transition	"We have five minutes until we get ready to ___."
2	Signal to gain student attention	"Ready to clean up in 5-4-3-2-1."
3	Clearly communicate instruction (*what*)	"Stop what you are doing and stand up."
4	Communicate behavioral expectation (*how*)	"Line up *quietly* at the door."
5	Specify a time limit for the transition with verbal and visual cues	"Stop what you are doing and stand up. Line up at the door in **10-9-8-. . . 2-1**."
6	Watch students for follow-through on expected behaviors	"I like how (student name) is lining up quietly."
7	Redirect by giving the same directions you initially gave and prompt, *as needed*	"I am waiting for (student name) to line up quietly."
8	Reinforce success	"Thank you (student name) and (student name) for following directions."
9	Signal the end of transition	"Great job everyone. Now we are ready to go to (next activity)."

Too often, adults may focus on the minority of children doing the wrong thing, rather than the majority of children doing the right thing. This can (i) neglect the children who are doing the right thing; and (ii) create a negative classroom environment (one with lots of "No!" "Stop ___ (student name)!") In fact, in school settings, evidence suggests that schools with positive behavioral interventions and supports reported higher levels of student and faculty understanding of behavioral expectations, stronger climates of trust and respect, and higher student academic outcomes (Houchens et al. 2017). Employing transition steps and focusing on positive reinforcement can contribute to a more positive classroom experience for all involved.

Interventionists working with children with autism in classroom settings may look to collaborate with classroom teachers to share this suggestion for transitions, as it can often be successful with general classroom management. If teachers respond that the steps are too time consuming, consider less helpful alternatives such as not all kids following directions and then the wasted time of frequently repeated instructions or punishment for student noncompliance. Done effectively, this transition schedule can actually help to minimize the time needed to transition between tasks and reduce both adult and child frustration with transitioning between activities.

Potential Goals and Interventions

Great goals to target in this area include communicating wants and needs (asking for a break) and increasing attention to tasks.

GOAL SPOTLIGHT

Student will verbally request for a break when needed in three of five opportunities given moderate prompts as measured by clinical data and/or teacher report.

What Might This Look Like in Practice?

A clinician might use visual cue cards and augmentative communication supports like sign language to prompt the student to make a verbal request. This type of target can significantly improve functional communication, which can reduce maladaptive behaviors and improve classroom performance. The clinician may first directly model "I want break" while signing and using hand over hand to help the child imitate the sign, followed by immediately giving the child a short, preferred task or activity. Gradually, the clinician can reduce the model, such as reducing from direct imitation, "I want a break" to just "I want ____" with only the sign for *break* to allow the child to complete the request. As the child improves, the clinician should reduce the cues appropriately such as less verbal modeling and less visual cues, as well as using a **token economy** to help the child increase the time spent in nonpreferred tasks.

Active Learning Task

Consider the token economy system below for an elementary school-age student with autism in the classroom setting. What do you think the student's preferred activity is? Role play with a peer on how you might introduce this system to a student and then employ it during intervention.

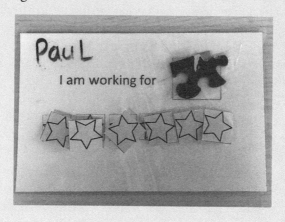

Literacy Tasks

Literacy tasks such as difficulty with oral narrative comprehension and production skills have been identified in verbal preschoolers with autism, which can persist to school-age years and adversely impact academic success (Westerveld and Roberts 2017). With potential difficulty retelling narratives, specific goals and tasks addressing these skills should be targeted in intervention. Wallach and Ocampo (2022) suggest modeling, exposure, and expansion to age-appropriate language structures and forms through books. In the early stages of preschool and kindergarten, intervention should facilitate reporting skills, while later elementary school grades should facilitate understanding of relationships among characters and events in addition to continuing to develop more age-appropriate and structured narratives (Wallach and Ocampo 2022). Interventionists working with students with autism may consider supporting literacy to facilitate academic success by using book shares consistently in intervention. We suggest thematic approaches to developing lesson plans to help reinforce content.

Therapy Golden Nugget

Tips for Supporting Literacy in Students with ASD
- Support story retell using *First, Next, Then, Last* by starting with simple three- to four-step sequences.
- Use wordless picture books and model as needed to help students with autism generate their own narratives.
- Try a picture walk with younger children. Instead of focusing on the words, have children describe the pictures they see.
- Promote inferencing by asking "What do you think will happen next?" before you turn the page.
- Target identifying emotions of characters. Ask questions like "How do you think __ feels?" "Why?" Begin with open ended questions and reduce to forced choice as needed.

Active Learning Task

Select a children's book and develop a 60-minute thematic plan that will address literacy, language, and articulation goals for an elementary school-age student with autism. Share plans with classmates and provide constructive feedback.

Group Work

Group Work can be challenging for children with ASD due to social skills deficits; however, group work is often an expectation for school-age children.

How Can Interventionists Support Children with ASD?

Interventionists might consider social skills lessons on active listening skills to help with success. When engaged in group tasks, clinicians might help by offering more explicit directions and checking in more frequently to make sure students are working together effectively.

Potential Goals and Interventions

Great goals to target in this area include turn taking and maintaining a topic of conversation.

GOAL SPOTLIGHT

- The student will independently demonstrate turn taking with a peer during a structured cooperative task as measured by clinical data and/or teacher report.
- The student will demonstrate appropriate conversation with a peer by maintaining a topic for a minimum of four conversational turns with a peer given minimal adult support as measured by clinical data and/or teacher report.

What Might This Look Like in Practice?

Rather than working with a student independently, the clinician might work with students in small group tasks to mirror the context in the classroom. The clinician might start by teaching appropriate social scripts like *Can I have a turn?* These types of structured classroom skills also translate well to social tasks like games with rules – imagine a child playing board games with a peer. We can sometimes assume that students automatically know how to do "simple" tasks. This is not true! We might need to directly teach skills like how to wait one's turn. Direct instruction via skill steps might aid in children with autism better understanding what and how to do the task, which can result in better peer engagement and academic performance.

Structured interventions targeting conversation can help highly verbal students with autism learn the rules of appropriate conversational turn taking including asking questions to extend conversation and appropriately employing methods of conversational repair (Muller et al. 2016). In intervention, clinicians may seek to use visual aids to support understanding of the cooperative nature of conversation. Some clinicians may use the idea of a conversation train that oscillates in colors, or give the analogy of a volleyball or ping pong game that visually demonstrates the importance of a back and forth engagement to be successful. In these examples, when one partner "drops the ball" the game ends. The same is true of conversation. Wiley et al. (2016) offer the use of a conversation train to prompt conversation maintenance, as exemplified in Figure 5.10.

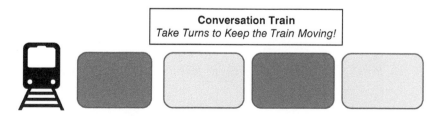

FIGURE 5.10 Use of a conversation train to prompt conversation maintenance.

Independent Tasks

Independent tasks can also be challenging for children with autism due to executive functioning deficits (Chan et al. 2009). Sometimes, children with autism can have difficulty organizing themselves, initiating tasks, and knowing when to ask for help. These challenges can make completing independent work difficult. At times, when these challenges prevent students with ASD from successfully completing assigned tasks, teachers can misinterpret this behavior as noncompliance or dismiss the student as forgetful or lazy. This assumption is incorrect and can negatively impact teacher perception of students with autism. Evidence suggests that students with autism can benefit from specific interventions to improve executive functioning skills (Weismer et al. 2018).

How Can Interventionists Support Children with ASD?

Again, providing more explicit directions can be helpful to add clarity. It may help to break up the activity into smaller tasks and use a checklist to help children mark off completed items. Similar to group work, more frequent check ins to make sure the child is on task and successful may also be helpful.

Potential Goals and Interventions

Great goals to target in this area include increasing executive functioning skills, Figure 5.11.

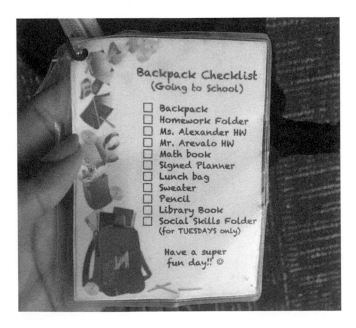

FIGURE 5.11   Checklist to support student executive functioning to aid with organization and independence for a 4th grade student.

> **GOAL SPOTLIGHT**
>
> The student will independently complete multistep tasks given one verbal directive in 8 of 10 opportunities, as measured by clinical data and/or teacher report.

What Might This Look Like in Practice?

Clinicians may work with students with autism on organizing and planning. Deficits in these areas of executive functioning can significantly adversely impact academic skills. Common reports from teachers are that students do not submit assignments on time or that academic work is not complete. Many times, these students report understanding class concepts, but simply unintentionally neglect to do the required work because they fail to effectively organize themselves. Imagine how frustrating that can be for students and teachers alike!

We once evaluated a highly verbal fourth-grade student with ASD who was earning failing grades. He achieved average scores on standardized speech and language assessments and had a typical IQ. However, he was not doing well in his general education classroom. After interviewing his teacher, it was revealed that the student had not turned in a single homework assignment for months, which was why his grades were poor. Upon investigation, most of the assignments were found crumpled at the bottom of his backpack or in his classroom cubby. Intervention focused on improving executive functioning skills, specifically organization and planning to complete tasks. This approach almost instantly improved his academic performance. The example checklist in Figure 5.11 helps to support student executive functioning by providing a visual support to promote organization and independence.

Active Learning Task

Finding Evidence-Based Practice to Support Intervention
Find two different peer-reviewed journal articles to support evidence-based practice for intervention with an elementary school-age client with autism.

A Note on Supporting Classroom Needs

Interventionists may consider using activities that support and reinforce academic tasks. For example, you might ask the classroom teacher about current activities and try to incorporate them into your sessions. This collaboration can help the student to better understand class concepts, especially since underlying difficulty with language may make academic tasks more challenging. Often, we will attempt to use reading assignments for class in our therapy sessions. If done beforehand, this practice can help to prime our students in the classroom setting so they feel more confident and capable in the large group setting in class with peers. If done afterwards, this practice can help to further explain concepts and identify areas our students may not fully understand.

For example, a student's parent once reported that her son was demonstrating significant frustration during class when the lesson was focused on counting money, a functional task. In response, we created a session task targeting the structure:

$$I\ see + quantity + noun + regular\ plural\ \text{-}s$$

since the student's goals included increasing mean length of utterance by using attributes like quantity and using regular plurals. We used coins to help the student complete the carrier phrase *I see* by counting the amount and then adding plural -s to the nouns (pennies, nickels, dimes, quarters). The teacher and parent immediately reported decreased maladaptive behaviors and frustration during tasks targeting counting money in the classroom context.

In addition, clinicians may consider collaborating with other allied disciplines if the student is getting other support services. Collaboration may look like working with colleagues in schools across contexts, discussing how your goals can be addressed in their setting, and/or training staff to stimulate speech and language and peer interaction in daily interactions. Such collaborative approaches have proven successful by offering training and live coaching to support promoting increased peer engagement, which is an area often targeted for children with autism (Daughrity et al. 2020). Overall, to support students with autism in schools, professionals should consider areas of synergy to support a team-based approach to intervention.

SUMMARY

This chapter reviewed common challenges for children with autism as they transition into the school district including ways to support behavior needs and academic and social difficulties. The chapter also included sample lesson plans to offer examples of treatment activities to address student goals with discussions on suggested modifications. Intervention goals must be functional and developmentally appropriate. In intervention, goals may often be similar to those of children without autism who have speech and language targets; however, treatment should include appropriate modifications specific to students with autism who may demonstrate different behavior and attention needs. Common challenges for students with autism in early school-age years include difficulty transitioning between tasks, following classroom instruction, engaging with peers during unstructured social interaction time, and asking for help appropriately, among other difficulties. Interventionists should work collaboratively with both parents, teachers, and appropriate professionals to support client needs to promote optimal student performance in the educational setting.

REFLECTIONS ALONG THE PATH

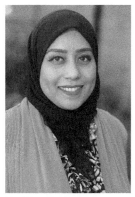

Nadhiya Ito, M.A.

Dear New Clinician,

First of all, congratulations on choosing a career path I consider to be truly fulfilling and rewarding! After being an SLP for over 16 years, I still feel as passionate about the work I do, as I did on the day I became one. What we do on a daily basis can be very impactful, and in return, it will also touch your heart. You might be one of the first people to witness a child say "Mama" for the first time in her life and you cry with the family because she had never uttered that word before and the mother waited for six years to hear it. Or, a child starts communicating his complex thoughts using his AAC (augmentative and alternative communication) device and tells you that he thinks "you are cool" because you always "believed in him." As an SLP, you will touch your clients' lives. You *will* make a difference.

I do, however, have to be honest and share that, while this career is rewarding, it will continue to require your hard work, dedication and commitment. Every day may not be as rosy as you would like it to be. There may be a lot of paperwork to manage (!) and "work and life balance" to consider. You may also work with clients whom you might find challenges making progress with or even bonding. You may feel "helpless" for not being "helpful" to your clients and their families. There may also be days where you question your clinical skills and wonder if you are doing the right thing. I want to let you know that you will learn the most from the most challenging situations. As a clinical supervisor, I tell all my supervisees, both clinical fellows and graduate interns, that the clients they have the most challenges with typically would become their most favorite clients in the end, and oftentimes, it is truly the case. Know that it is okay to seek support and help. Remember, it takes a village.

We learn and we grow, and in that process, I want you to value your uniqueness as a clinician. I'm not only talking about the uniqueness in clinical or therapy styles. Get to know who you are as a person, but also as a clinician. When I was a senior in college, I met Dr. Lily Cheng, who later became my mentor, at American Speech–Language–Hearing Association Annual Convention in Atlanta, Georgia. I attended the Asian Pacific Islander Speech–Language–Hearing Caucus meeting, where she chaired, and I was blown away by her passionate words. She said, "Because of your background, there will be people who can benefit from your services." It really resonated with me as a young SLP undergraduate student, and I slowly began to see the notion of being a "Minority" as my strength. We all do come from a variety of backgrounds: cultural, linguistic, family, socioeconomic, faith and belief, skill sets, life experience and so on. These influence and shape who we become as a person, but also as a clinician. On so many occasions, it brought me much joy to be able to advocate for my clients because of my unique background and I know it meant a lot for my clients, too. So, know that you are needed because of who you are. Know that you bring in the value because of your difference.

Last, but not least, I am so glad you are here! Now, go make a difference in the world!

Nadhiya Ito MA CCC-SLP
SLP and Clinical Supervisor
Los Angeles Speech and Language Therapy Center, Inc.
Vice President, Asian Pacific Islander Speech–Language–Hearing Caucus

TEST QUESTIONS

1. Goals for school-age children should be
   A. Functional
   B. Attainable
   C. Educationally relevant
   D. All of the above

2. Lesson plans are not as helpful after pre-professionals begin to work clinically. True or false?

3. Transitions between tasks can be challenging for children with autism; supports to help transitions can be helpful for both children with autism and their typical peers. True or false?

4. IEPs focus on the family in supporting the child with autism. True or false?

5. School-age students may qualify for a diagnosis of autism, but may not qualify for intervention services if they can adequately access their academic curriculum. True or false?

6. Which of the following unstructured tasks may be challenging for a school age student with autism?
   A. Recess
   B. English language arts
   C. Math
   D. Science

7. A special education setting is always best for students with autism. True or false?

8. Only behavior specialists should be familiar with positive behavior supports because that is their domain of expertise. True or false?

REFERENCES

Banda, D. and Grimmett, E. (2008). Enhancing social and transition behaviors of persons with autism through activity schedules: a review. *Education and Training in Developmental Disabilities* 43 (3): 324–333.

Banda, D., Grimmett, E., and Hart, S. (2009). Activity schedules: helping students with autism spectrum disorders in general education classrooms manage transition issues. *Teaching Exceptional Children* 41 (4): 16–21.

Bangert, K., Halverson, D., and Finestack, L. (2019). Evaluation of an explicit instructional approach to teach grammatical forms to children with low symptom severity autism Spectrum disorder. *American Journal of Speech-Language Pathology* 28 (2): 650–663.

Bopp, K., Brown, K., and Mirenda, P. (2004). Speech-language pathologists' roles in the delivery of positive behavior support for individuals with developmental disabilities. *American Journal of Speech-Language Pathology* 13 (1): 5–19.

Cappadocia, M., Weiss, J., and Pepler, D. (2012). Bullying experiences among children and youth with autism spectrum disorders. *Journal of Autism and Developmental Disorders* 42: 266–277.

Case-Smith, J., Weaver, L., and Fristad, M. (2014). A systematic review of sensory processing interventions for children with autism spectrum disorders. *Autism* 19 (2): 133–148.

Chan, A., Cheung, M., Han, Y. et al. (2009). Executive function deficits and neural discordance in children with autism Spectrum disorders. *Clinical Neurophysiology* 120 (6): 1107–1115.

Daughrity, B., Bittner, M., Ocampo, A. et al. (2020). Interprofessional collaboration with speech-language pathologists: training pre service adaptive physical education teachers to facilitate peer engagement among children with disabilities. *Perspectives of the ASHA Special Interest Groups* 5: 1313–1323.

Dean, M. and Chang, Y.-C. (2021). A systematic review of school-based social skills interventions and observed social outcomes for students with autism spectrum disorder in inclusive settings. *Autism* 25 (7): 1828–1843.

Gilliam, S., Hartzheim, D., Studenka, B. et al. (2015). Narrative intervention for children with autism spectrum disorder (ASD). *Journal of Speech, Language, and Hearing Research* 58 (3): 920–933.

Houchens, G., Zhang, J., Davis, K. et al. (2017). The impact of positive behavior interventions and supports on teachers' perceptions of teaching conditions and student achievement. *Journal of Positive Behavior Interventions* 19 (3): 168–179.

Iadarola, S., Shih, W., Dean, M. et al. (2018). Implementing a manualized, classroom transition intervention for students with ASD in underresourced schools. *Behavior Modification* 42 (1): 126–147.

Kretzmann, M., Shih, W., and Kasari, C. (2015). Improving peer engagement of children with autism on the school playground: a randomized controlled trial. *Behavior Therapy* 46 (1): 20–28.

Kurth, J., Love, H., and Pirtle, J. (2020). Parent perspectives of their involvement in iep development for children with autism. *Focus on Autism and Other Developmental Disabilities* 35 (1): 36–46.

Locke, J., Olsen, A., Wideman, R. et al. (2015). A tangled web: the challenges of implementing an evidence-based social engagement intervention for children with autism in urban public school settings. *Behavior Therapy* 46 (1): 54–67.

Lord, C. (2018). For better or for worse? Later diagnoses of autism Spectrum disorder in some younger siblings of already diagnosed children. *Journal of the American Academy of Child and Adolescent Psychiatry* 57 (11): 822–823.

Muller, E., Cannon, L., Kornblum, C. et al. (2016). Description and preliminary evaluation of a curriculum for teaching conversational skills to children with high-functioning autism and other social cognition challenges. *Language, Speech, and Hearing Services in Schools* 47 (3): 191–208.

Neitzel, J. (2010). Positive behavior supports for children and youth with autism spectrum disorders. *Preventing School Failure: Alternative Education for Children and Youth* 54 (4): 247–255.

Nuske, H., Hassrick, E., Bronstein, B. et al. (2019). Broken bridges – new school transitions for students with autism spectrum disorder: a systematic review on difficulties and strategies for success. *Autism* 23 (2): 306–325.

Otten, K.L. and Tuttle, J.L. (2011). *How to Reach and Teach Children with Challenging Behavior: Practical, Ready-to-Use Interventions that Work*, 1e. Jossey-Bass.

Ozonoff, S., Young, G., Brian, J. et al. (2018). Diagnosis of autism spectrum disorder after age 5 in children evaluated longitudinally since infancy. *Adolescent Psychiatry* 57 (11): 849–857.

Rotheram-Fuller, E., Kasari, C., Chamberlain, B., and Locke, J. (2010). Social involvement of children with autism spectrum disorders in elementary school classrooms. *Journal of Child Psychology and Psychiatry* 51 (11): 1227–1234.

Sheldrick, R., Maye, M., and Cater, A. (2017). Age at first identification of autism spectrum disorder: an analysis of two US surveys. *Adolescent Psychiatry* 56 (4): 313–320.

Vincent, L., Openden, D., Gentry, J. et al. (2018). Promoting social learning at recess for children with ASD and related social challenges. *Behavior Analysis in Practice* 11 (1): 19–33.

Wallach, G. and Ocampo, A. (2022). *Language and Literacy Connections: Intervention for School-Age Children and Adolescents*. San Diego, CA: Plural Publishing.

Weismer, S., Kaushanskaya, M., Larson, C. et al. (2018). Executive function skills in school-age children with autism spectrum disorder: association with language abilities. *Journal of Speech, Language, and Hearing Research* 61 (11): 2641–2658.

Westerveld, M. and Roberts, J. (2017). The oral narrative comprehension and production abilities of verbal preschoolers on the autism Spectrum. *Language, Speech, and Hearing Services in Schools* 48 (4): 260–272.

Wiley, P., Gentry, B.F., and Torres-Feliciano, J. (2016). *Autism: Attacking Social Interaction Problems – A Therapy Manual Targeting Social Skills in Children 4–9*. San Diego, CA: Plural Publishing.

CHAPTER 6

School-Aged Children Part Two: The Later Years

Learning Objectives

By reading this chapter interventionists will be able to:

1. Describe neurotypical social skills development for children of middle-school to high-school ages.
2. Define common challenges experienced by individuals with autism of middle-school and high-school ages.
3. Prepare a therapeutic setting and tasks that are age appropriate and engaging.
4. Plan activities for targeting pragmatic language goals. Develop appropriate objectives and plan therapy activities targeting pragmatic language differences.
5. Consider the role of maturation, sex, dating, and gender for teens with autism.
6. Prepare teens with autism for independence.

Blake is a 14 year old boy with autism. He loves everything dealing with literacy. He can read a chapter book, does well on his assignments in the classroom setting, and knows how to formulate age-appropriate sentences. His parents and teachers report that he is sweet and is not a challenge in the mainstreamed setting. He is a social loner at school and in the home setting. It is surprising

Autism Spectrum Disorders from Theory to Practice: Assessment and Intervention Tools Across the Lifespan,
First Edition. Edited by Belinda Daughrity and Ashley Wiley Johnson.
© 2023 John Wiley & Sons Ltd. Published 2023 by John Wiley & Sons Ltd.

though, because in the therapy room he loves to engage and show off his knowledge about trains to all of his therapists. In terms of progress, he is meeting his speech, occupational therapy, and resource specialist program goals. At this point, you are considering exiting him from your service. However, you know there must be more to work on. What is a newly-minted interventionist to do?

The above therapeutic depiction represents the challenge that many adolescents with autism face as they matriculate through the school-age years. Your traditional therapy goals are met and your client begins to demonstrate more novel and unique challenges. As an interventionist, it may make you question what exactly you should be focusing on in treatment sessions and how you can maximize your clients' potential to help meet the intervention goals.

Our advice during the planning stages is to be particularly aware of the scope of practice outlined by your national organization. As clients begin to meet most traditional therapy goals, the later school-age years typically calls for adjustments to your treatment approach. It is important to engage and create tangible, relevant, caregiver and client goals that make sense. These goals should be relative to your clients' life, self- and/or care.

To the planning stages, the execution stage is equally as important. Come to therapy with a clear targeted plan. Include at least two options for variation based on client response. We like to call this your **Oh goodness! plan**. The plan you have in your therapy tool belt to access quickly if you find that your original plan is not working. Regardless of how many years of practice you have, all prepared interventionists have an *Oh Goodness!* plan ready, just in case.

Well how will I know if I need to bring out my *Oh goodness!* plan, you may ask? Our answer is simple. Do you think a preteen or teenager will tell you when they don't like something? *Absolutely!* This is the same when working with an adolescent with autism. In fact, it is important to remember, whether your client has language or cognitive levels that are delayed, anatomically speaking, their bodies are maturing just like any neurotypical preteen or teenager. This factor must be taken into consideration with treatment planning and execution for adolescents, regardless of diagnosis.

Your clients will clearly let you know when something is not working, either through a meltdown, where maladaptive behaviors begin to show, or they will begin to tell their parents that they just feel bored and do not want to return, and you look around and notice that 50% of your group has stopped attending sessions. Either way, you don't want that to happen on your watch! And we don't want that for you, either.

While maladaptive behaviors and resisting treatment may occur as clients age, it is important to also note your therapy style and how that adjusts when working with students in the later school-age years. The primary purpose of this section is to explore many of the various needs of individuals with autism as they start to move into the later school-aged years and begin the process of maturation. From setting the tone in your therapeutic environment to being aware of common social pragmatic needs of adolescents, this chapter aims to prepare newly minted interventionists like yourself to be successful when treating adolescents with autism.

PARENTS AND THE ADOLESCENT REVOLUTION

Many parents of adolescents report that their role shifted when their children became teenagers, transforming from a smothering parent to a supportive parent (Van Bourgondien et al. 2014; Marcus et al. 2005). Smothering was further defined as unintentionally limiting independence, doing more for the child than the child does for themselves, and making decisions for the child independently. To be clear, this is not to look down on smothering parents; this statement is to highlight what was needed for the child at that time. As the child matures and hopefully meets goals, parents may feel a sense of moving into the role of guide and facilitator (Van Bourgondien et al. 2014) in an effort to help facilitate **self-determination**. This statement is also by no means suggestive that their job gets easier. In fact, many parents report that their role is even more hands-on as they transition to adulthood with their adolescent on the spectrum.

In addition to shifts in parenting style, parents of adolescents and adults with autism report that priorities also shift. This is the time when you may see shifts in therapy. Many individual with minimal challenges in our social skills program may stop coming for short periods of time, parents may focus on enrolling the child in a class to facilitate a hobby or allow the child to have time at home just relaxing. However, it is important to support parents during this time by asking them to consider that social skills are changing across the lifespan meeting goals today may not mean no need for service ever. As needs change, many students may need to stay engaged in some type of social skills training to ensure success. This even includes adults, who may be working a high-paying corporate job or a teen who cannot engage in typical social interaction but is a greeter at Walmart. Delayed social skills are a hallmark of autism. Consider the list of top parental concerns for their adolescent or adult with autism outlined in Table 6.1.

As an interventionist, you may not have answers to many of these questions for parents. However, our suggestion is to anticipate concerns and to ask parents about their current priorities. Ensure that the core areas you are focusing on help the client to ultimately get closer to providing a parent security and answers to the questions that they have. If you plan from a place of thinking of the patient's and parents' wants and needs, you will find that parents and clients will feel heard and included in the process of providing care.

SETTING THE TONE FOR SUCCESS

Consider the questions posed in Chapter 4: what would make you feel comfortable when going into a therapy session for yourself? We further discussed traits that one may value in any therapist. Now, consider the space in which you would feel comfortable telling your private thoughts and the workings of yourself and your life. What would be important to you? Maybe things come to mind like cleanliness, comfort, or privacy.

What you value or seek in a therapist may differ from person to person but what is consistent is that you have an opinion on what will help you to do what the therapist

TABLE 6.1   Top parental concerns for their adolescent or adult with autism.

Parent priority	Parent "realistic" concerns
Consistency of care	<ul><li>Who will work with my child?</li><li>Will this provider stay with us?</li><li>Who is on my child's care team?</li></ul>
Future and estate planning	<ul><li>How will I save to provide for my child for a lifetime?</li><li>What will my child do to be happy and fulfilled as an adult?</li></ul>
Guardianship	<ul><li>Who will care for my child when we are gone?</li></ul>
Transitioning to adulthood	<ul><li>What career is a good fit for my child?</li><li>Can they succeed in college?</li></ul>
Social opportunities	<ul><li>Will my child have friends?</li><li>Does my child have a hobby?</li><li>Will my child have something they can do to have fun?</li><li>Who will hang out with my child?</li><li>Will they live a life like a "normal" adult?</li></ul>
Independence	<ul><li>Will they live away from home?</li><li>How can I give them as much independence as possible?</li><li>What will my child do with their day? What type of job is a good fit?</li><li>Will my child have the skills to be successful?</li><li>Will my child know how to respond in an emergency?</li></ul>

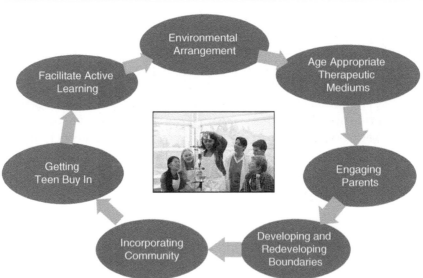

FIGURE 6.1   Components to successful adolescent therapy session implementation. Credit: Compassionate Eye Foundation/Steven Errico/DigitalVision/Getty Images

may be asking you to do. In our work as interventionists working with individuals with autism, our goal is to get them to open and start to change or develop key skills needed to be successful. It is especially important to consider environmental arrangement (Gentry and Wiley 2016): how you want your therapy room to look and feel.

When working with older children, you want to make the therapy room inviting. After all, your therapy may be one of five different therapies a client goes to in a week. While there is limited information on **environmental arrangement** and what works well for adolescents with autism, we offer you a few things to consider (Figure 6.1). We probed 10 therapists working with adolescents and this is what they offered:

- Your therapy space should not "feel" like school!
- You can't get social without enough space to socialize!
- Sometimes outdoors is a wonderful change of pace.
- Shift from children's chairs to adult or family style seating.
- Put up your students' work so they know the space is theirs.
- Hang some memes or inspirational posts; my students love to figure them out!
- Organize the space to be able to have two stations running if possible.

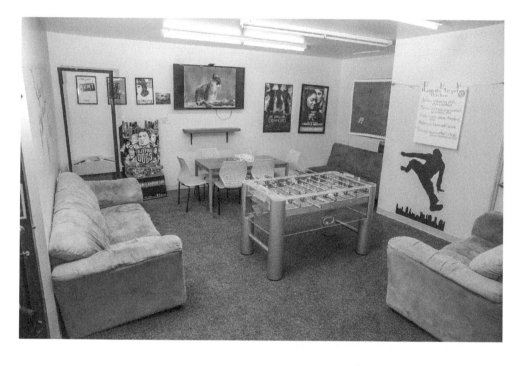

While we are suggesting making a therapy space feel more engaging to appeal to an older child, we are not expecting you to go out and spend your hard-earned money to outfit your office. Instead, we are encouraging you to think outside the box. As speech–language pathologists (SLP) serving adolescents, we look at our centers and see amazingly cool therapy spaces. We are proud that some of those items are items from our own homes donated to achieve a home feeling. Graduate-school couches, old televisions, POV, all can be found at one of our centers in our teen spaces. When choosing to repurpose, the one thing to ensure is that it is in good condition, has been sanitized, and is appropriate for use with clients. A wonderful reference is yourself; if you feel comfortable to be yourself in your space, your client most likely will as well.

Now that the mood for the scene is set for your adolescents, you must think through content. To teach a task or to accomplish your objectives, it is most useful to teach in multiple contexts so the brain can capture the task by tapping into more than one passageway. For example, in a birth of a word (Roy 2011), the speaker discussed how he was able to track how his son learned to say the word "water." Through 24-hour surveillance and significant time for analysis, he found that his son picked up words where he had the highest number of points of contact. He did not learn "water" one way, he learned it multiple ways finally, with practice and different points of exposure to the word, the child picked it up. This idea can be applied to how we can teach new or novel skills to adolescents with autism.

One strategy widely acknowledged in education is the process of active learning. Active learning is teaching a client something by having them involved in the learning process. It differs from "traditional" teaching methods where you are the expert and you are expected to give the person knowledge (Owens et al. 2020; Center for Educational Innovation 2022; Markant et al. 2016). Learning new tasks requires different types of memory and retrieval to be able to successfully learn. In the brain, memory is stored in many different parts. With active learning, the client can access memories and build new memories that will stick in other parts of the brain but will also build connections among all parts that have been accessed (Willis, 2018). In practice, this looks like a client using as many parts of their brain as possible to most efficiently and effectively learn the task you are trying to teach.

While therapy in general is an active process, we need our clients to respond to elicit a change or to observe progress. However, as therapists, we often do not acknowledge that even in our own practice, we can get stuck in our same way of "teaching." We want to avoid this, especially with teens and adults. Remember, when it gets boring to an adolescent or adult, self-determination will kick in and they will likely elect not to participate or will not feel motivated to be engaged.

Remember, self-determination is one's ability to make choices and decisions about one's own care. Incorporating active learning strategies in your own practice and consistently reminding yourself of the variety of strategies that can be used will be a key to success. Consider the strategies organized by degree of time and complexity it takes in treatment in Figure 6.2.

Reflect on the various components shared in the active learning chart (Center for Innovative Learning 2022). Notice that the most simple active learning strategy is writing and large group discussions. We urge you to remember, if you have a client who has autism and shows challenges with various concepts or skills, avoid taking the simple way out! Try to include some tasks that are more complex in an effort to reach the client the best way possible. Another tip is to avoid filling your session with pen and this paper tasks, can be daunting for individuals with autism. Consider challenges with fine motor development, self-regulation, literacy, comprehension, and attending to a task. Writing something down may be a challenge that brings up other deficits the client has making it more challenging to get what you are intending to be learned.

We are also not expecting you to be able to find different types of therapy materials that use varying active learning strategies to teach a certain skill. This is *not* what

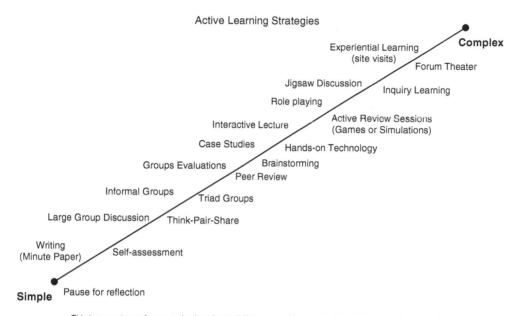

FIGURE 6.2   Active learning strategies.

we are encouraging you to do. We understand that task would be time consuming and unrealistic. However, may we suggest that you consider perfecting certain therapeutic mediums that will work with your style and the clients that you are working with. A therapeutic mediums is the means by which you deliver treatment. If you have a certain medium to use during your session, you can fill that medium with specific content, verbiage, or tasks (Table 6.2).

Video Modeling and Autism Spectrum Disorder

Think of a time where you were tasked with making a specific recipe. If you are like us, you will hop on your tablet, look at Food Network, and find a show that is making the recipe you are looking to try. As you watch these shows, you may do different things based on the task. For example, you may watch one step, do it and then go back into the video until you have completed the recipe. Or, maybe you watch the whole way through, execute the recipe, and start to visualize the steps you saw as you try them out in real time. Either way, that video helps to put life to the written words of a recipe so that we learn the more subtle methods of executing a new task.

This example is related to the helpfulness of **video modeling** to support a person with autism to achieve social pragmatic success. In fact, video modeling is an evidence-based instructional method that helps to improve performance and has been used extensively with people with disabilities (Green et al. 2017; Wertalik et al., 2016; McCoy et al. 2016).

TABLE 6.2   Therapeutic Mediums. Defined.

Therapeutic medium	Structural highlights	Active learning strategies (identified in Figure 6.2)
Hot potato	Clients sit in a circle; a bowl or basket with content is passed as quickly as possible. Each time a client has the bowl, they respond to the prompt.	• Pause for reflection • Role playing • Active review sessions
Peer-directed feedback	Students listen to a peer and provide feedback about what is seen or heard.	• Group evaluation • Hands-on technology • Peer review
Conversation partners	Students pair up with preidentified peer who has been identified as a conversation partner. Assignments can be given to call your partner or to meet with them virtually or in person. There is a specific task that must be accomplished with the conversation partner interaction.	• Think, pair, share • Hands-on technology
The "hot" seat	Students are in a circle, one chair is in the center of the circle that is called "the hot seat;" interventionist poses a question or task for participants to respond to. Instruct client who is in the hot seat to turn their chair to a peer of their choice to practice good eye contact and talking to someone specifically.	• Group evaluation • Role playing • Inquiry learning
Community-based outings	Students will engage in real-life activities stimulating the key skills taught in the therapy room. These activities will range from performance tasks (buying something from a store independently with a partner) to less structured social opportunities (going to a movie). The role of the therapist is to be a facilitator of the experience, a participant when needed, and an observer.	• Informal groups • Small group discussion • Inquiry learning • Experiential learning
Video modeling and discussion	Students watch a video targeting the correct and incorrect versions of tasks that are expected to be learned. Pausing throughout the video to check for understanding and attention is an important component of active learning. Students will discuss or recreate what was seen.	• Group evaluation • Think, pair, share
Small group discussion	Students are seated in a group of half or one third of the whole group size. Students will engage in a discussion guided by the interventionist. Key component of this is to encourage active listening and check for understanding.	• Interactive lecture • Brainstorming • Peer review

Sources: Laugeson and Ellingsen (2016); Gentry and Wiley (2016).

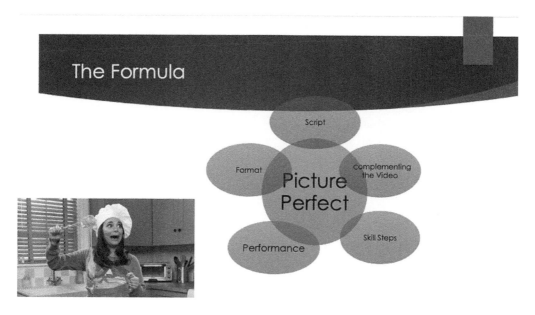

FIGURE 6.3   The formula to follow when leading social skills in a group setting.

It allows the student to observe the target behavior in a restrictive view and then practice what was modeled in the video as many times as needed until the desired outcome is obtained. This is particularly helpful in the treatment of individuals with autism who benefit from visual supports and incidental learning occurring while observing. This method is an effective evidenced-based practice that can also be fun to create.

This sounds great in theory right? But how is this done? And who exactly can it be used for? While it is suggested that video modeling is most effective with an individual with minimal challenges (McCoy et al. 2016), we found in practice that video modeling is a wonderful tool to use with all individuals with autism from early intervention age through young adulthood. Organization and planning are critical skills needed in the process to ensure successful implementations, especially with younger clients or with clients who present with more involved symptomology (i.e. presence of maladaptive behaviors). There is a formula we use in our center for interventionists to follow when leading social skills in the group setting (Figure 6.3). In 2018, we shared our practices with attendants at the American Speech and Hearing Association International Convention. During this presentation, we encouraged interventionists to create content for video modeling that was "picture perfect."

Taking time to think about the format of the video that you are producing is a critical component to success. When considering format, it is important to ask yourself what you are trying to achieve for the client as a result of watching the video you are creating? Depending upon your answer, one of the types of video modeling in Table 6.3 will be needed.

TABLE 6.3   Video modeling.

Type	Objective	What does that look like in practice?
Task based	Improve performance with a target skill or function.	Student learns the skills needed for joining a group effectively.
Situational	Respond appropriately in novel social scenarios.	Student learns how to respond when someone says hello to them.
Error analysis	Students will visualize areas of challenge or deficiency found in their own actions or within the group.	Watch for challenges in your population, identify opportunities to create a video model related to errors observed. Change domain if needed to avoid a student feeling "targeted."
Self-analysis	The students are videotaped applying the appropriate or even inappropriate execution of the skill step or target behavior. or Students are monitored in natural settings where the social demand includes a preidentified target behavior.	Allows interventionists to see the client perform a desired skill set. Take time to look for desired skills and take note of challenges or areas of growth. When watching and analyzing, it creates an opportunity to incorporate peer directed feedback.

Active Learning Task

Take a moment to come up with a social skill that you would like to teach a teen client with autism. Identify the type of video modeling that could be used. And, action! Create a first attempt at a video model. Share your picture-perfect video model with a peer. Take time and discuss whether this task was easy or challenging to complete. What challenges did you have along the way?

Once you have identified the type of video modeling you plan to create, take time to think through the key **social skill steps** needed to execute successfully. This may seem counterintuitive. However, remember that social skills challenges are a hallmark feature of autism. These things that may seem natural to one may feel unnatural to another. Therefore, taking time to plan out the activity and developing specific required skills that a client needs to experience success will be helpful. By doing this, you will provide clarity to your client and will help yourself to have clear measurable targets that can guide your decision of clients' progress and need. Remember, *your data drives therapy needs.*

In addition, the authors recommend creating a shell or **script** for your video. It is not natural to hop on camera and show your clients your talents. We understand that. However, when we take time to go through this process, we can check that all details are considered, and the final product is well thought out. This is the fun but necessary part of the process.

Therapy Golden Nugget

Video Modeling Outline
Type: Task based
Social skills unit: How to join a group
Objective: Students will learn the desired skills to effectively join a group of peers to complete a task or activity.
Social skills steps:

1. Think about what I want to say or do to show that I want to join the group.
2. Be close to the group so that people know you want to join.
3. Look interested in what is happening in the group by making eye contact or giving a social smile.
4. I need to do what the people in the group are doing if I want to join the group.
5. I will listen in the group so I can generate on topic comments and questions.
6. I will look at people's faces to understand if it is OK or not OK to join the group.
7. If the members look not happy or unfriendly, they may not want me to join in.

Script:
Background: Alexis sees her classmates playing at recess. She wants to play cards with them and is going to try to join the group.
Take a moment to complete this plan for your task-based video model. Once completed, shoot it and share it!

_____

_____

_____

_____

_____

ADOLESCENCE AND PRAGMATIC CONSIDERATIONS

When treating adolescents with autism, interventionists may likely find that the emphasis on treatment shifts from a standpoint of attacking deficits to a position of identifying and maximizing current strengths (Volkmar et al. 2016; Schall et al. 2016). Clients at this level are often accessing the academics the best they are able, whether this means accessing with ease or with significant accommodations. The subsequent focus as they get to adolescence is on functional skills for clients who may still have significant cognitive and language impairments or college readiness and career preparation for students with mild to moderate delays (Schall et al. 2016). Regardless of what the emphasis is for the client, there will still be a need for support with developing the social skills needed to navigate life in a meaningful way.

Regardless of level of functioning, many adolescents with ASD can be characterized as having poor friendships, lacking social engagement, and experiencing awkward social interactions with others resulting in peer rejection. You may read that and assume that you will experience higher degrees of challenge with the aforementioned areas as a client is more cognitively and language impaired. Right? Wrong! Both higher and lower functioning individuals with autism will experience social challenges as they become adolescents and experience maturation. In fact, we would say that, sometimes, you will see individuals with minimum challenges experience a higher degree of social communication challenges. This may be due to increased independence and ability to engage in more diverse social interactions.

For example, consider client Henry. He is a 17-year-old boy with autism who is in the general education setting. He enjoys anything related to transportation. He can navigate his bike and has recently been allowed to ride his bike to the local outdoor mall. Because Henry has poor friendships, he is often alone and will go there to find something to do. While there, he finds nice people and talks to them about his love for transportation. During these exchanges, people show different reactions ranging from finding him to be a sweet young man to feeling he is annoying and inappropriate. One day, Henry engaged a man who was not having a good day. Henry was unable to see the signs of annoyance on the young man's face. The man got upset and yelled derogatory phrases to Henry. Henry felt sad and decided never to return to that mall again.

The above example represents what can happen when a client presents as highly verbal but continues to struggle with the hallmark features of autism. On one hand, Henry appears to have all he needs to safely navigate the community. It even sounds that he has a solution for tackling loneliness associated with his poor friendships. However, with increased independence comes increased risk (Law 2017). Henry can experience present challenges because of his inability to filter, discern good from bad, and difficulty using the tools needed to generate appropriate social interactions. Add to that, he looks just like any typical 17-year-old boy.

While this situation resulted in just being talked to in an inappropriate fashion, it could have easily become dangerous. For example, one of our clients, a 17-year-old boy with an individual with minimal challenges, developed friendships with peers who were a negative influence. One day, his "friends" convinced him to take his bike onto a local bus and to ride around the city. As a result of not knowing his way, the client got lost on the bus. Authorities were engaged and search teams commenced. Three days later, the client was found at the local homeless shelter.

In this clinical case, the client had trouble inferring others' intentions via making social judgments. More specifically, the client had challenges understanding how to navigate various social scenarios, and had limited experience with independence. While his parents came in after the incident to begin social skills services, his social skills were significantly impaired, making it challenging to unlearn certain social thoughts and behaviors. Unfortunately, the client quickly became of age and elected to stop services against the family's wishes.

As an interventionist working with this population, engage social skill development as a critical area of emphasis as students get older. These important skills will support a student to obtain and maintain friendships, meaningful relationships, strong workplace skills, and to facilitate independence. Despite maturation, clients with autism may continue to experience delayed social pragmatic language and difficulty understanding social cues across the lifespan. As a result,

Therapy Golden Nugget

Conversation Sandwich

Objective: Clients will discuss the various components of a successful conversation through the lens of eating a hamburger. Students will role play an example of each component of the conversation sandwich.

Bun = Starting the conversation
- Greetings and openers

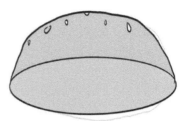

Meat = Conversation subject of intent
- Posing a question
- Making a comment
- Sharing a specific message

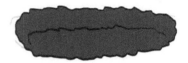

Toppings = Make a conversation taste good
- Nonverbal feedback
- Audible noises (i.e. mmhmmm)
- Body posturing

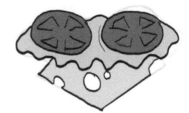

Bottom bun = Ending a conversation
- Salutation
- Final thoughts
- Well wishes

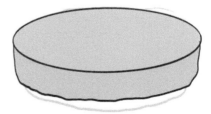

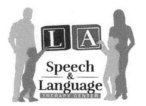

many adolescents with autism report feelings of loneliness and isolation (Lasgaard et al. 2009; Laugeson et al. 2014; Bauminger and Kasari 2000; Capps et al. 1998; Humphrey and Symes 2010).

It is important to include a curriculum that addresses *fostering positive mental health* and encouraging opportunities to *engage in experiences* important to peers their age. Remember, session emphasis will vary based on your specific discipline. However, your primary overarching objective can still address key areas of challenge. Consider the following list of common areas of deficit experienced by adolescents with autism. While there are suggested developmental milestones, it is important to remember the shift in treatment approach past developmental milestones and more toward key skills needed for the client to experience a fulfilled life and future. Our practice will shift from deficit focused toward planning and preparing for the future (Schall et al. 2016; Sundberg, 2008).

TOP ADOLESCENT SOCIAL SKILLS CONCERNS AND SOLUTIONS

Table 6.4 shows some common adolescent skills concerns.

TABLE 6.4   Common adolescent skills concerns.

Common adolescence need addressed	What skills does the client need to be successful?	How do I know my client understands this?
Active listening	• Body posturing • Self-regulation • Joint attention • Question posing • Comment • Generation retention of key details	Competency in this area results in a client's ability to demonstrate understanding and engage with information presented verbally.
Bullying	• Standing up for yourself • Reporting someone • Sharing self-experience with others • Defending and advocating for self	Competency in this area results in a client's ability to recognize and respond to being bullied by others. Client also understands perspective of all involved in scenarios where one is bullied.
Friendships	• Analyzing friendship development • Finding commonalities with others • Sharing experiences in multiple settings • Understanding right from wrong • Accepting and responding to rejection	Client has an emotionally intimate and reciprocal long-term relationship with someone who has shared interests and who they spend time with.

TABLE 6.4 (Continued)

Common adolescence need addressed	What skills does the client need to be successful?	How do I know my client understands this?
Presentation	• Vocal volume • Self-regulation • Responding to adult directives • Tackling • Social awkwardness • Responding to fears and anxiety	Competency will result in a client's ability to share/report information to a whole group in front of others.
Social interactions	• Addressing • restricted interests • On topic vs off topic, verbal and nonverbal responses • Turn taking • Eye contact • Vocal volume	Competency in this area results in a client's ability to know what to do to start or to engage in varying forms of social interaction.
Puberty	• Executive functioning for managing changes • Understanding emotions • Vocal tone and • Pitch • Private vs public displays	Competency in this area results in a client's working understanding of the events surrounding changes in their body.
Career interest	• Exposure to professions • Identifying interests and hobbies • Career preparedness • Job placement	Competency in this area results in a person's ability to match their strengths to find a career path appropriate for them.
Personal hygiene	• Grooming • Developing positive self-image • Theory of mind	Competency in this area results in a client's ability to develop an appropriate routine related to caring for their own body and clothing. This includes recognizing sign of when increased care is needed.
Loneliness	• Making friends • Accepting rejection • Standing up for yourself • Maintaining positive mental health	Competency will result in a client's ability to cope with and respond to peer rejection and to recognize appropriate social supports to address feelings of loneliness.

(continued)

TABLE 6.4   (Continued)

Common adolescence need addressed	What skills does the client need to be successful?	How do I know my client understands this?
Relationships	• Process awareness • Differentiating relationships • Do's and don'ts • Responding to novel • social scenarios	Competency will result in a client's ability to develop, navigate, and differentiate among family, acquaintances, romantic relationships, and friendship.
Persons of interest	• Eye contact • Vocal control • Accepting rejection • Overcoming anxiety • Social script • development	Competency in this area will result in a client's ability to approach a person of interest using appropriate verbal and nonverbal skills.
Executive functioning	• Organization and following directions • Task analysis and follow through • Navigating digital platforms • Formulating realistic goals	Competency results in learning and managing their own life on a daily basis to the best of the client's ability
Independence	• Personal hygiene • Cooking • Career preparedness	Competency will result in a client being able to manage their own care, health, and safety in the community.
Self-determination	• Advocating for yourself • Understanding your autism • Setting and achieving goals • Dreams for the future	Competency will result in a client's ability to make choices and decisions surrounding their own quality of life.
Conversations	• Understanding aspects of successful conversations • Role playing • Nonverbal communication • Overcoming social anxiety • Social script development	Being able to talk to someone in a fluid fashion demonstrating turn taking, topic maintenance, topic extension, adequate nonverbal communication.

Sources: Daughrity (2018); Schall et al. (2016); Laugenson and Ellison (2016); Laasgard et al. (2009); and Gentry and Wiley (2016).

DEVELOPING SOCIAL TARGETS

Neurodiversity Considerations

Interventionists may opt to target the areas below given client and/or parent report. It is important for interventionists to use their clinical judgment to determine whether targets are appropriate and functional for the client. Some clients may feel that they are **masking**, hiding things that they naturally cannot control (Mandy 2019). When a client expresses this or shows signs of resistance, it might be more appropriate for a client who fails to integrate eye gaze with verbal output to target self-advocacy in conversation such as, "I don't always look at your eyes when you're talking, but don't worry, I am paying attention!" Such advocacy approaches may be appropriate for highly verbal clients who report sustaining eye gaze as distressing and exceedingly difficult (Trevisan et al. 2017). In such cases, targeting self-advocacy may be more appropriate than targeting the goal of increasing eye gaze. Such an approach may serve to reduce social and occupational barriers, while preserving autonomy and accounting for client preferences.

Take note of the various challenges mentioned in the above list. Now look at the required social skills to be competent with the overarching goal. You may have noticed that many of the skills are repetitive. That is because critical social skills are needed to be successful with most types of novel social scenarios. In fact, in our practice, we call many of those skills **social targets**. Social targets are key skills that can support a student with most types of social interaction. During therapy, regardless of the topic or curriculum you are covering, you should engage social targets throughout the treatment sessions. When taught and emphasized through a variety of therapeutic mediums. (e.g., the hot seat, conversation partners, community-based outings), you will see that skills will generalize faster to the naturalistic setting. This is because you have worked on those specific skills throughout varying types of interactions in treatment sessions.

Common Social Targets for Adolescents with Autism

Eye contact	⟶	Client will make and sustain eye contact when engaging with others.
Clear voice	⟶	Client will use appropriate articulation to clearly relay message.
Loud voice	⟶	Client will modulate voice to minimally be at conversional level or louder.
Standing still	⟶	Client will regulate body to convey message and engage in social interaction.
Being on topic	⟶	Client will recognize and monitor on and off topic comments throughout social interactions.
Holding it in	⟶	Client will avoid maladaptive behaviors (e.g. interrupting and physical outbursts).

It is accepted that delayed social skills, poor friendships, and difficulty understanding and recognizing social cues are a challenge for many adolescents with autism. Now, imagine how those outcomes may shift if the client is able to master many of the targets. At the very least, it would improve the quality of the social interaction. That alone could lead to developing friendships or landing the job of their choice. And for some clients, that is more than enough!

Social targets are assigned to adolescent students at the beginning of their sessions. Ensuring that a client is aware of their targets is critical. When you observe a child not showing a target, you can discreetly remind them by saying, "Remember your targets!." This simple phrase will trigger a student to work on a few preidentified skills that you want them to master during social interactions. How will they know what you are expecting you may ask? Well, that is where teaching the task comes in. Consider basic behavioral principles to get a person to shift their behavior.

Before generalization of the skill, we recommend priming the clients by teaching the task and providing prompting (Figure 6.4). In the Therapy Golden Nugget below is one example of how to stimulate a client's awareness of the social targets.

Therapy Golden Nugget

Target Practice
Objective:
1. Students will gain awareness of desired social targets.
2. Students will use continuous speech to talk about a known subject.
3. Students will evaluate peer performance through providing feedback.
Preparation:
- Preidentified targets written out on a large piece of paper or whiteboard.
- Client chairs organized in a semicircle.
- Precut strips with hodge-podge topics (e.g., favorite movies, favorite food).
- Timer.
Procedures:
- Clients will be seated in a semicircle.
- Therapist reviews targets through self-modeling.
- Therapists poses question: "What are the things we like to do?"
- Students discuss the question.
- Therapist poses questions: "Can you do (social act) if you are (*opposite behavior from social target*)? That's why we want to work on our targets."
- Therapist introduces activity:
  - Clients will pick a strip with a hodge-podge topic.
  - They will say whatever they want to say about this topic to peers (use timer to add social pressure).
- Therapist poses question: "Did _____ work on his target?"
- Therapist leads students to provide peer directed feedback.
- Client will have another opportunity to practice with the same Hodge podge topic. Be sure client understands goal is to use what peers have said to improve. Fade tactile and verbal cuing as needed.

A NOTE ON PEER-DIRECTED FEEDBACK

In our therapeutic example of target practice, notice that there was no mention of providing the student feedback on performance as a therapist. Instead, feedback was suggested to be given by the students. Peer-directed feedback is an intentional strategy included because it works well with adolescents. In fact, studies show that adolescents respond to feedback received by peers better when it is posed in a positive or supportive way in comparison with negative feedback and rejection (Rosen et al. 2019; Butterfield et al. 2021). One study found that students with anxiety disorders ($n = 22$) responded better to positive peer-directed feedback in comparison with healthy youth ($n = 25$) in the study. This was captured through tracking pupil dilation (Rosen et al. 2019).

Another study focusing on teenage adolescent girls found that regardless of whether the feedback was positive or negative, adolescent girls showed increased response and arousal in comparison with neutral interactions. Listening to peer feedback induced an emotional subjective response from the female participants. These findings validated the fact that inclusion of peer-directed feedback tasks is positive for use working with adolescent girls and their peers (Butterfield et al. 2021).

While the sample sizes in these studies did not include students with autism specifically, autism, anxiety disorders, and even being female may share some similar features. For example, many students with autism may suffer from social anxiety or may experience anxiety as a result of sensory overload or being lonely. A client who is a female aged 16 years with autism is first, an adolescent girl. Both scenarios are more common than uncommon in practice. Future research should look toward discovering peer-directed feedback and its impact with students on the autism spectrum.

Despite its limited documentation and inclusion in research for people with autism, we think of one thing. If this can benefit our students, can we at least try it? Absolutely! We find it to be quite effective in my practice. We enjoy it because the students respond well, and it gives all students in the group a specific challenge to stay engaged and to pay attention and be ready to provide feedback when prompted. Our advice is when using peer-directed feedback:

- Be a guide by helping the students to understand how to give positive feedback.
- Set ground rules for being respectful and kind. Bullying and rejection will not be accepted.
- Support the student to formulate the structure of the feedback so it is clear. Remember, language may still be a concern for any client with autism.

Remember, for many clients, this is a new task, and it takes time to get comfortable speaking up and offering feedback or support to a peer about their performance. The following is an example of clients generated responses giving feedback.

"Good job Ashley! I can't hear you though. Can you do it again LOUDER?"

"Joey, I liked your eye contact but, you were moving around a lot while you talked; next time, try to stand still."

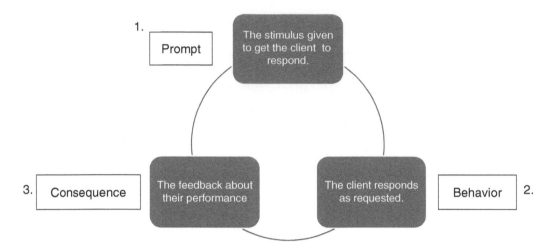

FIGURE 6.4   Teaching the task and providing prompting.

Relationships, Gender, and Sex

Like their neurotypical peers, it can be assumed many older school-aged children with autism have desires for romantic relationships. In addition to specific challenges, some also advocate for individuals with autism having sufficient information to make informed decisions in their own sexuality (Travers and Tincani 2010). While few studies explore this complex topic, limited findings indicate significant differences between adolescents with autism and their typical peers in abilities to engage in privacy, demonstrate knowledge of sex education, and display appropriate sexual behaviors (Stokes and Kaur 2005). Parents of adolescents with autism report increased fears of sexual victimization, in addition to concerns of others' misinterpretation their child's behaviors (Ballan 2012).

Take a moment to remember what was stressed in the start of this chapter; although your client may not socially be at age level, anatomically, they are developing like any neurotypical person. All people will mature; all people may start to develop interests in others (sexual and plutonic); it is on us as interventionists to take time to address it and support the client as they get to this place. Each year in our practice, our adolescents go through a unit on understanding the changing body, navigating relationships, and learning how to approach a person of interest. We chose to include various types of relationships so that students can feel comfortable to learn the material regardless of where they are maturity wise with wanting to approach people of interest. Our primary objective was to expose, bring awareness, focus on safety for self and others, and prime ability to differentiate "right" from "wrong" responses.

The dual challenges of ASD-specific social deficits and typical adolescent challenges of discovering sexual identity can contribute to particularly complex challenges for interventionists serving older school-age children with autism (Pask et al. 2016). Specific sex education programs that emphasize social interaction should be considered for adolescents with ASD (Stokes and Kaur 2005). Findings indicate sex education programs for individuals with intellectual disabilities have complex barriers, such as limited generalization to natural settings and increased intervention needed to maintain knowledge and skills (Schaafsma and Pfaff 2014). As such, interventionists with experience serving individuals with autism in middle- and high-school settings may be in a unique opportunity to support challenges during this period. Evidence suggests that manualized programs such as "Healthy Relationships and Autism" can yield positive outcomes on increasing sexual knowledge across children and adolescents with ASD of different abilities (Pask et al. 2016).

Interventionists should consider factors such as maturity, language level, comorbid conditions, and educational setting to determine how to address sexual education in a way that is most appropriate to the client's level of functioning. Importantly, any intervention on the sensitive topic should involve parents before implementation to solicit input regarding parent concerns.

Parent education interventions targeting sexuality education have been explored as methods to support teens with ASD navigate adolescence (Nichols and Blakeley-Smith 2009). If you work in a setting with older school-age clients with autism, you might consider asking parents whether they have concerns about their child navigating sexuality. While such conversations can potentially be uncomfortable, especially for new professionals, it is important to not avoid tough topics that may potentially help adolescents with autism avoid dangerous situations or face increased peer rejection due to difficulties with social interaction and navigating sexuality. You might also collaborate with allied professionals to address the topic. For example, nurse practitioners can help adolescents with ASD to navigate issues of sexuality and sexual health (Chan and John 2012).

Active Learning Task

How can you begin to address this complex topic with parents? Move past the uncomfortable feelings and ask! Ask parents:

- Are there any concerns you have right now as your teen is navigating sexual identity in middle/high school?
- Do you think your teen has the skills to safely navigate romantic relationships?
- Are you addressing these topics at home?
- Would you like me to address these topics in intervention?

ADOLESCENT GIRLS AND MENSTRUATION

Adolescent girls with autism present with differences than their male counterparts including sex-specific puberty issues (Cridland et al. 2014). Addressing topics like menstruation with adolescent girls with ASD can be accomplished by using social story interventions to target sexuality education (Tarnai and Wolfe 2008). Klett and

Turan (2012) used social stories and simulated conditions for visual support with adolescent girls with ASD to target increasing knowledge about reproductive development and independence in navigating periods.

You might question why this is important or if it fits into your domain? However, with your expertise in intervention with students with autism, if it is not your role, who would address it? If you find yourself struggling to answer "If not me, then who?" this topic might well be an area suited to your intervention with your experience with autism and awareness of its related social skills and/or language challenges.

As an applicable example, years ago, we worked with a wonderful teenage girl with autism named Asia. She was highly verbal and in a self-contained classroom. Upon entering an intervention session one afternoon after school, her mother reported Asja had spent the day in the nurse's offices after bleeding on herself during class. The mother was exasperated because she had repeatedly gone over how to use pads during her time of the month and thought Asja had regressed in her ability to successfully navigate her period independently. When the topic was brought up she said, "I know I needed to change my pad. I went to ask my teacher for permission to go to the bathroom, but she was helping another student, so I had to wait. After she helped the student, my teacher began the lesson, and I didn't want to get in trouble by leaving the room or interrupting her." In this case, Asja's report indicated a social skill difficulty of knowing how to interrupt appropriately and she was overgeneralizing class rules (e.g., don't leave the room without asking, and don't interrupt). To address her needs, we began incorporating role-playing tasks in intervention sessions to target how to interrupt an authority figure appropriately. We targeted scenarios when it would and would not be appropriate to interrupt.

Active Learning Task

Given the clinical scenario above, develop intervention session activities to address Asja's needs. Exchange your lesson plans with a peer and discuss your different clinical approaches.

Engaging Community

As adolescents continue to develop and shift their focus to future and independence, it is crucial to engage the community to assist the client to naturalize their skills. Remember the hierarchy discussed in Chapter 4. Figure 6.5 depicts therapeutic growth in a step-by-step fashion.

As a client gets to step 3 on our "Leading a Client to Success" chart, you will see that the goal is to observe their skills. It is important to remember this when in the community with a client. *You are not teaching the skills, you are observing and helping to facilitate the use of skills.* Our role as the interventionist is to provide the framework needed for the client to be able to naturally use the target skills taught in the treatment room, just in the community. Considering this, a true key to success is thorough planning and execution.

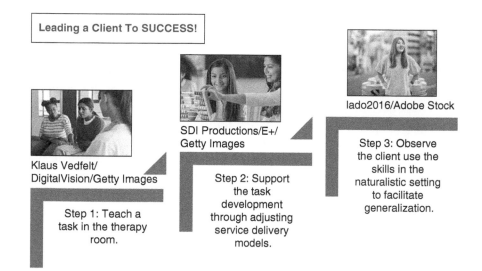

FIGURE 6.5 Basic behavioral principles.

When considering incorporating a **community-based outing**, we suggest looking for resources that are natural fits for the setting you are in. For example, in my practice, we have locations that are in the middle of the city and some locations that are a little more suburban. What that means in practice is that one group may be able to go to a mall to learn how to independently navigate a social setting with peers while our satellite students may be taking a walk to the office building café to practice the same skill steps just in a more convenient setting. When planning and executing a community-based outing, we offer the following tokens:

- *Less is more.* Keep your activity simple so that it can be well planned out and executed.
- *Make the experience as natural as possible.* Allow the client to engage in the activity as they naturally feel comfortable. In moments of comfort, you get to observe natural skills.
- *Take off the therapy hat in the community* by doing the social skill along with your client. If your client is showing you their tabletop chatting skills at a café, take time and be there in that moment with them. Sometimes your modeling can go a very long way.

SUMMARY

This chapter discussed the important information related to the treatment of individuals with autism when they reach adolescence. The key consideration was the shift from teaching things that the client is missing to a place of helping the client develop plans through focusing on areas like independence. Top parent concerns and common areas of social skills challenge for adolescents were highlighted. Suggestions for intervention are mentioned throughout the chapter. The chapter closes encouraging interventionists to use community-based outings as key moments to evaluate generalization of skills and continued areas of need.

REFLECTIONS ALONG THE PATH

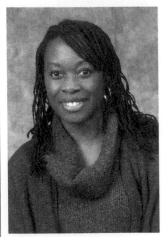

Danai Kasambira Fanin

This text, your courses, and clinical practicum will provide technical knowledge about working with autistic children, and I want you to also consider viewing autism through a non-traditional framework. The Americans with Disabilities Act of 1990 focuses on impairment, aligning its definition of disability with the medical model of how we treat our clients. Yet, there exists a diversity and equity framework of disability wherein autistics have a culture, akin to the Deaf community. I will describe examples of some things not to say to an autistic student to better fit the diversity and equity framework:

- Autism treatment: Treat communication deficits and not autism itself. Advocate for, support, or augment whatever voice(s) the child may have (e.g. sign, writing, pictures, speech generating device, verbalization).

- Low/moderate/high functioning: If these levels help you to organize, keep them in your head and, instead, talk about the level of supports needed. For example, a 'high-functioning' student might be included in the general education classroom and do daily activities independently, but may need moderate support for emotional regulation, like a visual strategy to get through unexpected changes in the schedule. Thus, just say they are an autistic student who needs a moderate level of supports.

- Student with autism: Sure, there are some autistic people and families who want to use person-first language, but you can contribute to the effort of destigmatizing autism by using identity-first language and not being fatalistic when a child is diagnosed. Listen to your student and their family to learn what term they are using but, if you are unaware and this is a first meeting, you are less likely to offend by leading with identity-first language.

- Inspirational: Calling anyone with a disability "inspirational" is annoying to many. It is fine to genuinely praise an autistic student for specifics like making the honor roll or being extra kind and supportive of peers. You can, however, save the "You are such an inspiration to us for being autistic!" because that can be demoralizing and embarrassing, even though you mean well.

- Training: Avoid saying "social skills training" or "AAC training". People find the word "training" to remind them of a dog being trained for the circus. Rather, replacing "training" with "education/teaching" works to where you can have "parent education sessions," not "parent training".

- Nonverbal: There have been different iterations of this term (e.g. minimally verbal) but some autistic adults say that pre-verbal is better. Although SLPs think of pre-verbal as an early childhood/infant level of typical communication development, pre-verbal can work for older autistic people because it presumes that they may be verbal someday.

Because the autism spectrum is not a linear scale, but more of a spherical, complex continuum of characteristics interacting with each other, the old saying attributed to autism advocate Dr. Stephen Shore of, "If you've met one person with autism, you've met one person with autism" holds true. Thus, all clients should be treated individually; yet we must not ignore neurodivergent populations as a culture. For instance, some social skills curricula aim to fit the child into typical society which might require them to pretend to be neurotypical or "mask" their true ways of interacting. Because there are several autistic socialization styles, I cannot say that zero autistic adults like social skills programs or that none want to learn to mask for specific purposes like asking a classmate to play or getting through a job interview. In fact, all people mask to get through job interviews or not lash out at customers at work. For autistic people, however, we should not assign a negative value to their way of socializing. We should remember that they may want to socialize with other neurodiverse people and, therefore, do not need to learn all of the social skills intervention. An SLP must find out what their autistic students want and customize intervention strategies to each student in a way that honors the student's wishes.

Danai Kasambira Fannin PhD CCC-SLP
Associate Professor, Department of Communication Sciences and Disorders
North Carolina Central University

TEST QUESTIONS

True or false?

1. When focusing on adolescents, your treatment goals should shift to focus on the future.

2. The final step when you are treating a client is seeing how well they do in the therapy room without your guidance.

3. When addressing tough topics like sex, or romantic relationships, ask the parent if there are any concerns they have right now as their teen is navigating sexual identity in middle/high school?

4. When using peer directed feedback in the group setting, it is important to be sure to encourage and guide clients to be kind as they tell others what they think of their performance.

REFERENCES

Ballan, M.S. (2012). Parental perspectives of communication about sexuality in families of children with autism spectrum disorders. *Journal of Autism and Developmental Disorders* 42 (5): 676–684.

Bauminger, N. and Kasari, C. (2000). Loneliness and friendship in high-functioning children with autism. *Child Development* 71 (2): 447–456.

Butterfield, R.D., Price, R.B., Woody, M.L. et al. (2021). Adolescent girls' physiological reactivity to real-world peer feedback: a pilot study to validate a peer expressed emotion task. *Journal of Experimental Child Psychology* 204: 105057.

Capps, L., Kehres, J., and Sigman, M. (1998). Conversational abilities among children with autism and children with developmental delays. *Autism* 2 (4): 325–344.

Center for Educational Innovation. (2022).Active learning. Available at `https://cei.umn.edu/active-learning` (accessed 30 January 2022).

Chan, J. and John, R.M. (2012). Sexuality and sexual health in children and adolescents with autism. *Journal for Nurse Practitioners* 8 (4): 306–315.

Cridland, E.K., Jones, S.C., Caputi, P., and Magee, C.A. (2014). Being a girl in a boys' world: Investigating the experiences of girls with autism spectrum disorders during adolescence. *Journal of Autism and Developmental Disorders* 44 (6): 1261–1274.

Daughrity, B.L. (2018). Parent perceptions of barriers to friendship development for children with autism spectrum disorders. *Communication Disorders Quarterly* 40 (3): 142–151.

Gentry, B.F. and Wiley, P. (2016). *Autism: Attacking Social Interaction Problems: A Therapy Manual Targeting Social Skills in Teens*. San Diego, CA: Plural Publishing.

Green, V.A., Prior, T., Smart, E. et al. (2017). The use of individualized video modeling to enhance positive peer interactions in three preschool children. *Education and Treatment of Children* 40 (3): 353–378.

Humphrey, N. and Symes, W. (2010). Responses to bullying and use of social support among pupils with autism spectrum disorders (ASDs) in mainstream schools: A qualitative study. *Journal of Research in Special Educational Needs* 10 (2): 82–90.

Lasgaard, M., Nielsen, A., Eriksen, M.E., and Goossens, L. (2009). Loneliness and social support in adolescent boys with autism spectrum disorders. *Journal of Autism and Developmental Disorders* 40 (2): 218–226.

Laugeson, E.A. and Ellingsen, R. (2016). Social skills training for adolescents and adults with autism spectrum disorder. In: *Adolescents and Adults with Autism Spectrum Disorders* (ed. F.R. Volkmar, B. Reichow and J.C. McPartland), 61–85. New York, NY: Springer-Verlag.

Laugeson, E.A., Ellingsen, R., Sanderson, J. et al. (2014). The ABC's of teaching social skills to adolescents with autism spectrum disorder in the classroom: The UCLA PEERS® program. *Journal of Autism and Developmental Disorders* 44 (9): 2244–2256.

Law, B.M. (2017). When autism grows up – and encounters cops. *The ASHA Leader* 22 (8): 54–57.

McCoy, A., Holloway, J., Healy, O. et al. (2016). A systematic review and evaluation of video modeling, role-play and computer-based instruction as social skills interventions for children and adolescents with high-functioning autism. *Review Journal of Autism and Developmental Disorders* 3 (1): 48–67.

Mandy, W. (2019). Social camouflaging in autism: is it time to lose the mask? *Autism* 23 (8): 1879–1881.

Marcus, L.M., Kunce, L.J., and Schopler, E. (2005). Working with families. In: *Handbook of Autism and Pervasive Developmental Disorders: Assessment, Interventions, and Policy* (ed. F.R. Volkmar, R. Paul, A. Klin and D. Cohen), 1055–1086. Hoboken, NJ: Wiley.

Markant, D.B., Ruggeri, A., Gureckis, T.M., and Xu, F. (2016). Enhanced memory as a common effect of active learning. *Mind, Brain, and Education* 10: 142–152.

Nichols, S. and Blakeley-Smith, A. (2009). "I'm not sure we're ready for this. . .": Working with families toward facilitating healthy sexuality for individuals with autism spectrum disorders. *Social Work in Mental Health* 8 (1): 72–91.

Owens, D., Sadler, T., Barlow, A., and Smith-Walters, C. (2020). Student motivation from and resistance to active learning rooted in essential science practices. *Research in Science Education* 50: 253–277.

Pask, L., Hughes, T.L., and Sutton, L.R. (2016). Sexual knowledge acquisition and retention for individuals with autism. *International Journal of School and Educational Psychology* 4 (2): 86–94.

Rosen, D., Price, R.B., Ladouceur, C.D. et al. (2019). Attention to peer feedback through the eyes of adolescents with a history of anxiety and healthy adolescents. *Child Psychiatry & Human Development* 50 (6): 894–906.

Roy, D. (2011). The birth of a word. *TED*, March. Available at https://www.ted.com/talks/deb_roy_the_birth_of_a_word (accessed 30 January 2022).

Schaafsma, S.M. and Pfaff, D.W. (2014). Etiologies underlying sex differences in autism spectrum disorders. *Frontiers in Neuroendocrinology* 35 (3): 255–271.

Schall, C., Wehman, P., and Carr, S. (2016). Transition from high school to adulthood for adolescents and young adults with autism spectrum disorders. In: *Adolescents and Adults with Autism Spectrum Disorders* (ed. F.R. Volkmar, B. Reichow and J.C. McPartland), 41–60. New York, NY: Springer-Verlag.

Stokes, M.A. and Kaur, A. (2005). High-functioning autism and sexuality: a parental perspective. *Autism* 9 (3): 266–289.

Tarnai, B. and Wolfe, P.S. (2008). Social stories for sexuality education for persons with autism/pervasive developmental disorder. *Sexuality and Disability* 26 (1): 29–36.

Travers, J. and Tincani, M. (2010). Sexuality education for individuals with autism spectrum disorders: Critical issues and decision making guidelines. *Education and Training in Autism and Developmental Disabilities* 284–293.

Trevisan, D.A., Roberts, N., Lin, C., and Birmingham, E. (2017). How do adults and teens with self-declared Autism Spectrum Disorder experience eye contact? A qualitative analysis of first-hand accounts. *PloS One* 12 (11): e0188446.

Van Bourgondien, M.E., Dawkins, T., and Marcus, L. (2014). Families of adults with autism spectrum disorders. In: *Adolescents and Adults with Autism Spectrum Disorders*, 15–40.

Volkmar, F.R., Reichow, B., and McPartland, J.C. (ed.) (2016). *Adolescents and Adults with Autism Spectrum Disorders*. New York, NY: Springer-Verlag.

Wertalik, J.L. and Kubina, R.M. (2018). Comparison of TAGteach and video modeling to teach daily living skills to adolescents with autism. *Journal of Behavioral Education* 27 (2): 279–300.

FURTHER READINGS

Children's Neurosychological Services. (2022). Children's developmental milestones. Available at https://www.childrensneuropsych.com/parents-guide/milestones (accessed 30 January 2022).

Freeman, S., Eddy, S.L., McDonough, M. et al. (2014). Active learning increases student performance in science, engineering, and mathematics. *Proceedings of the National Academy of Sciences* 111 (23): 8410–8415.

Mohammadi, F., Rakhshan, M., Molazem, Z. et al. (2018). Caregivers' perception of dignity in teenagers with autism spectrum disorder. *Nursing Ethics* 26 (7–8): 2035–2046.

Van Bourgondien, M.E., Dawkins, T., and Marcus, L. (2016). Families of adults with autism spectrum disorders. In: *Adolescents and Adults with Autism Spectrum Disorders* (ed. F.R. Volkmar, B. Reichow and J.C. McPartland), 15–40. New York, NY: Springer-Verlag.

CHAPTER 7

Autism and Adulthood

Pamela H. Wiley, Ph.D. H-CCC-SLP
Founder, The Los Angeles Speech and Language Therapy Center

Learning Objectives

By reading this chapter, interventionists will be able to:

1. Construct at least three therapy tasks to use with adults with autism.
2. Interpret the experience of adults with autism.
3. Understand meaningful employment and its impact on the life of an adult with autism.
4. Explain the value of role playing as an intervention task for young adults with autism spectrum disorder (ASD).
5. Analyze key areas of emphasis for independence development in adults with autism.
6. Provide at least three questions to pose to adults with autism and their families to promote partnered and family-centered intervention Figure 7.1.

INTRODUCTION

Since the end of the 20th century, there has been an increased understanding and awareness of children with autism, which has resulted in an earlier diagnosis and more students enrolled in special education departments across the country. The US Department

Autism Spectrum Disorders from Theory to Practice: Assessment and Intervention Tools Across the Lifespan,
First Edition. Edited by Belinda Daughrity and Ashley Wiley Johnson.
© 2023 John Wiley & Sons Ltd. Published 2023 by John Wiley & Sons Ltd.

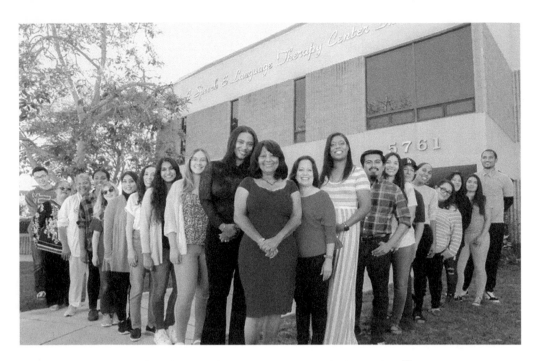

FIGURE 7.1   Dr. Pamela Wiley with her amazing interventionists and staff.

of Education indicates that figure to be 11% in 2019–2020 school year as compared with 5.8% 10 years earlier (Riser-Kositsky 2021). This figure represents the largest increase of all the eligibility criteria in special education. Despite this increase, consistent with previous findings, African American and Hispanic children were identified as having ASD less frequently than other groups, thus reducing or eliminating the benefits of early intervention services (Wiley and Gentry 2016; Pearson et al., 2021; Hannon et al. 2018).

Over the next decade, it is estimated that between 700,000–1 million teens will enter adulthood and age out of school-based autism services (Autism Speaks, 2020). Of those individuals, more than 50% will remain unemployed and unenrolled in higher education two years post-high school. Lastly, nearly half of 25-year-olds with autism will have never secured a paying job (Autism Speaks, 2020). What we do as interventionists today and in the future will shape the lives of not only our students and clients but families in general.

> "When we strengthen a child, we strengthen a family, and when we strengthen a family, we strengthen our society"
>
> Dr. P. Wiley.

We should be mindful to use the data to inform and shape our thoughts but to never limit or restrict our efforts. As practicing interventionists, we must be willing to look ***beyond the label*** of autism. This phrase, "beyond the label," has become an affirmation or belief in practice in all our centers.

This chapter shares current and previous data, as well as my personal and professional journey in response to the challenges and milestones achieved by these individuals, many of whom literally grew up in my center starting as young as 18 months of age. Today, many of my students are confident and hopeful young adults who embrace our belief that *"Autism is a label. It doesn't define your potential."* Parents' perspectives and cultural implications are also discussed, as we explore meaningful strategies to facilitate positive school and life outcomes for adults with ASD.

AUTISM, ADULTS, AND CURRENT KNOWLEDGE

Today, we are experiencing the first wave of young adults who have benefited from a range of services, which can include early intervention, speech–language therapy, social skills, behavior intervention, physical therapy, occupational therapy, and in some cases recreational services (Wiley and Gentry 2016; Volkmar, 2018). This does not include other types of interventionists like tutors, school shadows, and **tailor day workers**, who assist students with their daily living skills and needs.

The cost of care for these individuals in 2015 was approximately US$2.68 billion and is expected to increase to US$4.61 billion by 2025 (Wiley and Gentry 2016; Volkmar, 2018). Adult services account for many of the costs and are estimated to range from US$165 to US$196 billion/year. Despite the significant amount of money invested in their wellbeing, many of these individuals will remain unemployed or underemployed. **Sheltered employment** or employment that is restricted to one basic task is available for adults more impaired with autism. Sheltered employment is a term defined as a place where individuals with disabilities get job training and services with an objective of developing work-related skills and behaviors. While the name implies that it is a safe and protected space for an individual who presents with differences, it may not be fulfilling or stimulating for a an individual with autism who has higher levels of cognition. Even fewer jobs options exist for those in between (Wiley and Gentry 2016; Armstrong 2011).

Young adults with ASD continue to experience substantial challenges when seeking competitive **integrated employment opportunities** that are consistent with their skill sets and unique interests. It is important to note that an integrated setting is one where you find the individual with a disability (not limited to autism) is working and interacting with a range of individuals, mostly who are considered neurotypical. On the contrary, a **segregated job setting** is one where the employee is working with other individuals who have disabilities (Wiley and Gentry 2016). In fact, the 2017 National Autism Indicators findings of individuals who were able to be tracked as an adult with autism released a report to share employment outcomes (Roux et al. 2017). A summary of the report's findings are shown in Figure 7.2.

These and earlier research findings show that individuals with ASD have the lowest employment rate of all disabilities including intellectual disability, learning disability and speech and language delays (Shattuck et al. 2012). Additionally, individuals with ASD are at a significant disadvantage in the labor market that lacks understanding and support in the employment setting (Baldwin et al. 2014). Bennett and Dukes (2013) concluded that "individuals with ASD are ill prepared to obtain employment." Autistic individuals with college degrees are equally challenged to find employment. If they can find employment, many individuals are forced to settle for part-time or minimum wage positions (Pesce 2019).

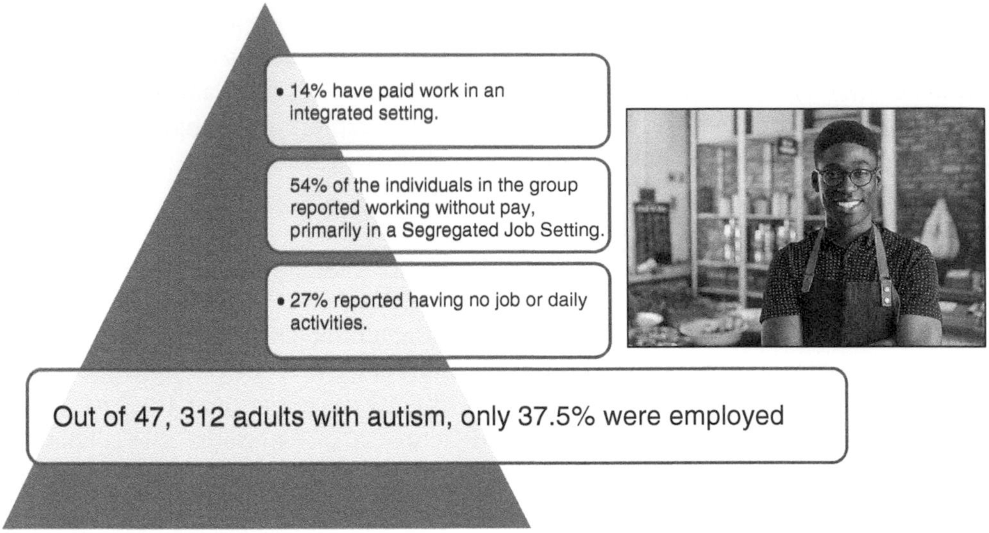

- 14% have paid work in an integrated setting.

54% of the individuals in the group reported working without pay, primarily in a Segregated Job Setting.

- 27% reported having no job or daily activities.

Out of 47, 312 adults with autism, only 37.5% were employed

FIGURE 7.2   Outcomes from the 2017 National Autism Indicators report. Source: Schall et al. (2020) and Volkmar (2018).

When considering research findings and our experience working, there are several key areas that are often an area of difference and challenge for an adult with autism as related to experiences surrounding the process of obtaining and maintaining meaningful employment (Figure 7.3).

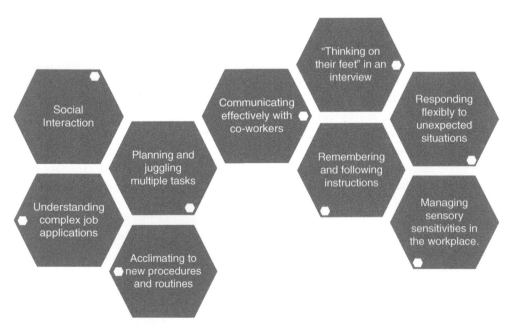

FIGURE 7.3   Areas of difference and challenges for an adult with autism. Source: Wiley and Gentry (2016) and Baldwin et al. (2014).

A NOTE ON ADULTS WITH AUTISM IN COLLEGE SETTINGS

Aligned with attaining meaningful employment, adults with autism may seek out higher education in pursuit of their unique vocational interests. In 2017, the US Department of Education and National Center for Educational Statistics reported that only 40% of individuals with autism graduate from post-secondary institutions compared with 60% of their neurotypical peers (Newman et al. 2011). University students with autism report a number of difficulties and little access to campus supports, suggesting a dire need for more effective transition support and curriculum designed to support neurodiverse strengths (Anderson et al. 2018). Evidence suggests that higher-education students with autism report high satisfaction with supports despite poor utilization, indicating potential needs in areas such as self-advocacy and awareness of support availability (Anderson et al. 2020). Peer mentoring at universities for students with ASD may be warranted if they include social, emotional, and psychological support to impact university success (Thompson et al. 2019). Evidence supports programs specific to students with autism that include training for social interaction and independent living as well as self-advocacy, emotional regulation, and adaptive skills (Elias and White 2018).

Some have suggested specific transition courses offered by high schools and universities to help students with autism accurately identify their strengths and weakness, so they can select an appropriate school and major suited to their skills and interests (Anderson et al. 2020). Remember that this transition time is a major life change for all students, and especially for students with ASD, who might be accustomed to more parental involvement.

Some universities may offer specific programs to support students with autism. Preliminary research on supporting the transition of students with autism from high school to college supports the development of programs with clearly documented, manualized procedures as well as sufficient flexibility to account for students' unique needs (White et al. 2017). For example, California State University Long Beach offers "Autism Ally," a program to teach both awareness to university stakeholders committed to helping students with ASD feel supported and welcomed, while educating about the strengths and limitations students with autism can experience in post-secondary education. Such programs can benefit college students with autism by training their faculty and peers to better recognize and support their needs. For college faculty, this may include pedagogical adjustments such as assigning students to groups rather than having them self-select, which can reduce the social demand on students with autism.

Research also suggests that individuals with autism have difficulties with adaptive behavior skills, which includes daily living, self-care, and functional communication. These skills are important and necessary for employment, independence, and quality of life (Volkmar, 2018; Meyer et al. 2018). To better understand daily living skills and the experience of individuals with autism, research has focused on understanding daily living skill development as an individual ages.

In 2015, Husp Bal et al. conducted a longitudinal study to assess the predictors and trajectories of daily living skills of individuals with ASD from childhood through adulthood. Their study revealed significant below age level expectations across the developmental period. In Smith et al. 2012, a study was conducted comparing individuals with ASD with those who have Down syndrome. They concluded that the daily living skills of those with ASD continued to improve during adolescence and then plateaued during their 20s. Individuals with Down syndrome continued to show growth in their daily living with no plateaus.

While these studies suggest an "atypical developmental trajectory of adaptive behavior in adolescents with ASD" (Meyer et al. 2018), future longitudinal studies are encouraged to provide a more comprehensive assessment of the developmental trajectories observed past the transition to adulthood. The authors further assert that interventions that focus on adaptive behaviors are needed to promote independent living and functional communication skills in adulthood. This area of study is particularly significant to ensure that as interventionists, we are addressing adulthood services in a comprehensive manner.

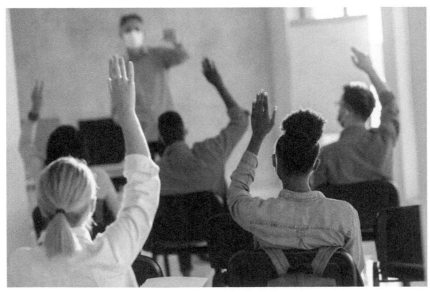

Drazen/Adobe Stock

Therapy Golden Nugget

With your adult client with autism, you can target video modeling to address adaptive behavior and living skills. Use the following activity.
Step 1: Objectives:

- Students will create video self-modeling of an adaptive skill or daily living skill they enjoy (see Chapter 6).
- Peers will watch and evaluate areas of strength and need.
- Students will ultimately create their own tangible objective related to showing improvements or advancing past the point shown on the video of themselves.

Step 2: Priming matters:
Share the below definition from Webster's Dictionary. Allow students to discuss the idea of "leaving the nest" and preparing for independence. Use the following independence rating scale for students to engage in self-reflection of their own levels of independence (adapted from Wiley and Gentry 2016).

> in-de-pen-dent, *noun*
> Not dependent; not depending or contingent upon something else for existence, operation, etc.

Step 3: Therapy sequence:

- *Explain to students* that as we move toward being independent, this also includes caring for yourself.
- *Pose the questions*, "What are ways that we can exist by ourselves?" "What do you do by yourself that you are good at or want to get better with?"
- *Empower active thinking:* Students will brainstorm together different strengths they have with daily living skills.
- *Give instructions:* Students will each make their own video showing a skill that they can do or would like to do at home that will help them to be independent in the future. Videos should be no more than five minutes in length.
- *Debrief:* Use videos to highlight each client's individual skill sets. Encourage clients to point out strengths and areas of weakness. Clients will ultimately develop their own personal goal related to this skill. Goals may focus on improving current skill or moving on to the "next" natural step. While the activity will end, remember that the goals should be brought back up and checked on often.

HOW "CHARGED" UP ARE YOUR INDEPENDENCE SKILLS?

Directions: Take time to think about your personal levels of independence in each area. Reflect on how much charge you have currently in the area? Remember, it is OK not to be 100% in each area.

Independence area	How charged are YOU?	Describe
I take public transportation or drive, alone.		
I oversee my own personal grooming.		
I can organize and go out by myself in the community.		
I wake up on my own.		
I pick out my own clothes.		
I do my own laundry.		
I can cook my own meals.		
I have my own bank account that I can access.		
I do specific chores at home by myself.		
I do my own homework assignments.		
I ask people when I want to go on dates with friends or people of interest.		
I know how to use my cell phone to call my family and friends.		
I make my own budget.		

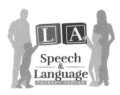

MY JOURNEY WITH AUTISM

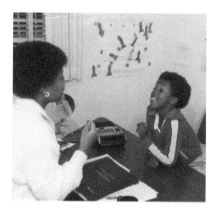

Dr. Wiley, young interventionist working with her first private practice client, c. 1977.

As a professional with more than four decades of experience, I too was challenged personally to identify what I deemed to be meaningful employment options for my young adults with ASD. Many of them, primarily males, had participated in my early intervention program, social skills, summer speech and drama camps, and individual speech–language therapy. They had blossomed under our care. My staff and I watched them develop from nonverbal or minimally verbal, fearful, and sometimes aggressive children to now becoming confident teens and young adults who could articulate their feelings, dreams, and hopes for their futures. But the reality for their futures was bleak with limited options available for meaningful employment!

There was an abundance of lower cognitive level jobs, typically made available for the masses of individuals with disabilities, but little that I felt challenged most of "my" students who had transcended the label of "autism." Despite the bleak outlook, I was determined to create a future for them that was consistent with their unique interests and skill sets.

In the summer of 2013, I reluctantly proposed to parents that because their teen-aged children had done so well, I thought it was time for them to matriculate in activities and programs with their neurotypical peers such as a "typical" summer camp program. Parents were mortified and asked if there was anything else I could do for or with them.

Not wanting to "banish" them from my center, I decided to invite a few of them to assist in our "Say N' Play" Summer speech camp as "speech buddies." Speech buddies were exceptional high-school volunteers who served as typical peer models for our adolescents and teens and as big brothers and sisters for our younger children. Needless to say, my parents were relieved and students were beyond excited to no longer be the "student in need," but serving in the same capacity as their neurotypical peers. We witnessed their self-esteem soar. They were more mature and walked with a greater level of confidence.

Client Profile 1

However, despite the growth, I also observed other areas of concern. For example, one young man was standing outside of his assigned classroom staring intently at the clock on the wall. When asked why he was standing outside he replied, "Ms. Nadhiya told me to wait until 12:00 for my lunch break."

Thus, his translation was literal, and he was patiently standing outside to observe the clock and wait until 12 noon.

Client Profile 2

Another young man overheard a parent speaking in a stern manner with his child and approached and reprimanded him for being so harsh with his son. The parent was taken aback and reported it to the speech–language pathologist, who followed up and asked our student why he would engage with the parent in such a manner. He responded, "I used to be that little boy. I was only trying to help. The dad is not helping his son!" While I was proud he showed **self-advocacy** and concern for others like him, it was not appropriate.

Client Profile 3

My third young man observed a group of female "speech buddies" exchanging cell numbers. He approached one of the girls and asked for her telephone number. Not wanting to be rude, she reluctantly gave it to him. The next day she came in crying and fearful and ready to quit. To use her words, "he blew my phone up and called me all night long." I calmed her down and then set off to find my guy. When I shared her comments with him, his eyes filled with tears and he said, "I only wanted to be her friend. She was pretty and nice to me."

Current literature shows that loneliness predicts depressive symptoms and thoughts of self-harm in adults with ASD, suggesting that there are mental health benefits of programs like community inclusion and social skills interventions (Han et al. 2019; Hedley et al. 2018). Among autistic individuals, online gaming, in moderation, has been found to decrease feelings of loneliness and offer opportunities for meeting more friends, but the activity does not typically indicate strong friendship quality (Sundberg 2018). Among adults with autism in their 20s and 30s, research indicates that those with more ASD symptomology and sensory aversion often report more anxiety and loneliness, suggesting that increasing sensory processing skills may help to mitigate such negative feelings (Syu and Lin 2018). In theory, we know that anxiety and experiencing loneliness may be a common experience of adults with autism, but in practice it may look like any of the clinical examples described above.

Active Learning Task

Take time with a partner. Match the student descriptions provided in Client Profiles 1–3 with the common social challenges outlined in Chapter 3. What similarities do you see? How do you think this may look different for an adult with autism?

As professionals, we know that missing social cues is pervasive across the lifespan. Regardless, innocent behaviors such as those witnessed in the clinical examples described above could be misinterpreted in a workplace setting with neurotypical individuals. Despite our belief that our students were good to go, we saw firsthand new areas in need of our support.

Therapy Golden Nugget

My advice to newly minted interventionists as yourself is to continue to push yourself to find areas of need in therapy. Your goal is to provide your client with the greatest foundation possible.

Thus, in 2014, I developed a targeted social skills program that essentially focused on the social skills needed to navigate effectively in the workplace. I selected eight students to be a part of my pilot program and worked with them free of charge for almost three years. After all, they had defied all of the "nos" and "nevers" often told to parents. My staff and I were determined to prepare them for the future and next phase of their lives. We needed everyone's buy-in, most importantly, their parents.

THE PROCESS OF STRENGTHENING: PARENT PERSPECTIVES

The continued strength and wellbeing of a child can be maximized with the support of the family. Often, we hear professionals say, "I can't get mom involved or the family is missing in action." *The success of the majority of "my" students is due in large part to the "true" partnership we have created with our families.*

Intervention consisting of family-centered training, individualized planning, and assistance with career exploration positively impacts self-determination ability and vocational decision making skills for young adults with ASD and their families (Hagner et al. 2012). A *"true" partnership* in my opinion, values and encourages parent input even if it defies our beliefs. It requires us to identify something positive to share about even the most challenging child. It also requires us to see the glass as half full rather than half empty, which means that we must see potential in each child. It also accepts "differences" without judgment. It requires us as professionals to genuinely humble and challenge ourselves to solicit and value parent input regardless of race or socioeconomic status. This last statement is often hard to accept. But the reality is that how we view and interact with others can be based on our perceptions of the individual or their group.

As I was planning for this next phase for our students, I believed it was wise to solicit the input and perspectives of parents whose children were already 21 years and older. I went in with their future and preparing for that in my mind (Volkmar, 2017). I also began with these three questions:

- What are your challenges?
- What are your hopes?
- What are your dreams?

I wanted to plan to ensure my students' continued growth and success consistent with the desires and support of the family unit.

Centered on Transition

Research clearly outlines the stress and unmet needs of families with ASD during the transition period from high school into young adulthood (Daughrity et al. 2021; Cheak-Zamora et al. 2015; First et al. 2016). In 2015, my colleague, Dr. Betholyn Gentry and I created a researcher-developed questionnaire: Transition or Departure: Parent Perspectives on ASD After age 21 (Wiley and Gentry 2015). Results were presented at the American Speech–Language Hearing Association, 2015 Annual Convention. Parents were emailed a link to respond to 20 questions related to their young adult in several areas, which included their age and types of educational services received, internships and employment experiences, personal goals for their young adult, social or behavioral challenges that might interfere with employment, parent access to information on services after age 21 and the types of post-secondary services needed or desired.

This small preliminary study revealed that 40% of the young adults had never been employed and 20% were seeking employment; 100% of the young adults had received speech–language therapy, 60% social skills, and 40% behavior management. Prior to age 21, behavior and speech–language were viewed as beneficial; 10% rated their social skills above average and 50% rated their young adults' social skills as poor.

Social challenges cited most frequently by the parents that could potentially interfere with employment were consistent. While these findings are in the process of being analyzed and more widely disseminated to increase sample size, there were three key areas observed initially to be mentioned by parents, illustrated in Figure 7.4; 100% of our parents responding agreed to the need for workplace social skills services, and 100% wanted guidance or assistance in helping to identify opportunities for their young adults.

The clinical implications indicate that 90% or a majority of those surveyed regardless of their child's level of functioning desired employment for them. Some could envision their young adults working independently while others saw employment with the support of a job coach. The most advantageous time to provide support services to our

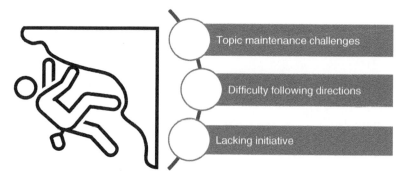

FIGURE 7.4   Three key areas of social challenge.

students is before they graduate from high school (Murray and Doren 2013; Test et al. 2014; Fong et al., 2013).

This small sample size provided us with clear goals and directives for the clients we serve in my centers. Our goal was to cultivate the skills necessary to fully prepare these young people to secure and maintain meaningful employment.

ADULTS AND CULTURAL CONSIDERATIONS

In the implementation of any functional adult social skills program, it is critical for the clinician to be familiar with individual and cultural group norms and values while allowing for intragroup differences. Consideration must also be given to sexual orientation and gender biases, as well as the unique culture of today's teens and young adults, which include the continuing influence of social media.

Cultural beliefs influence how autism is viewed and responded to by parents (Millau et al. 2018; Bernier et al. 2010). It also influences a parent's life's visions for their child as well as outcomes relative to their independence. To provide more effective services to multilingual and multicultural clients, we need to become more knowledgeable about their culture. Our awareness and acceptance are paramount to the success of social skills training that needs to be consistent with their individual and group social settings and norms.

Early in our program we ask our students to describe their culture; that is, their beliefs, preferences, customs/rituals, religion, and thoughts on "their" autism. As we are aware, something so basic as eye contact can vary among cultural groups. As clinicians, it is impossible to fully know and understand every client's culture. Therefore, it is important that we ask our clients and their families to seek out information from respected sources.

AUTISM IS A LABEL: IT DOES NOT DEFINE YOUR POTENTIAL

In 2018, we took our pilot employment readiness training program and opened it fully to the public. To date, we have served hundreds of adults with autism. Our success has been in part due to intensely addressing the critical social skills, identifying our students' unique interests and providing them with meaningful employment. Our program focuses on pivotal areas deemed appropriate and important for independence:

- vocational training
- social skills
- daily living skills
- personal development.

These are the first areas introduced to our adult students and what I personally consider to be the foundation on which the other skills are built. Students meet 16 hours/month.

The training provided includes many of the techniques that we have used throughout the years. The only difference is that it is focused on the social skills needed to navigate effectively in the workplace. We know that social skills are basic to all interactions and should be integral to any workplace training program (Kellems and Morningstar 2012). We continue to use video modeling, video self-modeling, role playing, socialization stories as well as computer research and community-based outings to facilitate carryover in the natural environment (Allen et al. 2010).

We also routinely include invited guest lecturers to discuss current events such as those illustrated in Figure 7.5. Conversation is had on topics ranging from civil unrest, current elections, the homeless or "unhoused" individuals in our communities, and COVID-19, and how to stay safe. Current events are important because such discussions allow us to observe their communication styles, which informs us of any unmet needs to be addressed, but more importantly, gives them the opportunity to engage in conversation.

GOAL SPOTLIGHT

Students will demonstrate appropriate conversation exchanges that occur in the workplace and in the community at large.

Additionally, we create social dilemmas and encourage them to role play with partners to resolve issues. Some of the dilemmas are situations shared or experienced by our students. The appropriate and safe usage of social media is also addressed

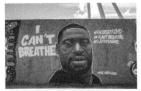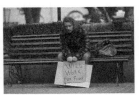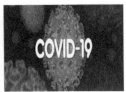

ZUMA Press/Alamy Stock Photo   prostooleh/Adobe Stock

FIGURE 7.5   Current events discussed: (left to right) George Floyd, homelessness, elections, the COVID-19 pandemic.

because it is an important part of today's culture. Adults with autism who use social media for engagement report more close friendships, despite offline engagement being a more accurate predictor of friendship quality and quantity (Mazurek 2013). Interestingly, adults with autism who engaged in social media in moderation reported higher levels of happiness than those who did not, suggesting that social media may have a positive impact and may serve as a protective factor against common mental health issues such as depression (Ward et al. 2018).

A common behavior observed in many individuals with ASD is their inability to continue conversations after the initial greeting, while others may dominate the discussion with their personal interests and obsessions. In response to this behavior, we host weekly chat rooms where students are placed in groups to discuss specific topics and propose solutions; specific rules, expectations, and boundaries are reviewed weekly as a condition of participation. Each group has a team leader whose role is to solicit the input of each group member, take notes, encourage balanced conversation, and finally report back to the group. This facilitates and strengthens their oral presentation skills, topic maintenance, listening, and leadership. We have observed significant improvement in their confidence and ability to speak fluently in group settings.

One young man who is gifted and terrified of speaking publicly shared the following: "When I'm asked to speak in class it feels like my brain encounters a wall with no way to resolve the situation." His solution to the problem has been to politely decline most social invitations and inconsistent attendance in our classes. His participation in our group was 25% and has now increased to 75% monthly attendance. Creating discussions and safe situations to address these types of social anxiety issues is important. The students in a group setting realize that they are not alone and will often gain strength from their adult peers with ASD.

THE IMPORTANCE OF ENVIRONMENT

Our headquarters is 16,500 sq. ft., which allows us the opportunity to provide designated areas specifically for our young adults. Our students have full access to a state-of-the-art "HollyRod Homework Helpers" computer lab, "RJ's Place," an area for relaxation, which includes a large-screen TV, a snack bar, an old-fashioned popcorn maker and cart, massage chair, and a ping pong/pool table. Many students arrive early to relax and engage with each other before our class begins. While staff are not physically engaged, we use this time to observe who gravitates to whom, as well as the quality of the conversations and interactions. We also observe the social loner who often prefers to observe others and sits quietly alone. In time, even this type of individual will connect with another peer, often because of a shared interest.

Our center also has the distinction of having three unique on-site authentic and functioning internship training centers: UPS Store, Outback Steakhouse and CVS Pharmacy training center (Figure 7.6). These training centers were sponsored by the individual corporations.

Upon completion of our classroom training program, students participate in a six-week paid internship opportunity and are supervised by our staff of

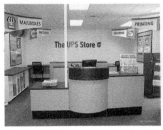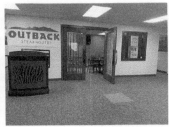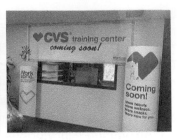

FIGURE 7.6   Employment Readiness Training Labratories, Los Angeles Speech and Language Therapy Center.

speech–language pathologists and program assistants, all of whom have worked closely with these students since the beginning of program training. Internships have been a proven key to successful employment outcomes for individuals with disabilities (Schall et al. 2020; Volkmar, 2018). Key components of a successful internship program in our center are as follows:

- Interns receive weekly feedback as well as a formal written evaluation identifying areas of strength and those in need.
- Interns are required to evaluate their experiences and performance at various intervals of the program.
- Self-identified challenges often become their personal targets and goals.
- Feedback informs any modifications needed to the training.

For example, several of our interns complained of fatigue. Although we gave them breaks consistent with California law, we failed to consider that work is "tiring" and requires constant focus, and that our students, most of whom had never worked or interned, may need more frequent breaks. As a result, we have changed our format to include breaks upon request, which allows them the opportunity to relax in whatever manner they desire.

Shifting Mindset from Job to Meaningful Employment

To date, we have successfully placed our students in various internship settings such as the public library for a young man who said "I don't like people but I love books. I am willing to do anything to be around books."

Another young man who is very engaging and rather "cool" was interested in social media and advertising. We assisted him in securing an internship and subsequent employment for a small medical clinic. They credit him with increasing their followers and business leads.

A young woman who started with us at an early age had always wanted to become a doctor. She has moderate receptive and expressive language delays but has always given us her best. We sought meaningful employment and with a little extra effort and creative thinking, we were able to place her at a medical clinic that specializes in treating individuals with developmental disabilities. She is an office assistant and is responsible for maintaining the environment, assisting in the preparation of patient files, and providing the nurses with specific tools needed. She was ecstatic, as were her parents!

Other students have been placed in more traditional settings such as CVS, Outback Steakhouse, and various corporate settings in a range of jobs. We also personally employ two students, who have taken community college classes and have expressed an interest in childcare. They are additional classroom assistants in our early intervention and typical preschool programs. *We practice what we preach and we lead by example.*

Despite the data and relatively bleak outlook, jobs are available, and employers want to get involved. As professionals who have invested time and effort into this population, I encourage us to use some creativity to help parlay our students' interests into internship opportunities and meaningful employment.

> Admittedly, it requires extra effort but the reward outweighs the effort expended.

Active Learning Task

Approach two different business in your community. Ask if they employ any individuals with disabilities like autism spectrum disorder. If they don't, ask if you can share information with them about the different abilities of autistic individuals to help increase their awareness. Often, the first step to creating more vocational opportunities for adults with autism is to increase community awareness to increase potential future possibilities and vocational opportunities.

Evidence-Based Approaches

While this information has been developed specific to the needs of the clients we serve, there are some evidence-based approaches, such as **Project SEARCH + ASD Supports (PS+ASD)** (Schall et al. 2020), which have been frequently cited in the primitive but growing body of literature surrounding working with adults with autism.

While authors mention the need for more specific data, and approaches found to be successful with this population (Volkmar, 2017; Schall et al. 2020) to be included in the growing body of literature, approaches such as PS + ASD offer interventionists a solid framework. This method was initially Project SEARCH, founded in 1996 at the Cincinnati Children's Hospital Medical Center. Project SEARCH has been proven to be effective in finding employment for individuals with disabilities. PS + ASD, a more recent program, has a specific emphasis for work with individuals with autism. Key components for success are shown in Table 7.1.

TABLE 7.1   Key components for success of the PS+ASD supports.

Component	Description
Instructional strategies	Evidenced-based teaching strategies are used to teach student key skills in the areas such as vocational, social, and communication skills. Common method used is ABA.
Internships	Over 700 hours of an on-site internship experience. Experience is centered around clients specific strength, preferences, and areas of need.
Vocational assessment practices	Continuing on-site assessment of skills and needs.
Resumé/work history	Students leave program with a completed resumé and key skills needed to increase employment odds.
Seamless transition to adult services	Supports, like key social services, are installed and implemented long before a student graduates from the program.
Meeting business needs	These positions are open positions within the organization that is currently not being filled by others.

Source: Adapted from Schall et al. (2020).

CORE TREATMENT AREAS

Personal skills development establishes the foundation for our program and has proven to provide the level of confidence and drive needed to persevere despite the odds that may be against us. An understanding and acceptance of "autism the label" is important for self-acceptance and ultimately future outcomes.

Through the years, we have observed many students and some parents shut down as we embark on "the ASD talk." In years past, we have observed that, sometimes, our clients have associated autism with:

- feelings of inadequacy
- being different and undesirable
- most importantly, feelings of being "special" in a negative way.

Parents have also harbored feelings of blame, failure, or misgivings about what they should or could have done differently, while others feel defeated from the outset. We also encounter parents who refuse to accept the diagnosis and discourage their children from accepting it as well.

One young man who joined us later in life was told by his mother that if a young woman became aware of his autism, she would not want him. While he wanted to learn about ASD, from a cultural perspective he was torn because he also wanted a relationship.

Parent education is important.

These parent concerns are typically discussed in a group setting during our **parent–professional partnership** sessions. Often, parents may reveal significant concerns about the transition into young adulthood (Daughrity et al. 2021). This model, developed specifically for various points of parenting a child with autism across the lifespan, is further discussed in Chapter 12. The vast majority of parents find this time to be helpful, transformative, and a safe space to be very helpful. With parents on board and in alignment with our goals, their young adults are more receptive to our subject matter and program design.

We approach the subject of autism with some caution, beginning with a discussion on autism in general, contrasted with autism myths, such as everybody has a little autism in them, or people with autism can never achieve in life. We follow-up by researching "autism notables." Students are amazed and feel empowered by the notables and to realize that others with their same profile have overcome this label. This therapy task is illustrated below.

Therapy Golden Nugget

STEP 1 Objectives:

- Students will identify positive traits in themselves.
- Students will describe autism on a personal level.
- Students will demonstrate an awareness of autism through the perspective of another person.

STEP 2 Therapy sequence:

- Explain to students. We are all unique and we have our strengths and weaknesses.
- Pose the question. What are some positive traits you see in yourselves? What are your interests? What are some of your accomplishments?
- Empower active thinking. Students will work as partners and discuss their strengths and accomplishments.
- Give instructions. Students will work as partners and become experts on an "autism notable." Some autism notable examples include Temple Grandin, Albert Einstein, Bill Gates, Anthony Hopkins, Tim Burton, Charles Darwin, Bobby Fischer, Satoshi Tajiri, Elon Musk. Each pair of students will have 20 minutes to research and complete the autism notables worksheet. Each pair of students will present to the whole class.
- Debrief.

STEP 3 Therapy activity
Directions: Print out pictures with names of various "autism notables" students may be familiar with. Divide students to work as partners and have each pair choose one autism notable picture. Students will research their autism notable and complete the worksheet below. Each pair will present their findings to the whole group.

Autism Notable

_____ is best known for ....

_____

_____

_____

Background	Important Events
Hometown: _____	1. _____
Family: _____	_____
_____	2. _____
Interests:_____	_____
_____	
_____	3. _____
	_____

I can relate to this person because.......

_____

_____

Lastly, we discuss everyone's "personal" autism and how it manifests itself in their lives. Understanding your personal autism is key to self-advocacy, self-determination, self-acceptance, increased self-esteem and social emotional development. An individual's personal development affects one's employability.

During this unit, students are administered the Sorenson self-esteem test, which provides a glimpse into how an individual sees himself and provides us an understanding of their collective fears and concerns regardless of level of functioning. Many of our students indicated feeling anxious in new social settings, not knowing who to trust and when to trust, fearful of making public mistakes, and lying to avoid criticism or rejection when telling the truth. Students use the results to develop their personal targets. This test is given annually to determine any changes in their self-esteem. Most of our students continue to demonstrate increased self-esteem.

In this unit, we also explore the mind, body, soul connection, which makes each student accountable for their individual happiness. Students are challenged to identify tools for happiness and to demonstrate an understanding of the importance of exercise and maintaining their mental health. Compared with their neurotypical peers, adults with ASD are less likely to meet standards for healthy behaviors like adequate exercise, diet, and sleep, increasing risk for poorer cardiovascular health (Weir et al. 2021). Each session begins with yoga and positive affirmations, which even the most resistant student today will participate in and enjoys.

Active Learning Task

Given the following objectives, create a fun and engaging activity and lesson plan for your group of 12 students between 18 and 22 years.
Objectives:

1. Students will identify positive traits in themselves.
2. Students will identify tools to relieve stress in their lives.
3. Students will explain the importance of good hygiene and positive social interaction.

Vocational readiness involves matching jobs to students based on their interests and skills. Most students with autism, unlike their neurotypical peers and many students with special needs, rarely engage or participate in internship opportunities during high school.

Internship opportunities provide students a chance to experience different types of employment without the risks of failure. Many young people, now prominent and practicing professionals, including the authors of this book, began as volunteers in my summer speech camp. As a result of the positive experience with this population, they have joined the ranks of our profession and are now licensed and practicing speech–language pathologists. The reality is that opportunities provided earlier in life oftentimes influence our career paths.

We begin this unit by administering the **RIASEC test.** This test was founded by John Holland in the 1950s and is also referred to as John Holland's Six Occupational Types of Personality. The RIASEC test identifies career interests based on 42 questions rated by how much you enjoy them on a scale of 1 to 5. It identifies six areas of primary occupational categories. Table 7.2 highlights the category and potential translation to career.

TABLE 7.2   Primary occupational categories, RIASEC test.

Scoring area	Career examples
Realistic	• Mechanical engineer • Health assistant
Investigative	• Chemist • Psychologist
Artistic	• Cosmetologist • Photographer
Social	• Teaching assistant • Public relations
Enterprising	• Retail store worker • Banker
Conventional	• Data analyst • Warehouse worker

A comprehensive list of additional occupations is taken from the **Department of Labor's O*NET database** and provides information of possible career choices as well as related pathways. This test serves as a good indicator and possible starting point as we identify internships and career possibilities. If students concur with the findings, they are required to conduct research using the database to gather information on possible salaries, different types of jobs, the availability of the jobs, and the education requirements. Students have found this to be very beneficial and, for us, it provides a glimpse into potential opportunities for our students, as well as the type of workplace culture that is consistent with our students' core values, beliefs, and tolerance levels.

Once we have identified possible job options, we begin to focus heavily on the *social skills needed to function in the workplace*. Inappropriate social interaction can ultimately positively or negatively impact employment outcomes. Regardless of how we would like to perceive the world as being all inclusive and kind, the reality is that people who present with status quo acceptable behaviors will be viewed more favorably in the workplace. Without these socially acceptable behaviors, individuals will run the risk of being isolated and excluded from the social aspects of work which is where relationships and connections are often made. Acceptance and respect in the workplace from co-workers, managers, and the boss are important on many levels.

Heavy emphasis is placed on the importance of making a good first impression. Often individuals with ASD exhibit what is called "social blindness," which means that they are sometimes unable to see themselves or the perspectives of others, so a "good first impression" may not initially be significant to them. Face-to-face interviews and now virtual interviews may be problematic as well. It is important for them to learn and appreciate the perspective of their peers and others. We have found video and video self-modeling to be very helpful as we contrast appropriate with inappropriate behavior.

Therapy Golden Nugget

To further assess their understanding of "first impressions," we introduce them to unfamiliar faces, both male and female, of different ages, race, personalities, and professional backgrounds, including human resources to serve as job interviewers. All students are engaged in the process as they observe and evaluate their personal behavior, as well as that of their peers. Each participant receives written and verbal feedback. Our interviews are also recorded to provide concrete visual feedback to each participant. Once again, students are challenged to identify personal goals.

How would you create tasks for mock interviews for your adult autistic clients? What skills and objectives would you target?

Executive functioning is another area addressed throughout our training. As professionals, we know that poor executive functioning impacts every facet of a person's life. We also know that many of our students with autism will have executive functioning deficits. This is supported by research that suggests the gap between students with ASD and their typical peers widens during the teen years (Rosenthal et al. 2013). Therefore, activities designed to challenge their reasoning, adaptability, focus, problem solving, and ability to pivot in response to unforeseen situations is important.

We also have fun learning about figurative language or idioms. It is estimated that the English language has at least 25 000 idiomatic expressions. Certain idioms are specific to certain groups or individuals. We identified 50 common workplace phrases and created a timed idioms test. Our students found it to be fun and challenging but for us it was an opportunity to identify additional areas to be addressed. Our program has specific group goals but also individualizes our goals based on each student's unique profile of strengths and areas in need of attention. As flexible and prepared as we are, we also can be blindsided!

A case in point was a situation that we experienced with a highly intelligent young man who received a degree in sociology from a top university. He was very frustrated because his classmates had received job offers and ultimately were gainfully employed. He was a nice young man but also had potential to ask intrusive questions. This had been identified as a personal goal for him and after a year in the program we were able to secure part-time employment at a major corporation. The corporate staff were trained and briefed on their new hire and were excited to receive him.

During his initial orientation, his immediate boss told him "loosely" to be sure and get to know his co-workers. I tried "tactfully" to let the boss know that our young man was very inquisitive and loved to talk. Therefore, I suggested that he become acquainted with his co-workers during breaks and the lunch hour. The boss said "Dr. Wiley, it's OK, we've got a close-knit unit. He'll be fine. We'll take care of your young man." I said "OK" but . . . in my heart of hearts I knew better. I told them that I would return in three weeks to follow up on my student.

In less than two weeks, I received a frantic call from the boss who said, "We need your help. My staff are going crazy because 'John' walks around all day long disturbing staff by asking them personal random questions. Despite the subtle hints that my staff give to him, he doesn't get it."

This situation required us to take a more proactive on-boarding process as we prepared our partners to work with our students. We also wrote a socialization story "Getting to Know my Co-workers," which included first asking, "Is this is a good time to talk?" The story included appropriate conversation and the appropriate action to be taken in response to their responses to him. We also prepared a daily schedule which included designated "times to get to know my co-workers," such as breaks, lunch time, and at the end of his workday, unless his co-workers were busy. The problem was ultimately embraced by all and resolved.

GOAL SPOTLIGHT

Partner with a peer to develop a creative lesson plan to achieve these objectives using a multimedia and sensory approach.
Objectives:

1. Participants will demonstrate an understanding of pre-interview readiness.
2. Participants will plan for the unexpected.
3. Participants will practice interviewing.
4. Participants will identify and decode workplace idioms.
5. Participants will become familiar with common workplace conversation starters.

Daily living skills are important to address as we prepare our adults for their independence. In our intake process, we have observed that many of our parents assume responsibility for just about all facets of their young adults lives, from managing their finances to shopping for their every need, including personal items. We also know that this group of young people are connected to the world through social media, which means that they have a broader world view of life. Many will want to leave home to experience life, consistent with their neurotypical peers. As professionals, we can also play a role to ensure their independence by creating opportunities through discussions and hands-on activities to increase their ability to live and function independently to whatever extent they envision and desire.

It is essential that we assist those students who demonstrate an ability or interest in living independently to develop an independence plan for life after high school. Students can be involved in rating their independence relative to basic household, financial, and community awareness, which increases their chances of living independently from their parents, as well as ensuring their safety in the community in general. This process should also enlist the support from the parents or caregivers. A component of daily living unit is safety awareness: general safety, such as when to call 911, and household hazards, safety in personal relationships, safety with law enforcement, and safety with social media. We are particularly concerned with safety in relationships and with law enforcement.

Adults with autism are at increased risk for sexual victimization than their peers without autism (Brown-Lavoie et al. 2014; Gibbs et al. 2021). Safety in relationships is important because it is reported that women with developmental disabilities have the highest incidence of physical, sexual, and emotional violence of all abused females (Wiley and Gentry 2016). Findings indicate that autistic females, regardless of sexual orientation, are more likely to have experienced unwanted sexual encounters (Pecora et al. 2020). Young women with autism might specifically benefit from personal safety training about positive adult relationships as their reports of difficulty with social inferences may increase their risk for sexual vulnerability (Sedgewick et al. 2019).

We approach this topic unit by identifying "red flag" situations. It is important for our students to know the difference between healthy and unhealthy relationships. Both people with autism and neurotypical adults perceive relationship intimacy similarly, but adults with autism experience more challenges with emotional and physical intimacy, suggesting interventions to support romantic intimacy are warranted (Sala et al. 2020). Since my students are feeling more confident, a few have developed same-sex, opposite-sex, and "polyamorous" relationships. Consistent with life, some are good, and others are not so good. Parents have called to solicit our support. We have recently begun to provide weekend-long single-sex retreats for our young adults. The groups are led by young adults, who can relate to their fears, concerns, and desires. Parents are relieved because many are uncomfortable having "the talk."

Also in recent years, we have seen an increasing number of students who are expressing an interest in driving. As a result, many of our young adults are engaged in their community and drive. While research indicates most teens with ASD in typical education settings have plans to drive, few have individual education plan goals specific to driving, indicating a potential area for interventionists working with this population to target in light of holistic needs in support of pending independence in young adulthood (Huang et al. 2012). According to a report issued by the Ruderman Family Foundation (Kaplan-Mayer 2016), one third to one half of all individuals killed by law enforcement have disabilities or mental health conditions. Another study conducted showed that Black and Latino people are more than 50% likely to experience some form of force in interactions with police. While there are no clear data specific to ASD, given the complexity and range of this population, we can surmise that they may be even more impacted (Fryer 2019).

In response to this, in 2016, we started a new program, Spectrum Shield, a weekend-long safety with law enforcement training program. Our students literally go to bed and wake up with police who volunteer their time to train our students. Goals of the program are to incorporate direct instruction and roleplay tasks to teach young adults with autism how to navigate encounters with law enforcement during traffic stops. Additionally, goals include training law enforcement officers on how to interact with individuals with autism by recognizing communication differences with the goal of increasing safe encounters.

A very positive but unexpected outcome was shared by 100% of police officers who all provide the same feedback, "They have had prior autism training but working with our students has made them more aware and committed to providing safer outcomes. Our students have been pulled over, and per parent reports, have calmly interacted with the police, followed our training and walked away with a handshake and a warning."

Our Collective Rewards

Today, after all our collective efforts and the hard work and dedication of our students, we have been successful in finding meaningful employment for them in various settings, which include the restaurant industry, convenience stores, health care, sports industry, corporate America, nonprofits, and soon the carpentry trade industry. Our young adults have a sense of independence and purpose.

Our targeted and comprehensive approach provides great rewards, to not only our students but also to corporate America, and society in general. Our young adults gain a sense of independence and purpose while also learning to become self-sufficient. Employment also provides them opportunities for increased socialization. I share with them that they are ambassadors, and their efforts will open doors for the children with ASD following behind them.

Our corporate leaders have become our partners and cheerleaders who believe in our mission; to help young adults with autism secure "meaningful employment consistent with their unique interests and skill sets." This phrase continues to be repeated throughout my chapter because I strongly believe that "meaningful" employment provides the same value and benefits to our young adults, the same as it does for each of us.

Corporations benefit by demonstrating tangible evidence of corporate responsibility to diversity and inclusion. Research shows that companies with greater diversity reap greater financial rewards. Staff become more sensitive and compassionate. We have had several chief executives independently thank me and say how our young adults have changed the culture of their company.

Lastly, society at large benefits because as our young adults gain employment and engage fully in our communities; they become contributors to our economy and society. Their presence will break down barriers of discrimination as they gain greater acceptance and inclusion in our communities.

As we continue our journey with these young adults, we will continue to be proactive in the continuum of services we provide, and our dedicated goal to help our students cross the finish line. Their growth and positive responses to life in general and the services that we provide, confirm my belief that autism is a label; it does not define their potential. As speech–language pathologists, we play a significant role in making a difference in the lives of these individuals.

As a newly minted interventionist yourself, I leave you with advice and real stories from real adults who are living and thriving as an individual on the spectrum. My sincere hope is that this will fuel you as you move forward into a path of supporting and treating individuals with autism.

Use your research to guide your thinking, but do not let it limit what you do. Follow the lead of the client and listen to what parents want and you will continue to make a difference in the lives of the people you serve.

–Dr. Pamela Wiley

SUMMARY

With available interventions and supports, many young children diagnosed with autism will become highly verbal young adults with a variety of support needs as they transition into young adulthood and prepare for higher education, employment, relationships, and independence. Interventionists working with adults with autism can support needs in adaptive behavior skills and social skills needed to thrive in vocational settings. Objectives should focus on meaningful employment to help adults with autism lead fulfilling lives with jobs matched to both passion and skill set. Interventions targeting use of social media and personal safety should be considered to support safe and fulfilling engagement in common social environments like social networking sites and intimate relationships. Planning for transition to adulthood with input from both adults with autism and their families, while also engaging community stakeholders such as business leaders and law enforcement, can help to mitigate challenges, while setting clients on a path for success.

REFLECTIONS: FIRSTHAND ACCOUNTS IN THEIR OWN WORDS

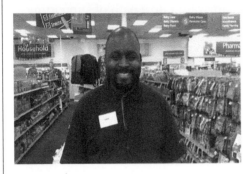

Hello too, new therapist, my name is Justin Sigler, I am 30 years old, currently live with my mom and her husband, and I go to West Los Angeles College. I hope we become good friends and you can become someone that I can talk to when things get hard. My life started when I was diagnosed with autism and Asperger's. At a very young age things started to get hard for me with my education and home life. When I was five years old simple things like learning how to do math was very hard for me even now. My teachers and my family tried to teach me basic addition, subtraction, multiplication, and division, but it was too hard for me. Even now, I struggle to do advance math in my college classes. Even today math is hard for me, but I still keep trying and never giving up!

As years pass, I've learned how to do basic math, but I still struggle to do advance math and how to express myself through singing. Singing has helped me through a little bit of my depression, especially when I had to live with my grandma, my little sister, and grandpa. Things got both very hard and scary for me. But I am getting better as I get older.

Right now, I work full time at CVS in Los Angeles, CA. I am living each day hoping to get better. I have a girlfriend I met in my employment readiness training program. I hope to start a family someday so I can love them. I hope to tell you more about myself one day soon.

Sincerely,
Justin

REFLECTIONS: FIRSTHAND ACCOUNTS IN THEIR OWN WORDS

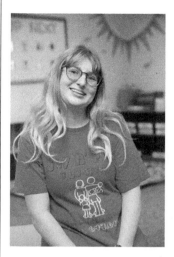

My name is Carrie, I am 27 and I was diagnosed with autism when I was 5. Some of the challenges I had growing up were making friends, expressing myself, and trusting others.

One reason I think it was hard for me to make friends was because on the outside I look like a "typical person" and others do not understand what they cannot see. People believe that autism is a "one size fits all," where if they meet one person with autism they think it is the same for everyone with autism, because they have very little to no knowledge of autism. When, in reality, people with autism are more like a rainbow since they have similar characteristics but also have their own personality and level of functioning.

Another reason it was hard for me to make friends was because I had to learn social skills. I have learned social skills through many social skills programs from various organizations and therapists. I had to work very hard to make and maintain friendships. I also needed help understanding phrases and idioms that my peers were using. It was hard for me to express myself because I did not understand other people's emotions including my own emotions. Through hard work with therapy, I am now able to express myself.

Lastly, when I was younger, I saw a play-based therapist. I did not know why or understand why I needed to go. I was very resistant and even spent a whole session sitting in a corner not talking. I feel that it is important for children to be informed about their diagnosis because then they will be less resistant to therapy and would also be more likely to trust others.

The type of therapies that worked best for me were dialectical behavior therapy (DBT) and cognitive behavioral therapy (CBT). DBT was very helpful because I learned strategies on how to handle conflict, control my emotions, and be mindful. CBT gave me the tools to help me rationalize my thoughts and have control over my anxiety. The types of therapy that I did not benefit from were group therapies, where most of the participants were boys and were lower functioning than me.

The college I attended had the support I needed to succeed and I graduated with honors. I now work full time at LA Speech and Therapy Language Center as a teaching assistant in a preschool classroom.

Overall, I was able to overcome many challenges and obstacles through hard work with therapy. It was helpful for me to get the support I needed when I was a child because I was able to improve on my social skills and understand emotions.

Sincerely,
Carrie

REFLECTIONS: FIRSTHAND ACCOUNTS IN THEIR OWN WORDS

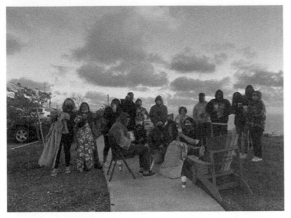 My name is Johnnie, I would like to share my journey of how I overcame obstacles/challenges as an individual with autism. At the age of three years old, I was diagnosed with autism and my mom was told that I would probably never talk. I was born in Los Angeles; however, when I was five years old, my mother and I relocated to GA. Not long after our relocation, I began to talk. My mother had high expectations of me, and she became my advocate; she always told me that autism would not define me, but I would define autism. My mom demanded of the school system that I would be placed in an inclusive educational setting and that I would graduate from high school with a diploma. Even though I was placed in general education settings with supportive teachers and documentation, I still struggled with being accepted by my peers.

As I aged, my peers seemed to notice my differences more and I began to feel socially isolated and invisible. I also felt bullied because I was misinterpreted by those around me due to my uniqueness. My coping mechanism – stimming – was often viewed as strange behavior by my peers and some adults in public settings. I stim whenever I am excited or overwhelmed. Stimming is a self-stimulatory behavior, a reiteration of physical movements, sounds, words, or moving objects. This type of behavior is mostly recurrent to those who are on the spectrum. I overcame my stimming by telling myself to remain calm.

For me to overcome these challenges, I began to become more involved in social and academic clubs in high school. I have carried the same practice now that I am in college. Currently, I am attending Marymount California University (MCU), a small, beautiful nurturing environment with wonderful professors and staff. Since MCU is a nourishing environment, I feel more comfortable, relaxed, and welcome from my peers. Additionally, an opportunity like this will expand my growth along the way with goals to reach back and be an inspiration to others.

Along the way, I gained support from family, friends, church members as well as social advocacy organizations. Since returning to Los Angeles in November 2018, I have received and benefited from many services of the South-Central Los Angeles Regional Center, the California Department of Rehabilitation, Los Angeles County Department of Social Services, Los Angeles Speech and Language Therapy Center, and the University of California at Los Angeles (*UCLA*)'s Center for Autism Research and Treatment.

In closing, I completed my first year at MCU with a 3.9 GPA for the Fall 2020 semester, and for the Spring 2021 semester, I got a 3.7 GPA.

Sincerely,
John

TEST QUESTIONS

1. Autism is largely a disorder of early childhood with fewer implications in adulthood. True or false?

2. Primary concerns for autistic individuals in adulthood include:

   A. Employment

   B. Friendships and relationships

   C. Independence

   D. All of the above

3. Adults with autism are at the same risk for cardiovascular health issues as their neurotypical peers. True or false?

4. Spectrum Shield is a program for adults with autism with the objectives of all of the following except:

   A. Increasing police officers' knowledge of autism and communication differences.

   B. Increasing the skills of adults with autism in safely interacting with law enforcement.

   C. Increasing cooking and life skills among adults with autism.

   D. Increasing awareness of traffic stops via role playing and direct instruction.

5. Adults with autism are at more risk for sexual exploitation than their neurotypical peers. True or false?

6. Intervention with adults with autism should involve (select all that apply):

   A. Input from autistic clients.

   B. Suggestions from family members.

   C. Perspectives of stakeholders like tailor day workers or job coaches.

   D. Evidence-based research.

REFERENCES

Allen, K., Wallace, D., Renes, D. et al. (2010). Use of video modeling to teach vocational skills to adolescents and young adults with autism spectrum disorders. *Education and Treatment of Children* 33 (3): 339–349.

Anderson, A., Carter, M., and Stephenson, J. (2018). Perspectives of university students with autism spectrum disorder. *Journal of Autism and Developmental Disorders* 48 (3): 651–665.

Anderson, A., Carter, M., and Stephenson, J. (2020). An on-line survey of university students with autism spectrum disorder in Australia and New Zealand: characteristics, support satisfaction, and advocacy. *Journal of Autism and Developmental Disorders* 50 (2): 440–454.

Armstrong, A.J. (2011). Sheltered employment. In: *Encyclopedia of Clinical Neuropsychology* (ed. J.S. Kreutzer, J. DeLuca and B. Caplan). New York, NY: Springer.

Baldwin, S., Costley, D., and Warren, A. (2014). Employment activities and experiences of adults with high-functioning autism and Asperger's disorder. *Journal of Autism and Developmental Disorders* 44 (10): 2440–2449.

Bennett, K.D. and Dukes, C. (2013). Employment instruction for secondary students with autism spectrum disorder: a systematic review of the literature. *Education and Training in Autism and Developmental Disabilities* 48 (1): 67–75.

Bernier, R., Mao, A., and Yen, J. (2010). Psychopathology, families, and culture: autism. *Child and Adolescent Psychiatric Clinics of North America* 19 (4): 855–867.

Brown-Lavoie, S.M., Viecili, M.A., and Weiss, J.A. (2014). Sexual knowledge and victimization in adults with autism spectrum disorders. *Journal of Autism and Developmental Disorders* 44: 2185–2196.

Cheak-Zamora, N., Teti, M., and First, J. (2015). 'Transitions are scary for our kids, and they're scary for us': family member and youth perspectives on the challenges of transitioning to adulthood with autism. *Journal of Applied Research in Intellectual Disabilities* 28 (6): 548–560.

Daughrity, B., Ellis, E., and Wiley, A. (2021). Parent perceptions of challenges for teens with autism spectrum disorder (ASD) transitioning to young adulthood. *Journal of the National Black Association of Speech-Language Pathology* 16 (1): 35–45.

Elias, R. and White, S. (2018). Autism goes to college: understanding the needs of a student population on the rise. *Journal of Autism and Developmental Disorders* 48 (3): 732–746.

First, J., Cheak-Zamora, N., and Teti, M. (2016). A qualitative study of stress and coping when transitioning to adulthood with autism spectrum disorder. *Journal of Family Social Work* 19 (3): 220–236.

Fryer, R.G. (2019). An empirical analysis of racial differences in police use of force. *Journal of Political Economy* 127 (3): 1210–1261.

Gibbs, V., Hudson, J., Hwang, Y. et al. (2021). Experiences of physical and sexual violence as reported by adults with autism without intellectual disability: rate, gender patterns and clinical correlates. *Research in Autism Spectrum Disorders* 89: 101866.

Hagner, D., Kurtz, A., Cloutier, H. et al. (2012). Outcomes of a family-centered transition process for students with autism spectrum disorders. *Focus on Autism and Other Developmental Disabilities* 27 (1): 42–50.

Han, G., Tomarken, A., and Gotham, K. (2019). Social and nonsocial reward moderate the relation between autism symptoms and loneliness in adults with ASD, depression, and controls. *Autism Research* 12 (6): 884–896.

Hannon, M.D., White, E.E., and Nadrich, T. (2018). Influence of autism on fathering style among Black American fathers: a narrative inquiry. *Journal of Family Therapy* 40 (2): 224–246.

Hedley, D., Uljarevic, M., Wilmot, M. et al. (2018). Understanding depression and thoughts of self-harm in autism: a potential mechanism involving loneliness. *Research in Autism Spectrum Disorders* 46: 1–7.

Huang, P., Kao, T., Curry, A., and Durbin, D. (2012). Factors associated with driving in teens with autism spectrum disorders. *Journal of Developmental and Behavioral Pediatrics* 33 (1): 70–74.

Kaplan-Mayer, G. (2016). *The Ruderman White Paper: On police violence, media and disability*. New York Jewish Week, 16 March. Available from `https://jewishweek.timesofisrael.com/the-ruderman-white-paper-on-police-violence-media-and-disability` (accessed 31 January 2022).

Kellems, R. and Morningstar, M. (2012). Using video modeling delivered through iPods to teach vocational tasks to young adults with autism spectrum disorders. *Career Development and Transition for Exceptional Individuals* 35 (3): 155–167.

Mazurek, M. (2013). Social media use among adults with autism spectrum disorders. *Computers in Human Behavior* 29 (4): 1709–1714.

Meyer, A.T., Powell, P.S., Butera, N. et al. (2018). Brief report: developmental trajectories of adaptive behavior in children and adolescents with ASD. *Journal of Autism and Developmental Disorders* 48 (8): 2870–2878.

Millau, M., Rivard, M., and Mello, C. (2018). Immigrant families' perception of the causes, first manifestations, and treatment of autism spectrum disorder. *Journal of Child and Family Studies* 27: 3468–3481.

Murray, C. and Doren, B. (2013). The effects of working at gaining employment skills on the social and vocational skills of adolescents with disabilities: A school-based intervention. *Rehabilitation Counseling Bulletin* 56 (2): 96–107.

Newman, L., Wagner, M., Knokey, A.M., et al. (2011). The post high school outcomes of young adults with disabilities up to 8 years after school. A report from the national longitudinal transition study-2 (NLTS2) (NCSER 2011–3005). Menlo Park, CA: SRI International.

Pecora, L., Hancock, G., Hooley, M. et al. (2020). Gender identity, sexual orientation and adverse sexual experiences in autistic females. *Molecular Autism* 11: 57.

Pesce, N.L. (2019). Most college grads with autism can't find jobs. this group is fixing that. MarketWatch, 2 April. Available from `https://www.marketwatch.com/story/most-college-grads-with-autism-cant-find-jobs-this-group-is-fixing-that-2017-04-10-5881421` (accessed 31 January 2022).

Riser-Kositsky, M. (2021). Special education: Definition, statistics, and trends. Education Week, 21 July. Available from `https://www.edweek.org/teaching-learning/special-education-definition-statistics-and-trends/2019/12` (accessed 31 January 2022).

Rosenthal, M., Wallace, G.L., Lawson, R. et al. (2013). Impairments in real-world executive function increase from childhood to adolescence in autism spectrum disorders. *Neuropsychology* 27 (1): 13–18.

Roux, A., Rast, J., Anderson, K., and Shattuck, P. (2017). *National Autism Indicators Report: Developmental disability services and outcomes in adulthood.* Philadelphia, PA: A.J. Drexel Autism Institute, Drexel University.

Sala, G., Hooley, M., and Stokes, M. (2020). Romantic intimacy in autism: a qualitative analysis. *Journal of Autism and Developmental Disorders* 50: 4133–4147.

Schall, C., Wehman, P., Avellone, L., and Taylor, J.P. (2020). Competitive integrated employment for youth and adults with autism: findings from a scoping review. *Child and Adolescent Psychiatric Clinics of North America* 29 (2): 373–397.

Sedgewick, F., Crane, L., Hill, V., and Pellicano, E. (2019). Friends and lovers: the relationships of autistic and neurotypical women. *Autism in Adulthood* 1 (2): 112–123.

Shattuck, P.T., Roux, A.M., Hudson, L.E. et al. (2012). Services for adults with an autism spectrum disorder. *Canadian Journal of Psychiatry* 57 (5): 284–291.

Smith, L.E., Maenner, M.J., and Seltzer, M.M. (2012). Developmental trajectories in adolescents and adults with AUTISM: the case of daily living skills. *Journal of the American Academy of Child & Adolescent Psychiatry* 51 (6): 622–631.

Sundberg, M. (2018). Online gaming, loneliness and friendships among adolescents and adults with ASD. *Computers in Human Behavior* 79: 105–110.

Syu, Y. and Lin, L. (2018). Sensory overresponsivity, loneliness, and anxiety in Taiwanese adults with autism spectrum disorder. *Occupational Therapy International* 2018: 9165978.

Test, D.W., Smith, L.E., and Carter, E.W. (2014). Equipping youth with autism spectrum disorders for adulthood: promoting rigor, relevance, and relationships. *Remedial and Special Education* 35 (2): 80–90.

Thompson, C., Bolte, S., Falkmer, T., and Girdler, S. (2019). Viewpoints on how students with autism can best navigate university. *Scandinavian Journal of Occupational Therapy* 26 (4): 294–305.

Ward, D., Dill-Shackleford, K., and Mazurek, M. (2018). Social media use and happiness in adults with autism spectrum disorders. *Cyberpsychology, Behavior and Social Networking* 21 (3): 205–209.

Weir, E., Allison, C., Ong, K., and Baron-Cohen, S. (2021). An investigation of the diet, exercise, sleep, BMI, and health outcomes of adults with autism. *Molecular Autism* 12: 31.

White, S., Elias, R., Capriola-Hall, N. et al. (2017). Development of a college transition and support program for students with autism spectrum disorder. *Journal of Autism and Developmental Disorders* 47: 3072–3078.

Wiley, P. and Gentry, B. (2015). *Transition or Departure: Parent Perspectives on ASD after Age 21.* Colorado: American Speech and Hearing Association National Convention.

Wiley, P. and Gentry, B.F. (2016). *Autism: Attacking Social Interaction Problems: A Pre-Vocational Training Manual for Ages 17+.* San Diego, CA: Plural Publishers.

FURTHER READINGS

Anderson, A.H., Stephenson, J., and Carter, M. (2017). A systematic literature review of the experiences and supports of students with autism spectrum disorder in post-secondary education. *Research in Autism Spectrum Disorders* 39: 33–53.

Anderson, C., Butt, C., and Sarsony, C. (2020). Young adults on the autism spectrum and early employment-related experiences: aspirations and obstacles. *Journal of Autism and Developmental Disorders* 51 (1): 88–105.

Autism Speaks. (2021). Autism statistics and facts. Available from https://www.autismspeaks.org/autism-statistics- asd (accessed 31 January 2022).

Bishop, H., Boe, L., Stavrinos, D., and Mirman, J. (2018). Driving among adolescents with autism spectrum disorder and attention-deficit hyperactivity disorder. *Safety* 4 (3): 40.

Fong, C.J., Taylor, J., Berdyyeva, A. et al. (2021). Interventions for improving employment outcomes for persons with autism spectrum disorders: a systematic review update. *Campbell Systematic Reviews* 17 (3): e1185.

Nagib, W. and Wilton, R. (2020). Gender matters in career exploration and job-seeking among adults with autism spectrum disorder: evidence from an online community. *Disability and Rehabilitation* 42 (18): 2530–2541.

Pearson, A. and Rose, K. (2021). A conceptual analysis of autistic masking: Understanding the narrative of stigma and the illusion of choice. *Autism in Adulthood* 3 (1): 52–60.

Volkmar, F.R. (2016). *Adolescents and Adults with Autism Spectrum Disorders*. New York, NY: Springer.

Wehman, P., Brooke, V., Brooke, A.M. et al. (2016). Employment for adults with autism spectrum disorders: a retrospective review of a customized employment approach. *Research in Developmental Disabilities* 53–54: 61–72.

CHAPTER 8

Autism and Echolalia

Learning Objectives

By reading this chapter, interventionists will be able to:

1. Learn historical perspectives of echolalia in research throughout the years.
2. Differentiate between immediate and delayed echolalia and gestalt language acquisition.
3. Understand the different ideas behind the functionality or non-functionality of the presence of repetitive speech.
4. Develop tools and strategies used to foster meaningful language development in echolalic children.
5. Identify various evidence-based approaches supporting and using the presence of echolalia.

ECHOLALIA 101

A newly minted speech pathologist walks into the room to evaluate a two-year-old who has a recent diagnosis of autism. As she interviews the parent, she shares primary concerns related to her child, including her inability to talk and engage with others. The parent says "It's like she's in her own little world."

Autism Spectrum Disorders from Theory to Practice: Assessment and Intervention Tools Across the Lifespan, First Edition. Edited by Belinda Daughrity and Ashley Wiley Johnson.
© 2023 John Wiley & Sons Ltd. Published 2023 by John Wiley & Sons Ltd.

The therapist looks at the client who is laying down looking at a train with one eye moving it vigorously back and forth. The client says "Alright, Mickey my pal! Let's go!" The therapist jumps and says "Oh, I thought he wasn't able to talk!" The mom responds "Oh yea, he can't talk, he just says that all day, it's from Mickey Mouse Club. He says other things from TV, too." She shakes her head and continues on to discuss her concerns.

What an interesting exchange between the parent and the interventionist, right? Well believe it or not, this may be a common occurrence for parents and also interventionists who work with children with autism. What was described in this scenario is called *echolalia*, which is the repetition of words in speech. Echolalia is a common occurrence typically until age two and a half and then it will disappear (Marom et al. 2018; Dobbinson et al. 2003; Howlin 1982; Stefanatos and Joe, 2008; Prizant and Duchan 1981).

While all children demonstrate repetitive speech during the development of language, children with autism are known to do it more than others (Van Santen et al. 2013; Gladfelter and Van Suiden, 2020). Echolalia is a hallmark feature of autism and is also one of the most recognizable characteristics that many students on the spectrum may exhibit. While all children hear something and then repeat it back, children with autism do so at a higher frequency. In fact, researchers suggest that roughly 75% of children with autism spectrum disorder (ASD) exhibit echolalia (Kanner 1943; Schuler 1979; Wing, 1971; Gladfelter and VanZuiden, 2020; Sterponi and Shankey 2014).

In practical terms, one may describe the speech to be "parodic," where you say something and then the child quickly repeats it back in the same style, tone, inflection, and rate. However, as an interventionist, we know that there must be more to it than just a child repeating what was heard. In fact, echolalia has long been the source of much controversy among researchers and practitioners in related disciplines.

Historically, the presence of echolalia was researched as early as 1825, according to Kanner. In 1943, Robert Kanner was the first researcher to write about echolalia through the lens of a child with autism. He described echolalia as dysfunctional and governed rigidly by asocial preoccupations (Kanner 1943; Sterponi and Shankey 2014). Adriana Shuler followed Kanner later in 1979, with the first analysis of issues and clinical application of echolalia. Her review of the literature stressed that echolalia is not easy to define or distinguish from more normal forms of repetition (Schuler 1979). The term echolalia was questioned as meaningless, considering the limited information that researchers had about it, and also that it was not used in the diagnosis of a medical disease.

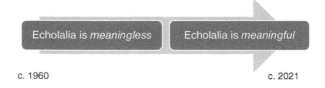

Echolalia is *meaningless*   Echolalia is *meaningful*

c. 1960   c. 2021

The limited knowledge of echolalia was primarily attributed to the confusion of terminology and lack of detailed description of behaviors that were seen in children exhibiting echolalia. Consequently, there was difficulty for researchers to form a firm belief in the identification and treatment of echolalia. One challenge noted was the inability to determine whether echolalia in children with autism was an intentional or unintentional behavior, citing that it may be a result of the child's excellent language memory.

Echolalia in a child with autism traditionally has been associated with inwardness, sameness, and limited communicative inventory (Sterponi and Shankey 2014). Some researchers continue to find it to be an interference as children develop language and lacking comprehension (Kenworthy et al. 2012). However, as our knowledge, understanding, and acceptance of autism has increased, echolalia is acknowledged more often as a viable pathway to meaningful, self-generated language that a child can use to intend to communicate. In fact, it supports many critical aspects of cognition, including rehearsal, self-regulation, and learning.

The American Speech–Language–Hearing Association takes the position that echolalia is a viable pathway to meaningful self-generated language (Stiegler 2015; American Speech–Language–Hearing Association 2006). In fact, this has long been the position of many speech–language pathologists working with individuals with autism. Consider the following statement from Sussman in the Hanen Centre's parent guide, *More than Words*:

> Echolalia is a good sign. It shows your child's communication is developing. Soon he may begin to use these repeated words and phrases to communicate something to you. For example, after he repeats what you say, he may look at you or move closer to an object. Or he may remember the words you use to ask him if he wants a drink, and later use these memorized words to ask a question of his own. The words your child learns from echolalia open the door to meaningful communication.
>
> (Sussman 2012)

A NOTE ON GESTALT LANGUAGE ACQUISITION

It has been highlighted throughout this chapter that all children may use echolalia as a bridge to developing meaningful language. Traditionally, children develop language by listening to what was said and then breaking it down into smaller units. For example, a mom may say, "Let's go to the store." A child understands the key word "store" and then says "store!" Those units start small and then gradually increase to reach the point of spontaneous production at the connected speech level.

However, research has pointed to the idea that many children with autism who use echolalia may be developing language in a different fashion, where their words come in longer chunked forms called "gestalt form". This style of language acquisition has been described as gestalt language, which begins with the production of multiple words and ends with novel utterance production (Stiegler 2015; Lowry 2018).

When a child develops language in the gestalt language acquisition style, they first begin to produce short multi-word productions. However, there is no distinction among the individual utterances or syntactic structure within the gestalt form. As development continues, the child then increases their understanding of the use and rules related to syntactic form; they are able to break down gestalt forms to produce more spontaneous utterances. This continues to increase as the child moves to creative production of language.

STAGES OF GESTALT LANGUAGE ACQUISITION

Table 8.1 shows the four stages of gestalt language acquisition. Understanding gestalt language is important when conceptualizing echolalia and also for determining ways to treat it. For example, if you have a child who is at stage one of gestalt language development, try to shift them to stage two by incorporating therapeutic tasks that strengthen cognitive growth and social experiences. This will help them to obtain the ability to break down and combine utterances. You continue this, and change objectives to support further development to move the client through more advanced stages.

Therapy Golden Nugget
For a client with autism using echolalia (stage 1 of gestalt language acquisition), interventionists can try to incorporate activities that help clients to break down and combine utterances. Intervention materials for the task: toy car, blocks. 1. Clinician models: (engine sound) "Crash car!" while crashing a car into the blocks. 2. Client imitates: "Crash car!" 3. Clinician repeats script at least three times to firmly establish the play routine. 4. Clinician sets up the task, but pauses unexpectantly before crashing the car into the blocks to allow the child to complete the verbal routine without the clinician model. If the child completes the script, offer verbal praise and positive affect. If not, return to modeling.

In our years of practice, we have seen some practitioners urge therapists to shape the behavior by using **verbal reprimands**, such as "Do not copy, do not repeat," in an effort to address and reduce echolalic behaviors produced during a treatment session. This method is one that has been researched and is used by practitioners (Stiegler 2015; Rapp et al. 2009) while other interventionists may turn echolalia into a meaningful statement using the echolalia as a tool. This form of recasting is also documented and used by researchers (Stiegler 2015). Personally, we use a mixture of both methods.

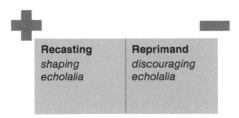

TABLE 8.1   The stages of gestalt language acquisition.

Stage	Term	Description
1	Echolalia	Utterances are largely echolalic and serve either a turn-taking function in conversation or a self-stimulatory function.
2	Mitigation	Cognitive growth and social experiences fuel echolalia that serves a greater variety of functions. Children's echoes evidence mitigation. They break down utterances and recombine shorter segments, or they use one- and two-word utterances.
3	Isolating words and recombining	Early semantic syntactic rules are acquired and echolalic utterances are broken down further. Spontaneous language increases and expresses functions previously fulfilled by echolalia.
4	Generation	more spontaneous and flexible language continues as semantic, syntactic, and morphological rules are acquired. Most communicative functions are served by spontaneously generated utterances. Echolalic utterances may be observed when an individual is tired, confused, or distracted.

Source: Lowry (2018).

Regardless of which train of thought you choose to ride on, we recommend ensuring that you support your decisions by looking at each client individually, staying informed about research and practices, and also engaging your colleagues to have thoughtful conversation around best practices. Echolalia is unique and has to be treated as such.

TYPES OF ECHOLALIA

Echolalia is often described in two major categories based on temporal latency (Sterponi and Shankey 2014; Powell, 2012; Steigler, 2015; American Speech–Language–Hearing Association, 2021). *Immediate echolalia*, which is repetitive speech observed within two conversational turns of the original language input, and *delayed echolalia*, which refers to repetitive speech that occurs after a significant delay. Take the following practical example, a client is in treatment with an interventionist:

> *Interventionist: OK Johnny, let's see if we can play Goldfish.*
> *Client: Play Goldfish. (Client sits at the table and folds his hands.)*

In this example, we see that the client produces immediate echolalia. The repetitive speech occurrence was within two conversational turns. The response following indicated comprehension of the directive and an appropriate behavior response. Let's take this same situation and change it slightly:

> *Interventionist: OK Johnny, let's see if we can play Goldfish.*
> *Client: OK Johnny, OK Johnny. (Client continues to run around the room.)*

In this adjusted example, we see another form of immediate echolalia. The repetitive speech occurred within two conversational turns. However, the output and behavioral response lacked comprehension of the adult directive and was less of an "appropriate" response. This example occurs to be less functional and complementary to the verbal exchange.

Active Learning Task

Considering the two practical examples of immediate echolalia, take a moment to answer the following questions;
- Did you note a difference in "functionality" of the echoic occurrences?
- How would your therapeutic response differ based on each example?
- Write a one-page reflection answering the above question. Compare and contrast responses of peers in the small group setting.

In addition to temporal latency, echolalia can also be evaluated through the lens of functionality and degree of echolalic occurrence (Shield et al. 2017; Schuler 1979; Marom et al. 2018; Stubblefield 2021). As speech–language pathologists, we see many interactions that include language as positive. However, considering functionality helps us to identify where to meet the client. Functional echolalia is attempted communication intended to be interactional, acting as communication with another person.

Understanding the functionality of the echolalia present in a client with autism is important to consider when choosing to target or not target during treatment (Schuler 1979; Sterponi and Shankey 2014; Stubblefield 2021). If you have chosen to target echolalia, remember that it should never be a source of strong emphasis where it can agitate or effect the client. When this occurs, the interventionist may experience the client withdrawing or increasing echolalic behaviors.

In addition to pure echolalia, which repeats the exact production, there is also *mitigated echolalia*, which differs in at least one way from the original utterance. Differences vary in pronominal substitutions, changes in prosody, semantic substitutions, expansions, or combinations of each of these Figure 8.1 (Shield et al. 2017; Bebko 1990). The quality of mitigated echoic responses are described as a more creative and productive use of language. In fact, some researchers have described it as a sign of recovery in other affected populations such as patients with aphasia (Shield et al. 2017).

CONSIDERING FUNCTIONALITY

Echolalia is a part of inclusion criteria when diagnosing autism. When present, it is considered an atypical behavior. When working with a client who exhibits echolalia, consider the type of echolalia the client presents with. Take note of the following practical examples of the various types of functional and non-interactional echolalia.

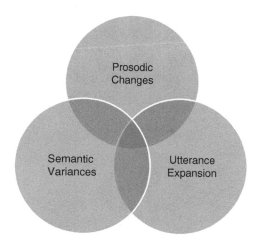

FIGURE 8.1   Differences in pronominal substitutions in mitigated echolalia.

Interactional (Fully Functional) Echolalia

Interactional or fully functional echolalia is seen when a person intends to communicate with others. While it may not demonstrate spontaneous and independently generated responses, it is often able to be recognized and understood by the listener in terms of relevance to the particular exchange.

- Requests: The person with echolalia may say, "Is it cake time?" to request for cake at a peers birthday party.
- Turn taking: Using phrases to fill in during an alternating verbal exchange.
  Parent: Do you want to go to the store?
  Client: The store. (Grabs bag and is ready to go.)
- Providing information: Speech may be used to offer new information, but it may be hard to connect the dots.
  Parent: Alex, what do you want for lunch?
  Alex: Sings "I'm loving it!" to signal a desire for a popular fast food brand.
- Verbal completion: Speech is used to complete familiar verbal routines that are initiated by others. Client repeats, "That's it, Jenny, you need to brush your teeth!" while brushing teeth, echoing what they are used to hearing from their caregiver each morning.

Non-Interactional (Limited Functionality) Echolalia

Non-interactional or limited functionality echolalia is limited communicative intent. It is often for personal use, like labeling or self-stimulation, which would be considered an atypical behavior.

- Rehearsal: The speaker may utter the same phrase softly to themselves a few times before responding in a normal voice. This may be practice for the coming interaction:
  - Client: Repeats, "OK, just calm down, you're almost up!" Client looks nervous while waiting for turn to kick the ball in his adapted physical education class.
- Non-focused speech: Saying something that is not relevant to the current situation experienced:
  - Client: Johnny is pacing back and forth on this toes. He belts out a repetitive phrase, "Alrighty, I've got you now!" Each time with the same level of vocal intensity and pitch.
- Situation association: Triggered by a particular influence, oftentimes situational, visual, by a particular person, or experience. This typically does not seem to be an attempt at communication:
  - Client, out in the community with a social skills group outing. Client sees a parent with baby and says "Hushhhhh little baby." Parent say's "Oh, he always does that when he sees babies!"
- Self-direction: Repetitive speech intended to aid oneself through a process:
  - Client is dismissed to find lunch box and stand at the door. They say "stand up, walk slowly, look for name, line up."
- Incidental: Occurs when the client is unable to filter what is occurring in the environment or in the background. It may present as impulsive and automatic.

THERAPEUTIC ACTION PLAN

As with anything, before addressing echolalia in treatment, you will want to take time and assess whether the client is using echolalia (Stubblefielfd, 2019; Steigler, 2015). The first thing you will want to do is to measure how severe the echolalia may be. When determining severity, we recommend using the chart in Table 8.2.

In addition to level of severity, you must also consider impact. Take note of the guided questions in the Therapy Golden Nugget below, as a means to stimulate thought surrounding this topic.

TABLE 8.2   Severity of echolalia.

Severity over time of treatment (%)	Severity rating
100–70	Severe
69–50	Moderate
49–25	Mild moderate
≤ 25	Mild

Therapy Golden Nugget

Guided Questions

1. Is this impacting the child's life? YES or NO
2. Is this a priority for parents? YES or NO
3. How does this impact communicative intent? YES or NO
4. Is it being used semi-meaningfully by the speaker? YES or NO
5. Is the client cognitively able to understand the behavior and its impact? YES or NO

If many of your answers are a strong YES, shaping echolalic behaviors will likely be an appropriate priority for treatment.

Echolalia can be considered a deficit due to lack of situational inhibitory control or an inability to effectively filter out incidental background noise in context (Grossi et al. 2012). While there are some treatments that are echolalia specific, an interventionist can also have a distinct set of behaviors or responses that are embedded throughout the course of the treatment session. This provides a natural way of targeting the behavior. In other words, when it happens, you address it.

Treatment of echolalia in individuals with ASD is promising (Table 8.3). Most effective approaches can include a behaviorally based approach using positive reinforcement for lower rates of behavior, verbal modeling, and visual cues (Neely et al. 2016). This section aims to assist interventionists such as yourself to employ the following methods:

- Working to be direct
- Teaching a client to pause
- Bringing reality and relevance to echolalic production
- Jumping into character.

Working to be Direct

With over 30 years of experience between the authors, we have seen that addressing echolalia in a direct manner that is respectful of the client is one of the best methods used to shift echolalic behaviors. This method is one that we use when the individual's echolalic behavior is interfering with ability to engage in social interaction with others.

TABLE 8.3   Treatment of echolalia in people with autism spectrum disorder.

Key strategy	Therapeutic presentation	Intervention suggestions
Facilitate verbal initiations	Offer opportunities for the client to initiate communication, rather than responding to questions.	Use activities with highly preferred items. Rather than asking "What's this?" try holding up items and waiting expectantly for the child to label the item.
Elicit careful observations	Make sure to track nonverbal indicators of comprehension like gaze, body language, and changes in facial expression. Note changes in types and frequency of echolalia to credit progress.	Note baselines and develop a system for consistent data tracking and informally review client progress at least bimonthly.
Facilitate low-constraint interactions	Avoid high-constraint utterances (questions, commands).	Create linguistic opportunities through play in a naturalistic setting.
Map language into known contexts	Use language the child already uses and change aspects to increase linguistic diversity.	If the child says, "Let's go!" try to make changes to one element such as, "Let's eat!"
Model useful gestalts	Model carefully selected, individualized, age-appropriate, high-frequency, and socially communicative utterances for the client to add to their current repertoire.	Target smaller, flexible units as a means to help generate more creative and meaningful utterances.
Provide opportunities to practice	Offer multiple repetitions to help the client learn the desired skill.	Target 10 opportunities per session. Once the client is successful in intervention, allow the client to practice with a peer when available.
Strengthen social closeness	Facilitate opportunities for social engagement.	Consider incorporating evidenced based approaches that emphasize joint attention and social engagement skills.
Develop opportunities to teach quiet behavior in specific settings	Teach the client to remain quiet in settings where echolalia is disruptive and/or inappropriate.	Try using a social skill steps with clients to respond appropriately in various target settings or social scenarios.

Source: Adapted from Stiegler (2015).

Active Learning Task

You have a new client Johnny and he seemed like he repeated most of everything you said during the session. Do you address it or not? Discuss with a peer.

For students who present with severe and moderate echolalia, consider approaching it directly. Literature suggests that, often, clients are unaware of the echolalic behavior but are intending to use it to develop relationships (Stiegler 2015; Lowry 2018; Sterponi and Shankey 2014; Stribling et al. 2006; Tarplee and Barrow 1999). Bringing a client's awareness into the fold may therefore shift the behavior – and that is what we want.

Earlier in the text, the phrase "Do not copy, do not repeat" was mentioned as a strategy to bring awareness to the client about their echolalia. This is a phrase that I will often use. However, it is hard for me to accept that this method is considered a *verbal reprimand*. I believe that it is direct, it is clear, and it gives the expected behavior for the client to use to be successful. While not all therapy is positive, it may result in positive outcomes when you give clear expectations to allow the client to easily shift the behavior and reach your target response.

When using this phrase, it is important to be consistent. Meaning, try to say the same phrase in the same fashion each time the behavior occurs. Once you say the phrase, you guide the client into saying something independent and not something repeated. Your support with this should be fading. The objective here is to produce relevant independent verbalization.

GOAL SPOTLIGHT

When given a verbal stimuli, client will produce an independent verbalization that is relevant to the social interaction.

Teaching a Client to Pause

Once the client has met this goal, the next objective should be to get the client to pause once a person says something to them. Being silent in conversation or when you hear conversation is something that is critical in many community, home, and educational settings. This is a critical objective to successfully treating a client with echolalia (Steigler, 2015). In therapy, this may manifest itself by teaching the client to pause. The cue that is used to elicit the behavior (pausing) can vary. Some types of fading cues that can be given include those shown in Figure 8.2.

Encourage the client to take time to process what is said and then give a response. During this time of pausing, the client will need to generate a response. Remember that these are two different tasks that must be individually addressed in treatment. We encourage interventionists to consider traditional language methods to teach a client to generate language. These traditional methods are discussed in Chapters 5 and 6.

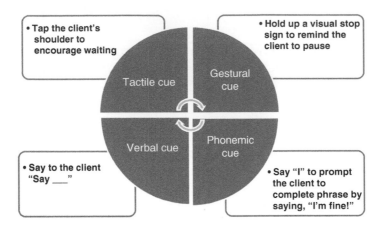

FIGURE 8.2   Fading cues.

Teaching a client to pause encourages (i) actively processing what is being said, and (ii) giving a contingent response. It is important to keep in mind that these are two distinct skills and should be evaluated respectively and addressed individually in treatment. Among children with autism using echolalia, the frequency of echolalic utterances reduces as linguistic competence and spontaneous utterances increases (Howlin 1982). Interventionists are encouraged to use traditional language stimulation methods to help clients increase expressive language skills.

Therapy Golden Nugget
Use visual supports plus a specific carrier phrase to strengthen a client's ability to produce novel sentences. First teach the carrier phrase "I+ see" then add a visual cue. Change the visual cue but keep the exact same carrier phrase structure. Imagine how much can be taught when you use "I+ see" as an anchor!

In promoting expressive language skills via direct language stimulation, some children may imitate the cue in addition to the target word or phrase. For example, an interventionist might show a picture or object and prompt language via "Say ___." A child with autism exhibiting echolalia might imitate the entire utterance including the command, rather than just the target. In this case, the cues–pause–point procedure has been shown to be effective to reduce imitations of the instruction prompt (Valentino et al. 2012).

In addition, it is important to consider that the linguistic demands placed on the client will influence the type and amount of echolalia that a client uses (Gladfelter and VanZuiden, 2020). Some researchers found that high constraint utterances like "wh. . ." questions and commands requiring the client to name and label often resulted in more echolalia.

In treatment, take a moment to consider what type of language you are presenting to your client. As you are teaching the skill of pausing, try teaching it in a simpler language context. Increase the language context as the client shows improvements and increased readiness.

Bringing Reality and Relevance to Echolalic Production

Consider the following example from Susan Stokes:

> If a child with echolalia gets angry at his teacher when recess is over, he might suddenly say "Go to h***, Lieutenant!" The teacher might later discover that the child had been watching A Few Good Men and had used a phrase he knew was tied to anger to convey his feelings in that moment.
>
> (Stubblefield 2021)

In the therapeutic setting, if you were to bring relevance to the statement you may say "I'm not lieutenant and we do not tell others to go to h***. That is not nice." You then will use the same step of helping the client to generate the response leading him through the process of saying "I am MAD" or "More recess please." This type of response is helpful for immediate echolalia, taking effect within two conversational turns. Additionally, response interruption and redirection by issuing vocal demands contingent on the occurrence of vocal stereotypy can help to suppress the behavior and increase appropriate communication in children with autism (Ahearn et al. 2007).

For delayed echolalia, you can bring reality to the echolalia by referencing where it may have come from. In practice, you may hear an interventionist say "Oh, are you talking like Daffy Duck, it's not time for Daffy Duck" or "That is not Daffy Duck, you are playing with a car." This will also be followed up by engaging the client to generate a more appropriate production. Remember, as a client improves with language functioning, it will be important to support the client to say what they really might like to say:

- Give a specific phrase that can be said.
- Provide the client with choices of example productions.
- Have the client spontaneously generate what they would like to say.

Bringing reality to echolalia will acknowledge the client's feelings and will shift the production to become meaningful and relevant. When using this strategy, you will find that you are teaching the client what can be said in certain situations. As with anything, the objective will be for this to generalize to similar interactions and various settings.

Jumping into Character

Current research suggests that students with autism demonstrate increased echolalia in the context of play-based tasks (Gladfelter and Van Zuiden 2020). With that being said, some of the most meaningful work to target echolalia can occur when you take a moment and meet the client to play. This may include jumping into the character that a child may be portraying. This works especially well for students who are known to use delayed echolalia stemming from media sources.

A highly memorable moment was working with a student who was known to recite slogans related to superheroes. I engaged the client in a play-based therapeutic task, we were playing with toys. As the client hums out the tune to *Batman* repeatedly, he moves his car back and forth and engaged in solitary interaction. In that moment he was demonstrating **vocal stereotypy**, when a client uses a feature of sound in an repetitive fashion in addition to delayed or immediate echolalia (Taylor et al. 2005; Steigler, 2015). Vocal stereotypy can be a diagnostic criterion for ASD and is more common in autism than in other disorders (Lewis and Bodfish 1998; Bodfish et al. 2000).

In addition to the sound, the client was displaying repetitive physical behaviors by rolling the car back and forth in an a typical fashion. I first attempted to join in his play by saying "OK. It's my turn to roll the car! Isn't that how one typically gets into a game?" However, the client made little eye contact, avoided interacting with me by turning his body, and continued the repetitive behaviors. Finally, I engaged again with the car, this time as he hummed his tune I took a moment and completed the theme song and said "Batman!" in the correct tone and pitch and melody. I grabbed a tree and made it lightly crash into his car. The client stopped. For that moment he made fleeting eye contact with me and had a puzzled gaze. Surprisingly, he looked bothered for one moment. If I could put words into his mouth he would say "What! This is MY world!" The engagement was gone, he turned back around quickly and attempted to continue his task.

At that moment, there was a display of joint attention and also a sign that you were able to stop a repetitive behavior. I did not give up, that was my new strategy I found. Join the clients world even for a split second through jumping into character with him. *As I continued to do this, after the third time, the client began to start to show interest in engaging with me.* With time, there was a reduction in echoic productions and an increased interest in joint attention with the clinicians during semi-structured play-based tasks.

Another alternative clinical option is to use less traditional approaches such as implementing a drama and theater with an intervention program. Pilot investigations evaluating such approaches using typical peers, video modeling, and behavior supports have shown that children with autism can improve in theory of mind and face identification, as well as socioemotional skills (Corbett et al. 2011). Drama therapy has become an evidence-based method for treatment for students with autism to increase friendship development, social interaction, emotion recognition, and language skills (Andersen-Warren 2013; Godfrey and Haythorne 2013; Beadle-Brown et al. 2018; Trudel and Nadig 2019).

Therapy for the Drama King or Queen

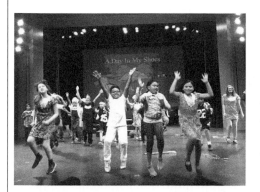

In 2007, as a young newly minted speech pathologist with an undergraduate degree in theater, I had taken my first job as the lead in a therapeutic speech camp program for children with autism. This world renown program included time where children could engage in typical hobbies to develop a passion and create a break in a normal therapy day.

During that time, I was tasked to come up with activities for my group of kids. I remember being fascinated with the students' ability to memorize information. They would see written information and be able to read it perfectly and then remember it verbatim later on in the day. In addition, many of the students engaged in scripting, where they would recite lines from movies or various media sources. I was always so fascinated by those two characteristics that many of our students had.

As a young person interested in the theater, I was curious whether the students would respond if we engaged in scripts through the lens of creation, rehearsal, and production. I introduced the project to the class and quickly saw that it motivated students and they were amazing with acting out different characters that we created as a group. In addition, it was a wonderful opportunity for students to practice conversation skills, turn taking, and also to develop a working understanding on when to assume a character and when not too. Some student would rehearse parts of the play during non-theater times during the camp day. When that occurred, we would make a point to discuss how the play was at a certain time and this was real life.

As a result of engaging in theater and intentional "scripting," students began to generalize skills. Particular gains were noted in social skill development, joint attention, confidence, and articulation skills. In addition to seeing therapeutic success, the students had fun and felt like we were building something together.

That year, parents and family members watched the students put on this play they created in an open park. Parents felt proud that their child found an amazing hobby and also had a moment to shine bright like the stars they each were. They also saw amazing growth in a very short amount of time. As a therapist, I felt like I was doing therapy, having fun, and seeing growth. My mission was accomplished but I realized it was far from over, I needed to continue to see this through because my clients were getting better. That is always my bottom line in decision making.

What I didn't realize at that time was that drama therapy would later become an evidence-based method for treatment of students with autism (Andersen-Warren 2013; Godfrey and Haythorn, 2013; Beedle-Brown et al., 2018; Brondino et al., 2015; Trudel and Nadig, 2019; Wiley, 2012). That also was the genesis of the Drama Kings and Queens summer intensive theater camp and social skills program serving children from ages 5–15. This program was established over 15 years ago and now serves children from all over the world. The program grew from a public park to being invited to perform in front of crowds of thousands of people at the opening of the 2016 World Special Olympics and putting on shows for crowds of hundreds of theaters alongside professional musicians in professional theater spaces.

As I take time to reflect, I realized that was a moment where my passion met my purpose which was to help people. Taking something like echolalia that often may be looked at as counterproductive, and using it to develop artistic talents is a skill that will always be useful to me. I encourage newly minted interventionists like yourself to incorporate your passion with your purpose as much as possible. You may never know when it will prove to be highly successful.

For more information on Drama Kings and Queens Summer Program, visit `https://speakla.com/drama-kings-and-queens/`.

SUMMARY

Echolalia is repeating the speech of others. This is a hallmark feature of ASD and impacts roughly 75% of children with an autism diagnosis. This chapter shared the historical background, understanding, and treatment of echolalia. As time and understanding has moved forward, our beliefs and use of echolalia has evolved. It is the position of the American Speech–Language–Hearing Association that echolalia can be used in therapy as a meaningful bridge to appropriate language production. The chapter highlighted overarching tools for practice when treating echolalia, specific strategies and ideas for treatment methods, and gave practical examples of what different forms of echolalia looks like in clients.

REFLECTIONS ALONG THE PATH

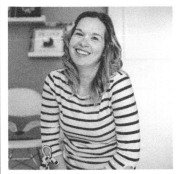

Clare Harrop, Ph.D.

I have always worked with children, but my focus in autism started during my doctorate at the University of Manchester. I trained within the Preschool Autism Communication Trial (PACT); a three-site randomized control trial for autistic preschoolers in the UK (Green et al., 2010). The PACT model was developed and implemented by speech–language pathologists.

I have spent the following years of my career working in multidisciplinary teams. I enjoy working with clinicians and clinician scientists and is the ultimate goal of my research, regardless of how far I step away from clinical settings with methods such as eye tracking and electroencephalography, is to inform diagnosis and treatment.

The PACT study provided me with in-depth and world-class research training and experiences to begin my career. Reflecting back now, my training was very much part of the medical model of ASD, which sees ASD as a deficit. I suspect that my training and research experiences would have been very different in 2021 compared with 2011. The neurodiversity movement (Kapp, 2020) has changed the way that I conduct research with autistic samples and how I interpret my findings. I hope that future clinicians can find a happy medium between historic medical models of ASD and the neurodiversity movement, recognizing that some individuals will need more support, but that autism is a different way of thinking, rather than the wrong way.

A clear example of my change in thinking has been how I study restricted and repetitive behaviors (RRBs) in ASD. My early work focused on comparing autistic samples with neurotypical samples, focusing on RRBs as something that needed to be changed or removed. Over time, I have shifted away from this viewpoint, largely influenced by the work of autistic scholars such as Dr. Kapp (Kapp et al., 2019). Instead, my team not only characterizes these behaviors, but also how parents respond to them, and what might be the underlying root of these behaviors. For example, removing or restricting certain RRBs may be detrimental to autistic individuals as some serve as a mechanism to control anxiety. Focused interests could be used as an entry into shared interests with peers or routes into employment.

Beginning in this field as a graduate student, first as a master's student and then as a doctoral student, I didn't have a clear idea where I would end up. I didn't think my plan would include moving countries, training in multiple new methods, or extending my work beyond young children to adolescence and now adulthood. Currently, I am an Assistant Professor in Allied Health Sciences at the University of North Carolina at Chapel Hill. While I am in a clinical department, I am a developmental psychologist by training. My research career has been embedded within multidisciplinary teams, spanning psychology, psychiatry, education, speech and hearing sciences, and occupational science. In line with this, my biggest advice is that it is okay to not have a concrete plan, and be open to change and new directions in your career with autism. You will always continue to learn and have a varied toolbox at your disposal!

Clare Harrop PhD
Assistant Professor, University of North Carolina at Chapel Hill

TEST QUESTIONS

1. Compare and contrast forms of interactive and non-interactive echolalia. Use one type of echolalia to describe what it may look like therapeutically. True or false?

2. In your own words, describe the four types of cues that can be given to teach a client to pause to avoid an echoic occurrence. True or false?

3. Discuss the key considerations needed to be made by an interventionist when choosing to target or not to target echolalia. True or false?

4. Echolalia in children with autism has a distinct pattern which matches the following style:
   A. Parrot speech
   B. Gestalt language
   C. Neurotypical language development
   D. Stuttering

5. When targeting echolalia in treatment, it is important to use low level language constraints. One example is:
   A. "Wh" questions
   B. Gestalt forms
   C. Commands
   D. All of the above

6. The percentage of children with ASD who demonstrate echolalia is:
   A. 85%
   B. 75%
   C. 50%
   D. 10%

7. A specific approach that targets, transforms, and builds upon echolalia is:
   A. Music therapy.
   B. Drama Kings and Queens.
   C. The Hanen approach.
   D. Cue–point-pause.
   E. All of the above.

8. Immediate echolalia happens:
   A. Within two conversational turns of the exchange.
   B. Within five to seven conversational turns of the exchange.
   C. After two conversational turns of the exchange.
   D. After three conversational turns of the exchange.

9. Complete the following chart (fill in the blanks):

Key strategy	Therapeutic presentation
Facilitate verbal initiations	Focus on opportunities for the client initiate language production rather than responding to questions and prompts.
Elicit careful and continual observations	
	Avoid using high constraint utterances like questions or commands.
Map language contents into known contexts	

REFERENCES

Ahearn, W., Clark, K., and MacDonald, R. (2007). Assessing and treating vocal stereotypy in children with autism. *Journal of Applied Behavior Analysis* 40 (2): 263–275.

American Speech–Language–Hearing Association. (2006). Principles for Speech–Language Pathologists in Diagnosis, Assessment, and Treatment of Autism Spectrum Disorders across the Life Span. Rockfield, MD: ASHA.

Andersen-Warren, M. (2013). Dramatherapy with children and young people who have autistic spectrum disorders: an examination of dramath 'rapists' practices. *Dramatherapy* 35 (1): 3–19.

Barrow, C.T.E. (1999). Delayed echoing as an interactional resource: A case study of a 3-year-old child on the autistic spectrum. *Clinical Linguistics and Phonetics* 13 (6): 449–482.

Beadle-Brown, J., Wilkinson, D., Richardson, L. et al. (2018). Imagining autism: feasibility of a drama-based intervention on the social, communicative and imaginative behavior of children with autism. *Autism* 22 (8): 915–927.

Bebko, J. (1990). Echolalia, mitigation, and autism: indicators from child characteristics for the use of sign language and other augmentative language systems. *Sigh Language Studies* 66: 61–78.

Bodfish, J., Symons, F., Parker, D., and Lewis, M. (2000). Varieties of repetitive behavior in autism: comparisons to mental retardation. *Journal of Autism and Developmental Disorders* 30 (3): 237–243.

Corbett, B., Gunther, J., Comins, D. et al. (2011). Brief report: theatre as therapy for children with autism spectrum disorder. *Journal of Autism and Developmental Disorders* 41: 505–511.

Dobbinson, S., Perkins, M., and Boucher, J. (2003). The interactional significance of formulas in autistic language. *Clinical Linguistics and Phonetics* 17 (4–5): 299–307.

Gladfelter, A. and Van Zuiden, C. (2020). The influence of language context on repetitive speech use in children with autism spectrum disorder. *American Journal of Speech-Language Pathology* 29 (1): 327–334.

Godfrey, E. and Haythorne, D. (2013). Benefits of dramatherapy for autism spectrum disorder: a qualitative analysis of feedback from parents and teachers of clients attending rounabout dramatherapy sessions in schools. *Dramatherapy* 35 (1): 20–28.

Grossi, D., Marcone, R., Cinquegrana, T., and Gallucci, M. (2012). On the differential nature of induced and incidental echolalia in autism. *Journal of Intellectual Disability Research* 57 (10): 903–912.

Howlin, P. (1982). Echolalic and spontaneous phrase speech in autistic children. *The Journal of Child Psychology and Psychiatry* 23 (3): 281–293.

Kanner, L. (1943). Autistic disturbances of affective contact. *Nervous Child* 2: 217–250.

Kenworthy, L., Wallace, G.L., Powell, K. et al. (2012). Early language milestones predict later language, but not autism symptoms in higher functioning children with autism spectrum disorders. *Research in Autism Spectrum Disorders* 6 (3): 1194–1202.

Lewis, M.H. and Bodfish, J.W. (1998). Repetitive behavior disorders in autism. *Mental Retardation and Developmental Disabilities Research Reviews* 4 (2): 80–89.

Lowry, L. (2018). *The Meaning Behind the Message: Helping Children Who Use Echolalia*. Toronto, ON: Hanen Centre Early Language Development Program.

Marom, M., Gilboa, A., and Bodner, E. (2018). Musical features and interactional functions of echolalia in children with autism within the music therapy dyad. *Nordic Journal of Music Therapy* 27 (3): 175–196.

Neely, L., Gerow, S., Rispoli, M. et al. (2016). Treatment of echolalia in individuals with autism spectrum disorder: a systematic review. *Journal of Autism and Developmental Disorders* 3: 82–91.

Prizant, B. and Duchan, J. (1981). The functions of immediate echolalia in autistic children. *Journal of Speech and Hearing Disorders* 46: 241–249.

Rapp, J., Patel, M., Ghezzi, P. et al. (2009). Establishing stimulus control of vocal stereotypy displayed by young children with autism. *Behavioral Interventions* 24 (2): 85–105.

Schuler, A. (1979). Echolalia: issues and clinical applications. *Journal of Speech and Hearing Disorders* 44: 411–434.

Shield, A., Cooley, F., and Meier, R.P. (2017). Sign language echolalia in deaf children with autism spectrum disorder. *Journal of Speech, Language, and Hearing Research: JSLHR* 60 (6): 1622–1634.

Stefanatos, G.A. (2008). Regression in autistic spectrum disorders. *Neuropsychology Review* 18 (4): 305–319.

Sterponi, L. and Shankey, J. (2014). Rethinking echolalia: Repetition as interactional resource in the communication of a child with autism. *Journal of Child Language* 41: 275–304.

Stiegler, L.N. (2015). Examining the echolalia literature: where do speech-language pathologists stand? *American Journal of Speech-Language Pathology* 24: 750–762.

Stribling, P., Rae, J., Dickerson, P., and Dautenhahn, K. (2006). "Spelling it out": the design, delivery, and placement of delayed echolalic utterances by a child with an autistic spectrum disorder. *Issues in Applied Linguistics* 15 (1): 3–32.

Stubblefield, H. (2021). Understanding echolalia. Healthline, 19 November. Available from https://www.healthline.com/health/echolalia (accesse3d 1 February 2022).

Sussman, F. (2012). *More than Words: A Parent's to Building Interaction and Language Skills for Children with Autism Spectrum Disorder or Social Communication Difficulties*, 2e. Toronto, ON: Hanen Centre.

Taylor, B.A., Hoch, H., and Weissman, M. (2005). The analysis and treatment of vocal stereotypy in a child with autism. *Behavioral Interventions* 20 (4): 239–253.

Trudel, C. and Nadig, A. (2019). A role-play assessment tool and drama-based social skills intervention for adults with autism or related social communication difficulties. *Dramatherapy* 40 (1): 41–60.

Valentino, A.L., Shillingsburg, M.A., Conine, D.E., and Powell, N.M. (2012). Decreasing echolalia of the instruction "say" during echoic training through use of the cues-pause-point procedure. *Journal of Behavioral Education* 21 (4): 315–328.

Van Santen, J., Sproat, R., and Hill, A. (2013). Quantifying repetitive speech in autism spectrum disorders and language impairment. *Autism Research* 6 (5): 372–383.

Wing, L. and Wing, J.K. (1971). Multiple impairments in early childhood autism. *Journal of Autism and Childhood Schizophrenia* 1 (3): 256–266.

FURTHER READINGS

Blanc, M. (2013). Echolalia on the spectrum: The natural path to self-generated language. *Autism Asperger's Digest*, March/April.

Hyams, P., Rae, J., and Dickerson, P. (2007). Two forms of spoken repetition in a girl with autism. *International Journal of Language and Communication Disorders* 42 (2): 427–444.

Peters, A. (1972). Language learning strategies: does the whole equal the sum of the parts? *Language* 53 (3): 560–573.

Roberts, J. (2014). Echolalia and language development in children with autism. In: *Beyond Echolalia: Promoting language in children with autism* (ed. J. Arciuli and J. Brock), 55–74. Amsterdam, The Netherlands: John Benjamins.

Schuler, A., Rydell, P., and Mirenda, P. (1994). Effects of high and low constraint utterances on the production of immediate and delayed echolalia in young children with autism. *Journal of Autism and Developmental Disorders* 24: 719–735.

CHAPTER 9

Autism and Social Justice

Learning Objectives

By reading this chapter, interventionists will be able to:

1. Define cultural competence and describe its importance in autism spectrum disorder (ASD) diagnosis and treatment.
2. List the steps of the cultural competence continuum.
3. Identify how individuals with autism from different cultural backgrounds may experience racism and prejudice.
4. Identify resources to continue to develop your cultural competence as an interventionist working with individuals with ASD.

This chapter starts by introducing concepts critical to understanding the intersection of autism and social justice. While this topic is not covered in depth, we do seek to introduce a cursory explanation on how interventionists might frame their professional work within a larger context. We hope this introductory framework will encourage clinicians to think holistically about their work with individuals with autism, especially clients with autism from minority backgrounds.

Autism Spectrum Disorders from Theory to Practice: Assessment and Intervention Tools Across the Lifespan,
First Edition. Edited by Belinda Daughrity and Ashley Wiley Johnson.
© 2023 John Wiley & Sons Ltd. Published 2023 by John Wiley & Sons Ltd.

CULTURAL COMPETENCE AND AUTISM SPECTRUM DISORDER

Professions that intersect both educational and health-related fields have a unique opportunity to help address social injustices by alleviating disparities contributing to existing inequities among marginalized communities (Horton 2021). The American Speech–Language–Hearing Association (ASHA) defines **cultural competence** as involving understanding and appropriately responding to the combination of cultural variables and the range of dimensions of diversity that the professional and client/family bring to interactions (Table 9.1). This definition is important because it specifies that both the professional and the client are key. Often, professionals may consider only the client perspective and fail to realize that, to demonstrate cultural competence, professionals must understand their own culture as well. Many may have a narrow view of culture, failing to grasp all its parameters, which include categories like race, sex, gender, sexual orientation, socioeconomic class, religion, age, and ability/disability. We encourage all clinicians to take time to identify their culture, recognize the values and perspectives influenced by that culture, and acknowledge the privileges that may be afforded some of those cultural identities. Completing the Matrix of Oppression exercise that can be found in *Teaching for Diversity and Social Justice* (Adams and Bell 2016) can be a very helpful activity to frame social identity through the lens of privilege.

Cultural competence is key in ASD diagnosis and treatment because diagnosis is largely influenced by caregiver report and perceptions of behavioral presentations. Clinicians must be able to use appropriate parent interview approaches to effectively discern the presence or absence of ASD symptomology, as well as appropriately interpreting parental concerns. When interpreting client behaviors, clinicians must be sure that cultural bias is not interfering with their clinical judgment. In intervention, treatment fidelity and parent buy-in might be significantly impacted by provider factors influencing the clinical interaction.

TABLE 9.1   Key Definitions according to the American Speech-Language Hearing Association (ASHA).

Term	Definition
Cultural competence	The knowledge and skill needed to address language and culture; this knowledge and skill evolves over time and spans lifelong learning.
Cultural humility	A lifelong commitment to engaging in self-evaluation and self-critique and to remedying the power imbalance implicit to clinical interactions.
Culturally responsive practice	Responding to and serving individuals within the context of their cultural background, and the ability to learn from and relate respectfully with people of other cultures.

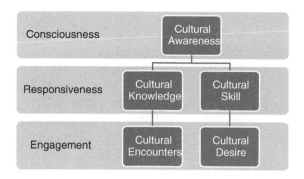

FIGURE 9.1   The cultural competence continuum.

Differentiating between key terms such as cultural competence and cultural humility is important for all clinicians who aim to conduct ethical care for culturally, linguistically diverse clients. The term "competence" can signal an idea of completion, which directly contradicts the spirit of cultural competence as a lifelong learning process. As such, some prefer the term "cultural humility," which connotes continuing acknowledgment that, because we never know it all, we continue to remain humble as we grow and improve our skills over time. Clinicians must acknowledge the assumptions and biases we hold so we can build our professionalism with diverse families and create clinical spaces of mutual respect and collaboration (Harry 2018). These skills contribute to our ability to demonstrate *cultural responsiveness*, where we acknowledge the important role of culture in our interactions and thus respond appropriately to our clients to provide them the best ethical care (Figure 9.1).

Cultural awareness is a critical first step in the cultural competence continuum because the ability to understand one's own culture is important to understand the unique perspectives and bias you bring to the interaction (Campinha-Bacote 2002; Hunt and Swiggum 2007). Scholar Kimberle Crenshaw explains the term intersectionality, which is important for clinicians to be aware of their own perspective of autism and disability when interacting with families, while noting how the intersection of their cultural identities informs that perspective.

Active Learning Task

Consider how your own cultural background impacts your interpretation of autism and how you think about best practices for treatment. Does your cultural background promote a medical or social model of disability? How does your culture perceive medicine in general? Do you tend to defer to science and trust professional expertise? Once you thoroughly understand your own cultural perspective, you can begin to understand how other cultures may present with wholly different perspectives.

Cultural knowledge and *cultural skill* are critical for responsiveness when working with individuals with autism. Interventionists should be aware of other cultures and perspectives so they can respond appropriately during clinical interactions. For example, when working with families with autism, it may be important to know how cultures perceive neurodevelopmental disorders like autism. As such, it might be appropriate to go about the diagnosis process in a less direct manner to allow the family appropriate time to process the diagnosis and seek out targeted intervention services.

Cultural knowledge may be challenging, considering that many clinicians may have limited experiences with culturally and linguistically diverse communities. However, it is important to note that clinical care should go beyond cultural sensitivity because clinicians must have specific knowledge and skills in distinguishing disorders from differences (Crowley et al. 2015). In working with individuals with autism, knowing about cultural norms is critically important, especially as much of the diagnostic criteria of ASD is behaviorally based. For example, if eye contact with adults is not an appropriate behavior in a particular culture, a clinician should not cite lack of eye contact as a key diagnostic indicator for a client, who may simply be following appropriate cultural norms. Research in allied health fields such as nursing indicates cultural competence can be promoted in pre-professionals via observations and clinical encounters to develop and expand interviewing techniques, the ability to become flexible with assessment procedures, and an appreciation for the client's perspective (Hunt and Swiggum 2007).

To be an effective clinician working with individuals with autism, a clinician should always be on a journey of cultural competence, understanding that there is always more to learn and space to grow. Cultural competence is not a point on a to-do list; rather, it requires interactions and cultural experiences to continually evolve (Hyter and Salas-Provance 2019). Evidence suggests that even brief learning modules delivered asynchronously can help to increase awareness among novel interventionists such as pre-professionals (Daughrity 2021).

Active Learning Task

Take a moment and respond to the following questions keeping your own culture, in mind.

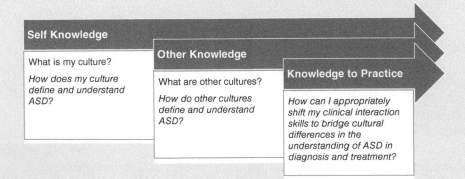

The arrows on the figure indicate a continuing process, rather than a finite ending.

When working with families with ASD, it is important to demonstrate cultural responsiveness when working with culturally, linguistically diverse families. It is *not* appropriate to treat all families the same, since every family will enter with different circumstances unique to their cultural background. Many clinicians make the mistake of saying, "I treat all families the same, so I do a great job because I treat them equally." However, it is important to recognize that our goal is *not* to treat each client and family equally. Our goal is to treat them *equitably* so we meet their unique needs to provide ethical and effective clinical care (Figure 9.2).

Cross et al. (1989) discuss the cultural competence continuum as a range of skills from cultural destructiveness to cultural proficiency (Figure 9.3). At the far extreme of

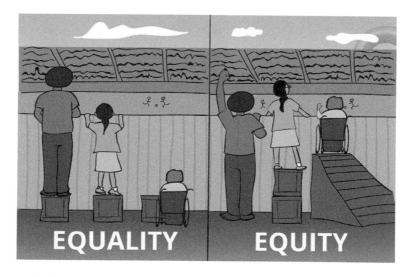

FIGURE 9.2   Equity, not equality.

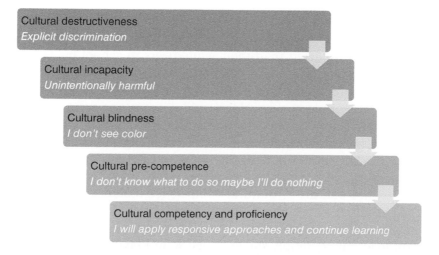

FIGURE 9.3   The cultural competence continuum.

the spectrum, *cultural destructiveness* includes explicitly discriminatory and harmful practices against groups that serve as points of future distrust of systems. Such practices can contribute to distrust of healthcare systems. For example, in our practice, some parents have expressed beliefs that vaccines caused their child's autism. The link between vaccines and autism has been firmly discredited (Taylor et al. 2014). Particularly for families of color, rather than simply dismissing their beliefs, consider *why* they might have a distrust of healthcare systems in light of historical medical abuses such as the case of the Tuskegee experiment.

Active Learning Task

Look up the following:

- Tuskegee experiment
- Mississippi appendectomies
- Madrigal v. Quilligan
- Relf v. Weinberger

Considering these historical cases, how might the family of a client with autism from a minority background respond with distrust of the healthcare system?

Cultural incapacity does not include intentional harm, but may include policies or practices that harm diverse communities. For example, among culturally, linguistically diverse families of clients with ASD, poor clinical experiences with interventionists who fail to apply interaction styles to engage families appropriately in assessment and intervention may contribute to less buy-in and use of available services.

Cultural blindness, while often well intended, also contributes to harm. Those who report, "I don't see color" often fail to recognize systemic inequalities that adversely impact communities of color. For example, research indicates Black and African-American students with autism and other language and learning disorders are more negatively impacted than their white peers in school by zero tolerance policies contributing to the school-to-prison pipeline and the overrepresentation of students of color with disabilities in the juvenile justice system (Johnson and Muhammad 2018). Failure to see color would prevent one from acknowledging disproportionality in school discipline between racial groups, allowing such mistreatment to continue without further exploration.

Cultural pre-competence reflects the desire of agencies and individuals to do better, although such attempts may not be successful if they do not reflect the need to continually learn and grow. Cultural competence includes *cultural proficiency* and *cultural humility* as professionals actively seek out knowledge and recognize that the journey of cultural competence is never complete because it is a lifelong commitment to learning. Simply stated, if you want to be better at serving diverse families with autism to deliver high impact and quality clinical care, you have to do the work!

Active Learning Task

Complete the online self-assessment and quiz below.

- ASHA Self-Assessment for Cultural Competence `http://www.asha.org/practice/multicultural/self`
- That's Unheard Of `www.thatsunheardof.org`

Once you have completed them, consider the following questions:
- What did I learn?
- What do I want to learn?
- How will I continue to learn to benefit my clients with autism?

THE INTERSECTION OF SOCIAL JUSTICE AND AUTISM

Although cursory evidence indicates individuals with ASD are not overly represented in the criminal justice system (King and Murphy 2014), forensic speech–language pathologists have recognized that individuals with autism and other communication disorders can be at increased risk of punishment due to misinterpretation of their communication deficits (Stanford 2019). Violence is not a core feature of ASD. Some suggest those with ASD who are violent may have difficulty empathizing with victims due to difficulty with theory of mind and understanding others' perspectives (Baron-Cohen 1988; Barry-Walsh and Mullen 2007).

Emerging research indicates that criminal judges and juries may encounter complex issues when considering individuals with autism and determining their culpability and appropriate sentencing in criminal proceedings (Berryessa 2014a, 2014b; Berryessa 2016; Allely and Cooper 2017). Evidence suggests that media portrayals inappropriately linking autism to violent behavior may adversely impact both members of the public and judicial system (Berryessa 2014a, 2014b). As experts in the presentation of individuals with autism, clinicians specializing in this disorder are uniquely positioned to offer critically needed education and professional advice during criminal proceedings to help inform ethical and appropriate judgments (Freckelton 2013). Further, it is recognized that those in criminal justice careers may benefit from training to better engage with those with low symptom severity autism and other disabilities, as poor understanding of ASD can often lead to misunderstanding, with catastrophic consequences for those with autism and their families (Browning and Caulfield 2011).

Active Learning Task

Listen to the podcast or read the transcript. Discuss how you might work with young adults with autism to navigate encounters with the police:

- Gray, J.D. (2019). ASHA Voices Podcast Premiere: Communication Disorders and the Justice System. *LeaderLive*, 11 September: `https://leader.pubs.asha.org/do/10.1044/asha-voices-cognitive-communication-disorders-and-the-justice-system/full`

Recall the discussion in Chapter 4 about clear disparities between healthcare providers and those they serve. It is important for clinicians to consider intersectionality and to consider the client's full existence during treatment. For example, considering the COVID-19 pandemic, more parents of color of children with autism reported vaccine hesitancy than their white counterparts (Chang and Kochel 2020).

Considering that the criminal justice system disproportionately impacts people of color as well as communities that are economically impoverished, it can be logically deduced that low-income, minority individuals with ASD may be even further at risk of potentially negative interactions with members of law enforcement and subsequently the criminal justice system. Factors that may place an individual at increased risk for criminal justice offenses include poor education, late diagnosis, and the presence of additional comorbid conditions (Dein and Woodbury-Smith 2010). It is important to note that factors such as late diagnosis of ASD and poor educational attainment disproportionately impact low-income communities of color, which indicates these particular individuals with autism may be especially at risk. There is evidence that many offenders with autism are only first diagnosed with ASD after incarceration, and such individuals may have experienced different outcomes had they received appropriate diagnosis and treatment (Mayes 2003). It is important for clinicians to understand that in the current education and criminal justice system, not all individuals are equally treated, nor do they have equal access to opportunities and supports.

ACCESS TO SERVICES AS A SOCIAL JUSTICE ISSUE

Clinicians working with culturally, linguistically diverse families with autism need to consider systemic barriers that adversely impact access to services. For example, as an example of cultural incapacity where systems are not intentionally culturally destructive but still lack the capacity to adequately assist minority clients, consider the 2017 report on disparities in services provided to clients with disabilities in California (Public Counsel 2017). Findings indicated that minority clients with autism and other disabilities received fewer intervention services than their white counterparts.

Consider how these disparities might impact a minority family of a child with autism. Findings indicate that these families might receive fewer services not related to severity of the diagnosis, but solely related to their racial and ethnic background. Overall, although the gap has narrowed, research indicates African-American and Hispanic children are more likely to be diagnosed with autism at a later age (Valicenti-McDermott et al. 2012). Additionally, considering that minority communities are overrepresented in poverty and jobs with lower wages with limited access to benefits like health insurance, minority families of children with autism may have reduced access to healthcare services and medical insurance to access targeted intervention services. As an interventionist dedicated to serving all families, these types of disparities should be particularly troubling for those specializing in ASD, since we know that early access to services and targeted interventions can significantly impact the trajectory of the disorder. If we consider the potential impact, we can certainly connect disparities for clients with autism to social justice because early intervention services promote optimal outcomes, which means lack of access can potentially reduce the opportunities of ideal results and quality of life for clients of color.

How Can Clinicians Make a Difference for Clients?

As interventionists, we must each do our very best to *adopt* culturally responsive clinical interaction practices that best serve our clients' unique needs, *assist* our clients in developing the social communication skills needed to interact appropriately with others, resolve conflicts peacefully, and ask for help as needed, and *advocate* on their behalf by making others aware of their language and social communication deficits that can be inappropriately interpreted, as well as helping to dismantle systems that prevent equitable access to care.

Interventionists might consider targeting the following areas to help support positive encounters between clients with autism and law enforcement, or to minimize negative outcomes with the social justice system.

Understanding Others' Perspectives and Nonverbal Cues

Understanding the perspectives and nonverbal cues of others is often adversely impacted in individuals with autism, who may display difficulty with theory of mind and may assume that their perspective is the only one. Activities that help individuals with autism understand different points of view are critical to addressing this social communication deficit.

Therapy Golden Nugget

Suggested intervention activities

- Try reading a book and talking about the different perspectives of the characters in response to the same event.
- Watch a movie trailer or short film and talk about the reactions of the different characters.
- Interpret nonverbal cues such as facial expressions to infer emotions.

Making Predictions

Making predictions can help clients to understand potential consequences of their actions, as in, "If I do X, the result may be Y." Some clients with autism may have trouble making predictions because they only consider the here and now. Tasks that help clients to understand what might come next can help them adjust their behavior to obtain a desired response.

Therapy Golden Nugget

Suggested intervention activities

Sequencing picture cards: Show clients two related picture cards and ask them to predict the next card in the sequence. For example, you might show related pictures and say:

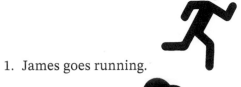

1. James goes running.

2. It starts to rain.

3. *What will happen next?*

Appropriate answers may be: "James will get wet," or "James will run home."

Make predictions through book or media share; ask the client, "What do you think will happen next?" Consider using visual cues. Once students make a prediction, continue the task to see the final outcome. Discuss whether the student was correct or incorrect. What clues might have been missed that would have predicted the next action?

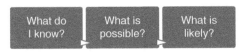

Following Directions

Following directions can help clients to follow verbal commands successfully, such as those that may be given during a traffic stop. Some clients may have difficulty processing, or they might have difficulty following directions without cues, challenges which may be perceived as non-compliance by law enforcement officers unfamiliar with receptive language deficits in autism or other disorders adversely impacting speech and language skills. This lack of understanding of ASD and language-related deficits may contribute to encounters being escalated due to a perceived threat.

Therapy Golden Nugget

Suggested intervention activities

Following directions tasks: Target following one- or two-step commands with fading cues.

Spatial concepts: Target following commands with spatial concepts, which might mirror encounters requiring clients to put their hands *on* the wheel or *behind* their back. This type of task might be particularly helpful for individuals with ASD who are more independent and engaged in tasks such as driving or walking around the community.

Role playing: Practice encounters with authority figures such law enforcement officers or campus police with your clients. It might be helpful to try this task with different tones of voice, since encounters may involve officers yelling commands and this behavior may be startling to clients and cause confusion.

Social Skills Groups

Social skills groups can be particularly helpful for individuals with autism to target increasing appropriate social interaction skills with peers, as well as prompting discussions about appropriate interactions with law enforcement officers, teachers, and other authority figures. In addition to directly teaching appropriate skills, groups offer increased prospects to develop appropriate peer relationships. For example, in cases of individuals with autism exhibiting stalking behaviors, direct intervention approaches using evidenced-based practices like video modeling, social stories, scripts, and visual supports can be helpful to reduce and redirect such behaviors, while also offering opportunities for appropriate social integration (Post et al. 2012). Overall, establishing friendships may serve as a support for individuals with autism in preventing isolation and loneliness, providing companionship, and offering opportunities for positive, productive social interaction Figure 9.4.

HARD TRUTHS: CASES TO EXPLORE

Consider some of the cases of individuals with autism and the criminal justice system that received national news coverage such as Matthew Rushin, Neli Latson, Preston Wolfe (see box), and Charles Kinsey and Arnaldo Rios Soto.

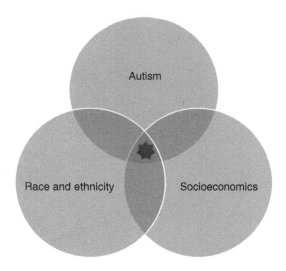

FIGURE 9.4   Disparities that impact a minority family of a child with autism. * Maximum impact.

The Case of Preston Wolfe

By Minyvonne Burke. NBC News, April 23, 2021.

A California father accused a police officer of being unnecessarily aggressive during an incident involving his teenage son, who has autism. The father said a Vacaville officer threw his son, Preston, 17, to the ground and punched him in the face during a citation Wednesday afternoon.

"I am pro police, but I am not pro ABUSE," Adam Wolf wrote in a Facebook page on Thursday. "This individual and department must be held accountable for their actions. NO child, disability or not, deserves to be treated like this."

Police said an officer was dispatched to the area around 2:30 p.m. for a report of a possible stabbing or assault with either a knife or a pipe. The officer found the victim of the assault, a 16-year-old boy, who had minor injuries that did not require medical attention, the department said in a press release.

The officer then found the suspect, a 17-year-old boy, police said.

"The officer asked the suspect to sit down, which he did. When the police officer took out his handcuffs, the suspect actively began resisting arrest, trying to get up and run. In response, the officer forced the suspect to the ground and onto his stomach," the press release states.

The incident was captured on a Ring doorbell video, which Wolf shared on his Facebook page.

In the footage, the officer is heard telling Preston to sit down. "I'm not going to tell you again, sit down," the officer says.

Preston sits on the curb. The video shows the officer grabbing something from the teen and throwing it.

The teen then gets up and appears to run away, but the officer grabs him and slams him to the ground, the video shows. A second doorbell-camera video shows what appears to be a scuffle between the officer and Preston.

"You're going to get hurt," the officer says. "Don't make me hurt you more."

Wolf said in his Facebook post that his son has autism and ADHD and "looks and acts younger than he is."

He accused the officer of throwing his son's scooter and said Preston tried to leave because he was scared.

"My son became fearful, as would any child with Autism. The officer went to touch Preston, at which point Preston moves away. At this point, Preston was confused and afraid and moves away from the officer even more," Wolf wrote. "At that point the officer felt it was a good idea to THROW Preston to the ground. Once on the ground, the officer climbed on top of Preston and PUNCHED him in the face."

Wolf could not be reached by NBC News on Friday. He told NBC Bay Area that he thought the officer's actions were "sickening and it shouldn't have happened."

Police said the teen was arrested and detained for about an hour before he was cited and released to his stepmother. The officer, who has not been identified, was unaware that the teen has special needs, the department said in its release.

"We understand the video posted on social media can appear very disturbing," said acting police Chief Ian Schmutzler. "When we receive a 911 call involving an assault with a deadly weapon and potential stabbing, we respond immediately to ensure we keep those in the vicinity safe. Our officer had a clear description of the suspect and the minor who was arrested fit this description."

The Vacaville Police Department is handling the investigation into the incident.

Reproduced with permission from NBC News.

Active Learning Task

1. Imagine you are the interventionist for the client described above. While we cannot predict outcomes, what types of skills would you target that might have improved outcomes?

2. Now imagine you are called to give a statement to a court regarding your clients above. What would your statement include?

3. Next, imagine you are called to give a training presentation on autism to either law enforcement or members of the court (judges, jury members, etc.). What would your presentation include to help better inform criminal justice stakeholders about ASD?

4. Research and investigate another case of an individual with autism encountering law enforcement. Once the chart below is completed, exchange it with a peer for discussion

Name	What are the case details (when, where, who)?	How might ASD symptomology be involved?	How might bias be involved?

When Individuals with Autism Encounter Law Enforcement

For all clients with autism, but particularly for young men of color with autism, it may be appropriate to directly address expected behaviors when interacting with law enforcement officers. While this type of topic might be uncomfortable for clinicians, many of whom have not experienced negative encounters with police officers themselves, such topics addressed in intervention may prove life altering for clients with autism. Interventionists might discuss the benefits of disclosing an autism diagnosis during encounters with law enforcement. Disclosure may help an officer to be more sensitive to atypical behavior that can be misconstrued as aggressive. Some states may have autism disclosure cards for clients to use during police encounters. By disclosing and asking for help, individuals with autism may benefit from the presence of a parent or guardian or appropriate advocate to consider their best interests when engaging with law enforcement.

In addition to reviewing social skill steps about these encounters, role-playing events may be helpful to provide additional practice so that individuals with ASD have experience of thinking about their actions and practicing appropriate engagement. Unfortunately, these practices do not guarantee that negative encounters will be avoided. As such, clinicians should continue to seek to address bias within systems themselves, in addition to engaging in their clinical practices with clients.

Active Learning Task

A Case for Comparison

Client A   Client B

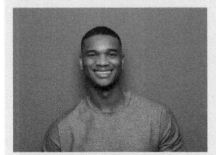   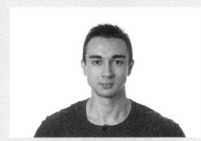

mimagephotos/Adobe Stock   Axel Bueckert/Adobe Stock

1. Considering the life points mentioned at the start of this section, and in particular that case of Preston Wolfe (Box 9.1), how might a client with autism who is also a student of color have different experiences than a white peer?

2. Assuming that ASD symptomology is equal, what systemic inequalities might exist for the student of color? How is "I don't see color" harmful?

Diagnostic Process   Community Experiences
                            Transitioning to Adulthood

Intervention Experiences in School

SUMMARY

Cultural competence is important to effectively diagnose and treat individuals with autism from culturally, linguistically diverse backgrounds. Clinicians should seek to demonstrate cultural responsiveness in their intervention with clients with autism and their families. Unintentional bias may play a role in disproportionate service delivery and support to clients with autism from diverse backgrounds, while flawed educational and criminal justice systems may exacerbate disparities for communities of color. While helping clients to improve their skills, clinicians should continually seek to advocate for clients individually and, when possible, to make improvements to systems more broadly to improve equity and provide ethical, quality care to all clients. For professionals working with clients with autism, in addition to cultural competence that considers the intersectionality of oppression, care should be given to actively employ anti-racist practices in assessment and intervention.

TEST QUESTIONS

1. Explain and define your own culture. What various intersectionality do you encompass? Why is knowledge of your own culture important to serve clients with autism from diverse backgrounds?

2. Why is cultural competence relevant for assessment and intervention practices with ASD?

3. How can poor cultural competence contribute to disparities in ASD diagnosis and treatment?

4. How will you continue to develop your cultural competence as a professional working with individuals with autism? Identify specific resources and professional continuing education you will pursue.

5. How is cultural responsiveness clinically useful for clients with and without autism?

REFERENCES

Adams, A. and Bell, L.E. (2016). *Teaching for Diversity and Social Justice*. Hoboken, NJ: Routledge.

Allely, C. and Cooper, P. (2017). Jurors' and Judges' evaluation of defendants with autism and the impact on sentencing: a systematic preferred reporting items for systematic reviews and meta-analyses (PRISMA) review of autism spectrum disorder in the courtroom. *Journal of Law and Medicine* 25 (1): 105–123.

Baron-Cohen, S. (1988). An assessment of violence in a young man with Asperger's syndrome. *Journal of Child Psychology and Psychiatry* 29 (3): 351–360.

Barry-Walsh, J. and Mullen, P. (2007). Forensic aspects of Asperger's syndrome. *The Journal of Forensic Psychiatry and Psychology* 15 (1): 96–107.

Berryessa, C. (2014a). Judicial perceptions of media portrayals of offenders with high functioning autistic spectrum disorders. *International Journal of Criminology and Sociology* 3: 46–60.

Berryessa, C. (2014b). Judiciary views on criminal behavior and intention of offenders with high functioning autism. *Journal of Intellectual Disabilities and Offending Behaviour* 5 (2): 97–106.

Berryessa, C. (2016). Brief report: judicial attitudes regarding the sentencing of offenders with high functioning autism. *Journal of Autism and Developmental Disorders* 46 (8): 2770–2773.

Browning, A. and Caulfield, L. (2011). The prevalence and treatment of people with asperger's syndrome in the criminal justice system. *Criminology & Criminal Justice* 121 (2): 165 180.

Campinha-Bacote, J. (2002). Cultural competence in the delivery of healthcare services: a model of care. *Journal of Transcultural Nursing* 13 (3): 181–184.

Chang, J. and Kochel, R. (2020). Vaccine hesitancy and attributions for autism among racially and ethnically diverse groups of parents of children with autism spectrum disorder: a pilot study. *Autism Research* 13 (10): 1790–1796.

Cross, T., Bazron, B., Dennis, K., & Isaacs, M. (1989). *Towards a Culturally Competent System of Care: A Monograph on Effective Services for Minority Children Who Are Severely Emotionally Disturbed*. Washington, DC: CASSP Technical Assistance Center, Georgetown University Child Development Center.

Crowley, C., Guest, K., and Sudler, K. (2015). Cultural competence needed to distinguish disorder from difference: beyond Kumbaya. *Perspectives on Communication Disorders and Sciences in Culturally and Linguistically Diverse (CLD) Populations* 22 (2): 64–76.

Daughrity, B. (2021). Exploring outcomes of an asynchronous learning module on increasing cultural competence for speech-language pathology graduate students. *American Journal of Speech-Language Pathology*.

Dein, K. and Woodbury-Smith, M. (2010). Asperger syndrome and criminal behavior. *Advances in Psychiatric Treatment* 16: 37–43.

Freckelton, I. (2013). Autism spectrum disorder: forensic issues and challenges for mental health professionals and courts. *Journal of Applied Research in Intellectual Disabilities* 26 (5): 420–434.

Harry, E. (2018). Cultural reciprocity in special education: building bridges to cross-cultural understanding with parent. *Journal of Early Childhood Studies* 2 (2): 383–396.

Horton, R. (2021). *Critical Perspectives on Social Justice in Speech-Language Pathology*. Hershey, PA: IGI Global.

Hunt, R. and Swiggum, P. (2007). Being in another world transcultural student experiences using service learning with families who are homeless. *Journal of Transcultural Nursing* 18 (2): 167–174.

Hyter, Y.D. and Salas-Provance, M.B. (2019). *Culturally Responsive Practices in Speech, Language, and Hearing Sciences*. San Diego, CA: Plural Publishing.

Johnson, S. and Muhammad, B. (2018). The confluence of language and learning disorders and the school-to-prison pipeline among minority students of color: a critical race theory. *American University Journal of Gender, Social Policy and the Law* 26 (2): 691–718.

King, C. and Murphy, G. (2014). A systematic review of people with autism spectrum disorder and the criminal justice system. *Journal of Autism and Developmental Disorders* 44 (11): 2717–2733.

Mayes, T. (2003). Persons with autism and criminal justice: core concepts and leading causes. *Journal of Positive Behavior Interventions* 5 (2): 92–100.

Post, M., Haymes, L., Storey, K. et al. (2012). Understanding stalking behaviors by individuals with autism spectrum disorders and recommended prevention strategies in school settings. *Journal of Autism and Developmental Disorders* 44: 2698–2706.

Counsel, P. (2017). *Assuring Equitable Funding of Services for Children with Developmental Disabilities*. Palo Alto, CA: Lucile Packard Foundation for Children's Health.

Stanford, S. (2019). Casualties of misunderstanding: communication disorders and juvenile injustice. *The ASHA Leader* 24: 44–53.

Taylor, L.E., Swerdfeger, A.L., and Eslick, G.D. (2014). Vaccines are not associated with autism: an evidence-based meta-analysis of case-control and cohort studies. *Vaccine* 32 (29): 3623–3629.

Valicenti-McDermott, M., Hottinger, K., Seijo, R., and Shulman, L. (2012). Age at diagnosis of autism spectrum disorders. *Journal of Pediatrics* 161 (3): 554–556.

FURTHER READINGS

Derr, A. (2003). Growing diversity in our schools: roles and responsibilities of speech language pathologists. *Perspectives on Language Learning and Education* 10 (2): 7–12.

Ebert, K. (2013). Perceptions of racial privilege in prospective speech-language pathologists and audiologists. *Perspectives on Communication Disorders and Sciences in Culturally and Linguistically Diverse (CLD) Populations* 20 (2): 60–71.

Hampton, S., Rabagliati, H., Sorace, A., and Fletcher-Watson, S. (2017). Autism and bilingualism: a qualitative interview study of parents' perspectives and experiences. *Journal of Speech, Language, and Hearing Research* 60: 435–446.

Ijalba, E. (2016). Hispanic immigrant mothers of young children with autism spectrum disorders: how do they understand and cope with autism? *American Journal of Speech-Language Pathology* 25 (2): 200–213.

Keller-Bell, Y. (2017). Disparities in the identification and diagnosis of autism spectrum disorders in culturally and linguistically diverse populations. *Perspectives of the ASHA Special Interests Groups* 2 (14): 68–81.

Pearson, J., Hamilton, M., and Meadan, H. (2018). "We saw our son blossom": a guide for fostering culturally responsive partnerships to support African American autistic children and their families. *Perspectives of the ASHA Special Interest Groups* 3 (1): 84–97.

Riquelme, L. (2013). Cultural competence for everyone: a shift in perspectives. *Perspectives on Gerontology* 18 (2): 42–49.

Wiley, P., Gentry, B.F., and Torres-Feliciano, J. (2016). *Autism: Attacking Social Interaction Problems – A Therapy Manual Targeting Social Skills in Children 4–9*. San Diego, CA: Plural Publishing.

CHAPTER 10

Autism and Augmentative and Alternative Communication

Learning Objectives

By reading this chapter, interventionists will be able to:

1. Define augmentative and alternative communication (AAC).
2. Identify at least one high- and one low-tech AAC system that could be employed with a minimally verbal individual with autism.
3. Describe the importance of caregiver buy-in for AAC success for students with autism.
4. List the four different considerations for communicative competence for individuals with autism using an AAC system.

A new classroom assistant was facilitating a book-share task with a small group of young children with autism spectrum disorder (ASD). During the reading, she occasionally stopped to ask comprehension questions to the children. She had her nonverbal client point to pictures in the book. When the lead teacher entered the room, she asked about the student's iPad to communicate. The assistant responded, "Oh I didn't think we needed it for this." The teacher immediately responded, "You need it for everything! The device is the student's voice!"

Autism Spectrum Disorders from Theory to Practice: Assessment and Intervention Tools Across the Lifespan,
First Edition. Edited by Belinda Daughrity and Ashley Wiley Johnson.
© 2023 John Wiley & Sons Ltd. Published 2023 by John Wiley & Sons Ltd.

AAC is a mode of communicating in addition to or in place of verbal speech. This approach may be helpful for individuals with autism who have significant difficulty producing verbal speech or who might present with significantly reduced speech intelligibility when using verbal communication, which results in reduced communicative competence. While this population of children with autism who are minimally verbal are typically highly heterogeneous due to widely variable symptom presentation, augmentative methods are often identified as helpful approaches to improve communication skills (Tager-Flusberg and Kasari 2013). As such, individuals with autism can significantly benefit from incorporating AAC when unable to use typical speech (Ganz 2015). It is important to remember that the overall goal is to facilitate effective communication; AAC may be a way to help achieve that goal so messages are more effectively conveyed to a communication partner. Evidence supports the use of speech-generating devices (*SGDs*) with children with ASD while employing behavioral and naturalistic intervention approaches (Meer and Rispoli 2010). Individuals with ASD using AAC often demonstrate improved speech, although use of AAC continues to exceed verbal output (White et al. 2021).

AAC can often be misunderstood by many professionals, especially those with less clinical experience, indicating less confidence and limited experience in supporting students with AAC (Light and Drager 2007; Sanders et al. 2021). Among early career speech–language pathologists (SLPs), many reported a need for more explicit training in AAC, particularly as it relates to morphology and syntax (Kovacs 2021). It is important to recognize that nonverbal does not mean noncommunicative, as these students may just expressively communicate in diverse ways other than verbal speech.

NONSPEAKING ≢ NONTHINKING!

Nonspeaking does not mean nonthinking! Many individuals without verbal speech can have average receptive language skills, which is why it is important to explore alternative modes to verbal speech if that modality is not successful. For example, in our years of practice, we have often encountered clients who are nonverbal but can communicate wonderful ideas once given a modality to facilitate expression. While AAC implementation itself benefits from specialized expertise and instruction, ultimately, we hope that this chapter helps to clarify some misconceptions and encourage practitioners to consider this approach if appropriate for your minimally verbal client with autism.

NONVERBAL AND MINIMALLY VERBAL CLIENTS WITH AUTISM

"Nonverbal" and "minimally verbal" are frequently used in clinical practice and in research literature, although definitions often vary, indicating a need for more consistent descriptive practices to better understand the significant heterogeneity among this population (Koegel et al. 2020). It should be noted that some families and/or clients with autism may prefer using the term "preverbal" or "minimally verbal" to acknowledge the presence of limited speech or the possibility of future speech, rather than "nonverbal."

Some individuals classified as nonverbal may present with some limited verbal speech. For the sake of this text, we define **minimally verbal** as individuals demonstrating less than 10 intelligible single words across contexts. These individuals with autism often present as significantly heterogeneous because ASD is a heterogeneous disorder and this particular population may present with additional comorbid conditions such as intellectual disability and/or motoric challenges. Often, these individuals may present with maladaptive behaviors due to significant frustration at being unable to successfully communicate wants and needs. "**Preverbal**" may be used as a term for younger children with autism who have yet to develop verbal speech, while minimally verbal or nonverbal may be used for children who have not developed verbal speech and are unlikely to use verbal output as a primary expressive communicative modality in the future. Young preverbal children with autism are candidates for AAC to readily promote communicative effectiveness and facilitate the development of verbal communication skills. For example, a former client was classified as preverbal at age three as he had no intelligible speech; however, after introducing AAC via signs while also targeting verbal output, he later developed typical verbal expressive communication skills.

TYPES OF AUGMENTATIVE AND ALTERNATIVE COMMUNICATION

High-Tech Options

It is important to distinguish between the different types of AAC before considering assessment and intervention. AAC can be categorized in different ways. One way of categorizing AAC is high tech or low tech. "High tech" often references text to talk speech-generating devices (SGD) like Dynavox or speech-generating applications such as Touch Chat or Proloquo2Go, which are compatible with devices like iPads (Figure 10.1).

Decades ago, such devices were often inaccessible for a number of reasons including high costs and device cumbersomeness. Technological advances have helped to ease such concerns, especially since devices have become considerably lighter and more durable. While devices have significantly decreased in cost, financial barriers can often prevent clients from lower socioeconomic backgrounds from accessing such devices to assist with communication.

Low and No Tech Options

Low-tech AAC options include modalities such as writing with a pencil and paper, using communication boards, and using a picture exchange communication system (PECS). Such modalities are often cost effective and may be used to help quickly ascertain an individual's understanding of AAC as a viable communicative system. For example, an interventionist might try a simple option board incorporating core vocabulary (Figure 10.2). Such systems can be quickly created by hand with simple drawings. How might you use them with a client?

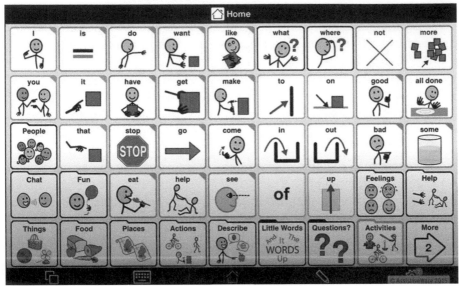

Augmentative and Alternative Communication (AAC) - ASHA

FIGURE 10.1   An example of a speech-generating application.

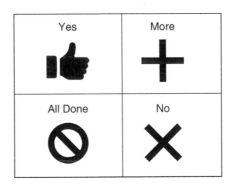

FIGURE 10.2   A simple option board incorporating core vocabulary.

Therapy Golden Nugget

1. Introduce a simple *yes/no* or *more/all done* task. You can introduce pre-ferred items like blowing bubbles or, for children less engaged, physical manipulation like tickling if the client has a preference.
2. Engage in the preferred activity with the child, then stop.
3. Clearly point to the picture/text of "more" and then continue the task. Repeat this at least three times.

4. On the fourth trial, stop and wait for the child to indicate. If the child does not initially respond, you can push the paper closer the child to indicate for them to use it to communicate. If the child continues to not respond, you can take the child's index finger and point to the target word and then continue the activity before allowing the child another trial to execute the task independently.

As the child masters the task, you can add additional options and/or make the icons/text smaller. If a child is having difficulty, you might consider making the icons bigger, reducing choices, placing them further away from each other, and/or including colors as another marker of difference.

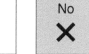

Visual representations have strong evidence of supporting communication in individuals with autism (Quill 1995; Meadan et al. 2011). Sign language is also an option for children with autism who continue to struggle with verbal communication output and may benefit from a visual representation of expressive language as an alternative to verbal speech. Interventionists might consider incorporating signs with verbal output as a method to encourage communicative success for clients with autism who are minimally verbal.

Active Learning Task

Look up signs for the following words to incorporate into your intervention sessions. After looking up the signs, practice with a partner.
- More
- All done
- Play
- Yes
- No

In considering AAC effectiveness, one should consider the different types of competence for communication success (Figure 10.3; Light and McNaughton 2014).

Operational competence includes the ability to effectively navigate the AAC device, such as using operational functions like turning the device on and using functions like back buttons to delete. For students with autism with motoric challenges, this consideration is particularly important because the interventionist should consider motor deficits when implementing AAC, which should influence the type of system implemented so the student can be most successful.

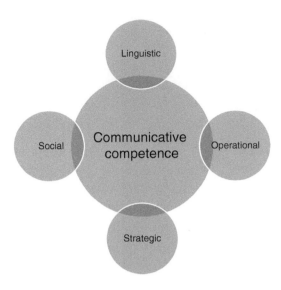

FIGURE 10.3   The different types of communicative competence.

Therapy Golden Nugget

Operational Areas to Evaluate and Target in Intervention

- Locating and accessing a picture symbol on the device.
- Demonstrating use of navigational tools (e.g. *on, off, clear, delete, back*).
- Selecting a category folder to navigate appropriate symbols.
- Using an index finger to select appropriate symbols on device.
- Activating a message bar.
- Erasing messages.

Linguistic competence includes knowledge of the linguistic code unique to the AAC device and a core vocabulary. A common goal in this domain is to increase mean length of utterance. Intervention may consider a total communication approach that includes an SGD, gesture or sign language, and/or verbal approximations, as appropriate. Evidence suggests that minimally verbal school-aged children with autism can make gains in spontaneous language using interventions that focus on targeting joint engagement and play while also incorporating an SGD (Kasari et al. 2014). In clinical practice, this might look like making sure the child readily has access to their AAC device in natural contexts like recess to offer opportunities for social initiations during play.

Therapy Golden Nugget

Social Areas to Evaluate and Target in Intervention

- Using AAC to *share*.
- Increasing intentional communication.
- Using AAC to comment on a shared activity.
- Increasing rate of initiation.
- Increasing rate of responsiveness

Social competence includes skills of social interaction to initiate, maintain, and terminate communication interactions. An important aspect to target in this domain is pragmatic use of language, as some minimally verbal AAC users often use language predominantly to make requests. This skill is often targeted early to get the client to use communication to ask for wants and needs, which, when used successfully, can significantly reduce the presence of maladaptive behaviors. However, this success does not target the other pragmatic domains of language, such as using language for the more social functions such as sharing information. Intervention may focus on creating communicative opportunities and increasing client productions via direct modeling. These opportunities should be motivating and engaging to increase the likelihood of the client wanting to initiate comments about the task.

INTERVENTION SUGGESTIONS

To target increasing linguistic and social competence in intervention with clients with autism using AAC:

- Make sure that the child's SGD is easily accessible throughout the activity.
- Establish a clear routine: consider at least three completed trials as an established routine.
- Model comments on the activity by pointing and making a statement.
- Offer communicative opportunities by limiting questions: try making statements to prompt initiations instead.
- Incorporate nonverbal communication cues (eye gaze, directed facial expressions) to encourage social engagement.

Therapy Golden Nugget

After establishing a play routine with a client with puzzles, you can begin to point at a puzzle piece and say, "Look!" or "Wow!" You can then model by saying, "Look! I see ____" while showing the item to the child. Give opportunities for the child to imitate these behaviors. Make sure to incorporate high affect into the task by smiling and using directed facial expressions. Incorporate gesture by clearly pointing while modeling. As appropriate, model comments on the child's device so the child sees how to initiate such comments for the purpose of sharing.

Strategic competence includes compensatory strategies for individuals who use AAC to cope with some of the interaction limitations. Intervention targets should focus on increasing client persistence to repair communicative breakdowns. For example, an interventionist might turn away from the client and ignore a communicative bid from the client's AAC to prompt the client to include other ways of gaining attention appropriately, such as tapping on the shoulder and/or repeating messages. These types of tasks are important to help clients learn to use a variety of methods to successfully gain attention and convey communicative messages. Such skills translate well into the natural environment where students might need to learn persistence to successfully engage with a partner in various conditions. After targeting this domain in your session, consider incorporating the natural environment to address this area in natural contexts, which are much less predictable than typical clinic therapy rooms.

> Think of a young child struggling to talk to a peer on a noisy playground where the SGD is not readily heard on the first attempt. Later in life, if this skill is not targeted, the challenge could persist over time such as older clients communicating in a crowded restaurant or getting the attention of a store clerk who is busy stocking shelves when the client is seeking help.

Overall, consider which of these domains will most help your client to make the most significant impact in *communicative competence* skills. It is important to note not only areas of growth, but also areas of relative strength. Interventionists should seek to identify competencies in clients' communicative output, as well as recognizing their own behaviors that encourage more positive interactions (Stiegler 2007). Remember, the goal is communication effectiveness and success.

INTRODUCING AUGMENTATIVE AND ALTERNATIVE COMMUNICATION

All interventionists naturally employ no-tech AAC approaches such as gesture, body language, and facial expressions during communicative interactions with clients. Many interventionists also employ simple signs such as "more" or "all done" as a visual representation of verbal output. While previously AAC was only introduced after years of failed attempts at eliciting verbal speech production, current practices advocate introducing AAC much sooner during early intervention for young children at risk of reduced intelligibility or lack of verbal output (Romski et al. 2015; Cress and Marvin 2003). Adults with autism using AAC advocate for early introduction of AAC to promote communication choice, rather than only introducing AAC as a final option after sustained failure of verbal output (Donaldson et al. 2021). While the development of an AAC program might be in the primary domain of an SLP, collaboration is key for client success and generalization of skills. The primary interventionist should seek out the other key stakeholders to share AAC approaches to allow the client the opportunity to use AAC across multiple domains and environments. Such interprofessional collaboration significantly improves the client's use of the communication modality and creates consistency between settings.

Caregiver Buy-in and Cultural Considerations

Perhaps one of the most significant factors in successful AAC use is support of caregivers and key stakeholders. Incorporating caregivers is important because parents can often elicit more communication at home than can be elicited with trained practitioners in a clinic setting, indicating that involving parents is a critical component of promoting communication across contexts for minimally verbal children with ASD (Barokova et al. 2020). For AAC to be successful, the client must use it consistently across contexts and communicative partners. For African-American and Black families, as well as other families of color, cultural views toward disability and communication can impact if interventionist recommendations are adopted (Parette et al. 2002). As such, SLPs and other individuals serving clients with autism using AAC must prioritize training both parents and teachers on device use to increase AAC use (DeCarlo et al. 2019). Too often, children are reduced to only using their SGD during formal intervention time like during speech therapy sessions; however, AAC should be implemented throughout the child's day to offer the most communicative opportunities. This includes daily activities like play, mealtime, and community based-outings. Keeping this in mind, interventionists should prioritize parent training to promote use of AAC across settings. For example, findings indicate training and coaching via telepractice can increase family members' modeling and use of the SGD, prompting increased device use among AAC users (Douglas et al. 2021).

In promoting use of AAC, clinicians should be keenly aware of parent perceptions of SGDs. Early communicative competence, facilitated through the use of AAC, may contribute to more optimal outcomes for individuals with ASD who struggle to master verbal communication skills. Research acknowledges that a student's use of an AAC impacts the entire family and positive outcomes in AAC are heavily dependent on family support (Angelo 2000; Parette et al. 2000; Mandak et al. 2017). In promoting AAC to potential families of children with autism, interventionists should consider the family's preference, because their support is integral to the client's communicative success. Clinicians should be careful to explain the purpose and use of AAC, as many families may perceive it as an indication of "giving up" on verbal speech. To the contrary, introducing AAC early can facilitate communicative success, reduce maladaptive behaviors as children increase communicative competence, and provide models for speech production. Families initially reticent to embrace an AAC approach might be amenable to a total communication approach that employs a mix of verbal approximations, AAC, and/or gesture. Such an approach supports the child's efforts in a range of modalities to successfully convey an intended message. In fact, evidence suggests interventions including visual-graphic symbols, sign language, and/or an SGD via total communication had the most successful outcomes for individuals with autism using AAC (Nunes 2008). Often, we find that families demonstrate the most buy-in when they can witness communicative success firsthand. In such cases, inviting parents into therapy sessions can be helpful to both include them in the intervention process and to directly show them the success of the AAC approach in supporting communicative attempts.

A NOTE ON ASSESSMENT

For clients with autism using AAC, special consideration should be given during assessment procedures. Namely, when evaluating, you should be sure your assessment is an accurate reflection of the client's skills, rather than a reflection of expressive limitations. For example, clients using high-tech AAC devices might not have access to icons to readily identify items in pictures or respond to questions. Failing to account for response differences may significantly distort your evaluation results and may paint a much more restricted picture of the client's abilities. You might consider beginning with receptive language tasks that use pointing and/or *yes/no* responses for clients with restricted verbal output. To assess expressive skills, you might consider using a thorough language sample analysis to capture the client's abilities. Your evaluation should note the client's ability to use AAC modalities independently to inform intervention approaches.

INTERVENTION CONSIDERATIONS

Regardless of what kind of AAC system you are working on with an individual with autism, session preparation is particularly important with this population. You must be thoughtful and intentional about session tasks and activities to allow for the most communicative opportunities during the intervention session. We recommend considering increasing opportunities for modeling, timing responses and clinical feedback, incorporating peer models, planning environmental arrangement and task selection.

　　When working with children with autism using AAC for functional communication, modeling has proven effective in teaching children symbol comprehension and

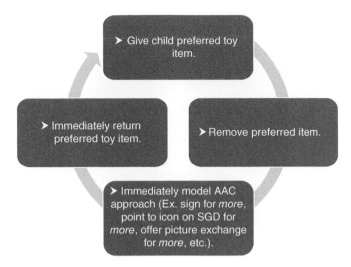

FIGURE 10.4   Example modeling intervention.

production using communication boards (Drager et al. 2006). When working with this population, modeling interventions should be employed to clearly indicate how to use AAC systems effectively. For example, consider the approach in Figure 10.4.

Timing is key, as the return of the item must be immediately following the communication bid to clearly establish the connection of the effectiveness of communication. This is particularly important for clients displaying behaviors as the client must learn that their AAC modality is more effective than maladaptive behaviors (crying, throwing tantrums, etc.). Additionally, for the task to be motivating, the toy or activity being used must be one that interests the child. This is important because every child may be motivated by different items. We have seen some children who love being tickled and others who detest it. Some children may like bubbles, while others may be ambivalent. The clinician must use what is appropriate for that particular client. To find an appropriate toy or item, the interventionist might ask parents about preferred items at home. Alternatively, the clinician may place a variety of toys in the room and note what the client elects to play with. In employing modeling interventions, it is important to determine client understanding before fading out models to allow the client to demonstrate use more independently (Figure 10.5).

Along with modeling as a prompting strategy, interventionists should employ an approach working from least to most prompts to facilitate a positive increase in producing multi-symbol messages among children with AAC using multimodal communication strategies (Figure 10.6; Finke et al. 2017). Such an approach includes strategies of verbal prompting by asking a question, verbal cueing by requesting for production, and graphic modeling by encouraging imitation of device use, in addition to verbal models and expectant delay (Finke et al. 2017).

While collecting data and assessing treatment effectiveness, interventionists must consider the amount of prompts and cues that a child requires to be successful. Keeping in mind that the ultimate goal is independence, a client requiring consistent

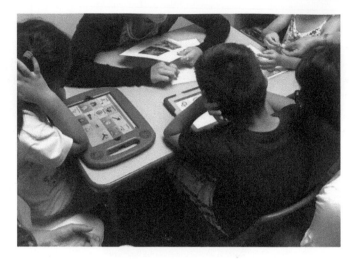

FIGURE 10.5   Using communication devices in small group intervention settings.

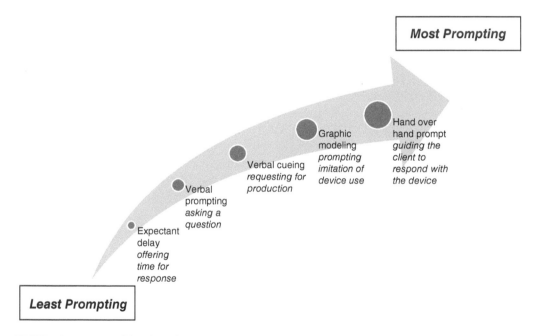

FIGURE 10.6   Working from least to most prompts.

maximum prompts over an extended period of time may need to be considered for an alternative intervention approach. While you should evaluate the success of each session, it may be appropriate to consider the success of intervention each month or two at most. Such reflection allows you to determine whether the client is making steady progress with the approach being employed, which provides an opportunity to review evidenced-based practices and determine whether a new approach should be attempted or the client is responding to the current method(s).

Some approaches may be more appropriate than others. For example, facilitated communication is a controversial approach that has been discredited by professional associations such as the American Speech–Language–Hearing Association (2018), while some parents continue to advocate for the approach that involves physical support such as directing the hand or wrist to direct communicative messages. Direct attempts to counter against misinformed practices must be led by professionals working with children with ASD, which includes parent education and effective evidence-based intervention strategies (Trembath et al. 2016). Selecting appropriate and effective treatment approaches, in addition to consistent culturally responsive parent counseling, is critical to avoid parent adoption of discredited approaches. As such, interventionists should be sensitive to caregivers throughout the intervention process, prioritizing parent engagement and education, as well as adapting evidence-based practices to select treatment approaches that best meet the needs of clients and their families.

Incorporating Peer Models

Interventionists should consider the importance of neurotypical peer models when promoting use of AAC. Often, a child using AAC may be the only person not using verbal communication in their classroom, home, and community. Incorporating neurotypical peers can help to increase communicative acts among children with autism using SGD, while also equipping typically developing peers with the tools to support device use by their peers with ASD using AAC (Trottier et al. 2011). Consider incorporating peer-mediated intervention strategies where appropriate. For example, you might educate peers without autism on how to support their peers using SGDs in the hope of increasing communicative attempts in the classroom setting. Research indicates that training typical peers on SGDs promotes more reciprocity during communication exchanges with children with ASD using AAC and their peers, including more frequent requests for objects and actions as well as some increases in comments (Figure 10.7; Bourque and Goldstein 2020; Thiemann-Bourque et al. 2017; Thiemann-Bourque et al. 2018).

If working in a school setting, interventionists might consider doing a presentation to students about diverse communication and including an introduction of AAC. While most children associate tablets with game play, the interventionist can illustrate how tablets may also be used for communication. We often tell children about their peer using AAC "the tablet is the voice for ___." This can help to discourage peers who are often intrigued by the client's use of AAC from taking it away to explore. Try asking, "How would you feel if someone took your voice away?" Simultaneously, you want to teach the child with AAC self-advocacy so the children learn to take ownership of their voice.

Incorporating typical peers with children with autism using AAC can be helpful, not only among those using SGD but also across different AAC modalities such as for those using PECS. Including neurotypical peers by training them to use PECS can help them to increase their communication with their peers with autism and facilitate social skills, while also assisting their peers with ASD using AAC increase their social engagement (Thiemann-Bourque et al. 2016).

Environmental Arrangement

In working with individuals with autism with AAC, environmental arrangement is key. In intervention, make sure that the child's device is readily accessible at all times (Figure 10.8). Treating the device as an extension of the child is critical, as we

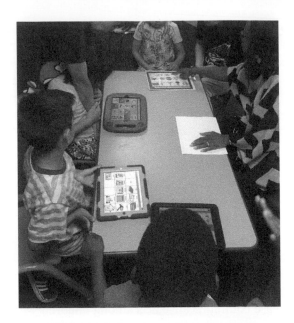

FIGURE 10.7   Using communication devices in the classroom setting.

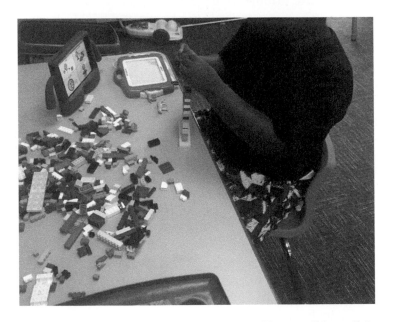

FIGURE 10.8   Ensure that the communication device is readily accessible at all times.

recognize the device offers the child an additional means of expressive communication. Interventionists should consider the environment when working with children using AAC and selecting treatment activities (Table 10.1). For example, a clinician could substitute sensory play with water activities or shaving cream with sensory tasks that are less likely to impede AAC use.

TABLE 10.1   Examples of clinician intervention activities adapted for AAC users.

Activity target	Initial task selected	Adjusted task
Labeling animals using carrier phrases, (e.g., I + see +_____)	I will hide toy animals in shaving cream to incorporate a sensory element.	Hide toy animals in dry beans or pasta to engage in the same task that won't adversely impact AAC use.
Increasing comments during play	I will use finger paints because it is fun and interactive.	Use crayons or colored pencils to accomplish the same task and leave fingers free for AAC use.
Increasing functional play skills	I don't need to have the child's AAC available since we are just targeting play.	Place the AAC within reach to allow for communicative opportunities within natural tasks like play.
Here, create your own target and adaptation		

Therapy Golden Nugget

Intervention Suggestions

Minimally verbal children with autism made more improvements in spontaneous communicative utterances when using interventions that employed evidenced-based approaches focusing on play and joint attention with SGDs, rather than omitting SGDs (Kasari et al. 2014). You might also consider creating an AAC-rich environment. How? Add picture symbols to your setting to help create more inclusivity for complex communicators. Such practices can enhance the environment for all communicators. It makes AAC users see their communication modality used in their daily environment, while exposing those using verbal speech to AAC modalities employed by their peers. This practice exposes all students to text representation, which can be used to support letter sound correspondence and offer opportunities to support reading and spelling in natural contexts. Consider adding picture and text icons to objects in the environment to help increase familiarity with device symbols. You can also encourage families to do this at home as well. As much as possible, use images that replicate your client's modality (picture representations, signs, etc.).

Active Learning Task

Identify three items in your environment to create symbols for and label. Depending on items available, you can use pen/pencil and paper, color, or print and laminate items.

Therapy Golden Nugget

Attempt to incorporate AAC into activity tasks. Copy a page of the client's SGD in black and white and have the client color the icons to match his/her device. This matching task gives the client the opportunity to become more familiar with the device icons, while engaging in an active intervention task.

Therapy Golden Nugget

Evidence suggests interventionists can use a strategy of prepare, offer, wait, respond to increase social communication of students with autism (Douglas and Gerde 2019; Douglas et al. 2013; Douglas et al. 2014). Steps are outlined below:

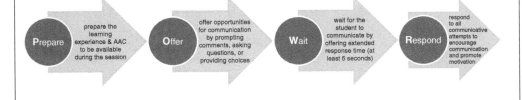

Therapy Golden Nugget

Consider frontloading reading tasks. When making intervention plans that incorporate a book share, make sure to add key vocabulary to the child's device (or have caregivers add symbols) and teach them ahead of time so the child has more opportunities to actively engage in book-share activities. Also, consider completing extension tasks before or after the reading task that allows the child to use the same vocabulary. Setting up thematic sessions can be helpful for both the interventionist and for the child with AAC to allow multiple communication attempts with the same targets.

Often, you can find children's books on YouTube. Consider doing book shares in multiple modalities to help increase engagement as many children may engage more actively in activities involving digital media. Offering both options for engagement also offers multiple communicative opportunities (Figure 10.9).

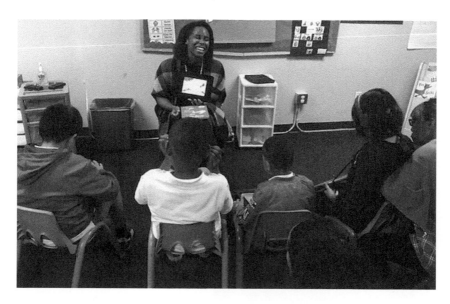

FIGURE 10.9   Dr. Belinda reading a book using a standard book board and the same story on YouTube shown with a tablet.

Active Learning Task

Consider a traditional children's book that you could use in intervention. What key vocabulary would you attempt to frontload to provide the most communicative attempts for the child? Select up to 10 words and/or phrases. Next, create representations of that vocabulary that a potential client could use to communicate.

SUMMARY

AAC should be considered for clients with autism who are not readily successful with verbal speech as an expressive communication modality. In selecting an appropriate system, interventionists should consider linguistic, operational, social, and strategic competence skills. Cultural and linguistic differences should be respected to ensure the client and family are supportive of the use of AAC and understand how to use the system across contexts, which promotes optimal outcomes. Appropriate integration of AAC can significantly help to increase communicative competence for minimally verbal individuals with autism, which can help to reduce maladaptive behaviors as clients can more readily express their wants and needs. In many cases, a total communication approach using multiple expressive communication methods like signing, verbal approximations, gestures, and an SGD can yield the most positive results. Interventionists considering AAC for a client should take time to research the literature to determine best practices and approaches. Interventionists working with children with autism with AAC should seek out professional continuing education to increase the effectiveness of their practice and confidence implementing intervention.

REFLECTIONS ALONG THE PATH

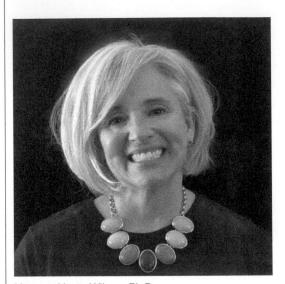

Margaret Vento-Wilson, Ph.D.

As you well know by now, ASD is a life-long neurodevelopmental condition with communication as a locus. For many individuals with ASD, natural speech can be either minimally present or completely absent (Tager-Flusberg and Kasari 2013), with obvious connotations. As our field has evolved over the decades in concert with shifts in the views of disability, rather than labeling this profile as severely communicatively impaired, individuals with this profile are viewed as having complex communication needs. Addressing these needs is an important role of SLPs across clients and settings.

My clinical experience with ASD was gained as an SLP at an elementary school with an ASD-focused special education program. The students in this program required very substantial levels of support and many demonstrated no natural speech or limited natural speech, to such an extent that there was a significant gap between their need to communicate and their ability to communicate. Much of my daily clinical work was geared toward closing the gap, which frequently involved the introduction of AAC.

When I consider what I wish I had known when I walked into my office that first day as an SLP, I offer the following suggestions to future practitioners so they can start their careers with some central tenets that took me years to develop:

- Mind the gap: This focus has the potential to shape long-term outcomes and logically implicates the introduction of an AAC system as soon as young children begin to demonstrate a high level of need for support in communication or as soon as individuals with ASD and complex communication needs find their way to your office.
- Presume potential: There are no prerequisite skills required before AAC can be introduced to someone, regardless of their age or profile. Because AAC systems are multidimensional, there is an option for every individual. Bringing this philosophy into your clinical work validates the principle that communication is not a privilege, but a basic human right that should be accessible to all.
- Explore the participation model: This model parallels the International Classification of Functioning, Disability and Health, and the social model of disability, but with an AAC flavor. Although it may initially appear labyrinthine,

adopting it into your practice guides your work with individuals with ASD and complex communication needs and supports improved outcomes.
- Go the distance: AAC is a long game. Individuals with ASD and complex communication needs must master both the AAC system and their own language. As a result, progress can often be incremental. However, over time, those incremental steps add up. Regardless of when AAC is introduced, be patient and maintain fidelity to the process.
- Cultivate clarity: The presence of limited language or the absence of natural speech do not equate to having nothing to say. Conversely, lack of access to a reliable method of communication often results in not being able to say anything. Be wary of confusing these two paradigms.

I hope these suggestions are helpful to you as a new practitioner – they would have been to me. However, I recognize that each of you must forge your own path, make your own mistakes, and experience your own achievements, which is how learning is internalized. Perhaps what these suggestions really offer is a set of information you can revisit at some point when you are not sure how to proceed or when *you have tried everything else*. Regardless, I wish you luck in your clinical work, because what we do matters in ways both big and small.

Margaret Vento-Wilson PhD CCC-SLP
Assistant Professor, Speech-Language Pathology
California State University, Long Beach

TEST QUESTIONS

1. With children with autism using AAC, interventionists should employ a most to least prompting approach. True or false?
2. The ability to effectively navigate the AAC device is known as:
   A. Operational competence
   B. Linguistic competence
   C. Social competence
   D. Strategic competence
3. Teaching your client to persist to repair communicative breakdowns when they occur is an example of:
   A. Operational competence
   B. Linguistic competence
   C. Social competence
   D. Strategic competence
4. AAC should only be used after attempts at verbal communication have failed for at least one year. True or false?

5. Incorporating typical peers can encourage children with autism using AAC to produce more peer-directed communication and increase peer engagement. True or false?

6. AAC modalities include:
    A. SGD
    B. PECS
    C. Pencil and paper
    D. All of the above

7. AAC is:
    A. Alternative augmentative communication
    B. Augmentative alternative communication
    C. Alternative augmentative competence
    D. Adjusted alternative communication

REFERENCES

American Speech-Language-Hearing Association. (2018). *Facilitated Communication.* Rockville, MD: ASHA. doi:10.1044/policy.PS2018-00352.

Angelo, D. (2000). Impact of augmentative and alternative communication devices on families. *Augmentative and Alternative Communication* 16 (1): 37–47.

Barokova, M., Hassan, S., Lee, C. et al. (2020). A comparison of natural language samples collected from minimally and low-verbal children and adolescents with autism by parents and examiners. *Journal of Speech, Language, and Hearing Research* 63 (12): 4018–4028.

Bourque, K. and Goldstein, H. (2020). Expanding communication modalities and functions for preschoolers with autism Spectrum disorder: secondary analysis of a peer partner speech-generating device intervention. *Journal of Speech, Language, and Hearing Research* 63 (1): 190–205.

Cress, C.J. and Marvin, C.A. (2003). Common questions about AAC services in early intervention. *AAC: Augmentative and Alternative Communication* 19 (4): 254–272.

DeCarlo, J., Bean, A., Lyle, S., and Cargill, L. (2019). The relationship between operational competency, buy-in, and augmentative and alternative communication use in school-age children with autism. *American Journal of Speech-Language Pathology* 28 (2): 469–484.

Donaldson, A., Corbin, E., and McCoy, J. (2021). "Everyone deserves AAC": preliminary study of the experiences of speaking autistic adults who use augmentative and alternative communication. *Perspectives of the ASHA Special Interest Groups* 6 (2): 315–326.

Douglas, S. and Gerde, H. (2019). A strategy to support the communication of students with autism Spectrum disorder. *Intervention in School and Clinic* 55 (1): 32–38.

Douglas, S., Light, J., and McNaughton, D. (2013). Teaching paraeducators to support the communication of young children with complex communication needs. *Topics in Early Childhood Special Education* 33 (2): 27–37.

Douglas, S., McNaughton, D., and Light, J. (2014). Online training for paraeducators to support the communication of young children. *Journal of Early Intervention* 35 (3): 223–242.

Douglas, S., Biggs, E., Meadan, H., and Bagawan, A. (2021). The effects of Telepractice to support family members in modeling a speech-generating device in the home. *American Journal of Speech-Language Pathology* 30 (3): 1157–1169.

Drager, K., Postal, V., Carrolus, L. et al. (2006). The effect of aided language modeling on symbol comprehension and production in 2 preschoolers with autism. *American Journal of Speech-Language Pathology* 15 (2): 112–125.

Finke, E., Davis, J., Benedict, M. et al. (2017). Effects of a least-to-Most prompting procedure on multisymbol message production in children with autism spectrum disorder who use augmentative and alternative communication. *American Journal of Speech-Language Pathology* 26 (1): 81–98.

Ganz, J. (2015). AAC interventions for individuals with autism spectrum disorders: state of the science and future research directions. *Augmentative and Alternative Communication* 31 (3): 203–214.

Kasari, C., Kaiser, A., Goods, K. et al. (2014). Communication interventions for minimally verbal children with autism: sequential multiple assignment randomized trial. *Journal of the American Academy of Child and Adolescent Psychiatry* 53 (6): 635–646.

Koegel, L., Bryan, K., Su, P. et al. (2020). Definitions of nonverbal and minimally verbal in research for autism: a systematic review of the literature. *Journal of Autism and Developmental Disorders* 50 (8): 2957–2972.

Kovacs, T. (2021). A survey of American speech-language Pathologists' perspectives on augmentative and alternative communication assessment and intervention across language domains. *American Journal of Speech-Language Pathology* 30 (3): 1038–1048.

Light, J. and Drager, K. (2007). AAC technologies for young children with complex communication needs: state of the science and future research directions. *Augmentative and Alternative Communication* 23 (3): 204–216.

Light, J. and McNaughton, D. (2014). Communicative competence for individuals who require augmentative and alternative communication: a new definition for a new era of communication? *Augmentative and Alternative Communication* 30 (1): 1–18.

Mandak, K., O'Neill, T., Light, J., and Fosco, G.M. (2017). Bridging the gap from values to actions: a family systems framework for family-centered AAC services. *Augmentative and Alternative Communication* 33 (1): 32–41.

Meadan, H., Ostrosky, M., Triplett, B. et al. (2011). Using visual supports with young children with autism Spectrum disorder. *Teaching Exceptional Children* 43 (6): 28–35.

Meer, L. and Rispoli, M. (2010). Communication interventions involving speech-generating devices for children with autism: a review of the literature. *Developmental Neurorehabilitation* 13 (4): 294–306.

Nunes, D. (2008). AAC interventions for autism: a research summary. *International Journal of Special Education* 23 (2): 17–26.

Parette, H.P., Brotherson, M.J., and Huer, M.B. (2000). Giving families a voice in augmentative and alternative communication decision-making. *Education and Training in Mental Retardation and Developmental Disabilities* 35 (2): 177–190.

Parette, P., Huer, M., and Wyatt, T. (2002). Young African American children with disabilities and augmentative and alternative communication issues. *Early Childhood Special Education* 29 (3): 201–207.

Quill, K. (1995). Visually cued instruction for children with autism and pervasive developmental disorders. *Focus on Autistic Behavior* 10 (3): 10–20.

Romski, M., Sevcik, R., Barton-Hulsey, A., and Whitmore, A. (2015). Early intervention and AAC: what a difference 30 years makes. *Augmentative and Alternative Communication* 31 (3): 181–202.

Sanders, E., Page, T., and Lesher, D. (2021). School-based speech-language pathologists: confidence in augmentative and alternative communication assessment. *Language, Speech, and Hearing Services in Schools* 52 (2): 512–528.

Stiegler, L. (2007). Discovering communicative competencies in a nonspeaking child with autism. *Language, Speech, and Hearing Services in Schools* 38 (4): 400–413.

Tager-Flusberg, H. and Kasari, C. (2013). Minimally verbal school-aged children with autism spectrum disorder: the neglected end of the Spectrum. *Autism Research: Official Journal of the International Society for Autism Research* 6 (6): 468–478.

Thiemann-Bourque, K., Brady, N., McGuff, S. et al. (2016). Picture exchange communication system and pals: a peer-mediated augmentative and alternative communication intervention for minimally verbal preschoolers with autism. *Journal of Speech, Language, and Hearing Research* 59 (5): 1133–1145.

Thiemann-Bourque, K., Guff, S., and Goldstein, H. (2017). Training peer partners to use a speech-generating device with classmates with autism Spectrum disorder: exploring communication outcomes across preschool contexts. *Journal of Speech, Language, and Hearing Research* 60 (9): 2648–2662.

Thiemann-Bourque, K., Feldmiller, S., Hoffman, L., and Johner, S. (2018). Incorporating a peer-mediated approach into speech-generating device intervention: effects on communication of preschoolers with autism Spectrum disorder. *Journal of Speech, Language, and Hearing Research* 61 (8): 2045–2061.

Trembath, D., Paynter, J., Keen, D., and Ecker, U. (2016). "Attention: myth follows!" facilitated communication, parent and professional attitudes towards evidence-based practice, and the power of misinformation. *Evidence-Based Communication Assessment and Intervention* 9 (3): 113–126.

Trottier, N., Kamp, L., and Mirenda, P. (2011). Effects of peer-mediated instruction to teach use of speech-generating devices to students with autism in social game routines. *Augmentative and Alternative Communication* 27 (1): 26–39.

White, E., Ayres, K., Snyder, S. et al. (2021). Augmentative and alternative communication and speech production for individuals with ASD: a systematic review. *Journal of Autism and Developmental Disorders* 51 (11): 4199–4212.

FURTHER READINGS

O'Neill, T., Light, J., and McNaughton, D. (2017). Videos with integrated AAC visual scene displays to enhance participation in community and vocational activities: pilot case study with an adolescent with autism Spectrum disorder. *Perspectives of the ASHA Special Interest Groups* 2 (12): 55–69.

CHAPTER 11

Scope of Practice Considerations and Service Delivery Models

Learning objectives

By reading this chapter, interventionists will be able to:

1. Define interprofessional education (IPE) and interprofessional practice (IPP).
2. Describe methods of collaboration with other professionals involved in the therapeutic process with children with autism spectrum disorder (ASD).
3. Contrast the pros and cons of individual and group services for clients with autism.
4. List at least two different modalities for delivering intervention services for clients with autism.
5. Explain the importance of determining the appropriate service delivery model for clients with autism and their families.

Understanding the importance of collaboration is key in the success of effectively serving individuals with ASD and their families. **Interprofessional Practice (IPP)** supports allied health professionals collaborating to best serve clients with needs across multiple domains of functioning such as those with ASD (Johnson et al. 2016; Morrison et al. 2011). **Interprofessional Education (IPE)** includes colleagues across related disciplines educating and learning from one another to generate shared decisions to best serve clients

Autism Spectrum Disorders from Theory to Practice: Assessment and Intervention Tools Across the Lifespan,
First Edition. Edited by Belinda Daughrity and Ashley Wiley Johnson.
© 2023 John Wiley & Sons Ltd. Published 2023 by John Wiley & Sons Ltd.

(World Health Organization 2010; Johnson et al. 2016; Neubauer et al. 2014). For students with complex needs such as those with autism spectrum disorders, IPE establishes clarity of one's own scope of practice and where it overlaps with other professional roles, which combats treatment redundancy (Christopherson et al. 2015; Neubauer et al. 2014). Because collaboration seeks to develop a common knowledge base, IPE provides a shared vocabulary and context for decision making and communication in professional contexts (Christopherson et al. 2015; Lytle et al. 2003; Neubauer et al. 2014). When working with students with autism, especially those who might be receiving multiple services from a variety of professionals, it is especially important to seek collaborative practice that removes the traditional siloed approach to intervention.

Active Learning Task

How well do you know the related disciplines who support individuals with autism? Find professionals in the following fields and ask, *What do you do and how do you support individuals with autism spectrum disorders*?

Professional	How long has the person been working in the profession?	How long has the person worked with individuals with autism?	How does the person support individuals with autism?
Speech-language pathologist			
Adapted physical education teacher			
Special education teacher			
Occupational therapist			
Psychologist			
Applied behavior analysis therapist			
Student choice			

Reflection: What did you learn about how various professions support individuals with autism? What did you know before and what did you learn that was new to you? Considering your current or future work setting, what professionals can you envision working with to provide comprehensive, collaborative intervention services to individuals with ASD?

IPP refers to two or more professionals cooperating to improve outcomes and quality of care for their client without a preconceived professional hierarchy (World Health Organization 2010). One might venture to say that IPE precedes IPP; you need to know what other professionals do with clients with autism to be able to identify where

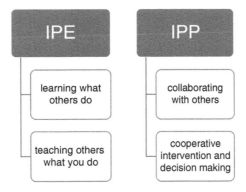

FIGURE 11.1   Interprofessional education compared with interprofessional practice.

your expertise might best support the client's total needs and where your domain might intersect with a colleague's domain (Figure 11.1).

Active Learning Task

In Chapter 1, you were given the active learning task to consider your professional scope of practice. Using that information, create an in-service presentation and/or handout designed to inform other disciplines about your role with individuals with autism. Make sure you use appropriate language that someone outside of your discipline would understand by avoiding professional jargon.

Once completed, share your finished product with a colleague in another field and ask for a rating from 1 to 5 (1 being unclear and 5 being perfectly clear) on the information you presented. What suggestions would make it better?

COMMUNICATION CONSIDERATION

Communication is key when collaborating with professionals. How can you keep your collaboration meaningful and effective?

- *Vibe check:* Are you personable and welcoming with a truly collaborative mindset? Or are you thinking you are "in charge" and hoping everyone else falls in line? Your vibe matters! When it comes to collaboration, everyone plays a key role on the team. Make sure you remind yourself that everyone has value and something to contribute. Everyone has the same goal – making intervention a success for the child with ASD. Put that goal first.
- *Less is best:* As a professional, it can be tempting to share *every single bit* of information you know. Do not do that! Often, that can be overwhelming and people can shut down when provided with excess information. More is not

always better. Instead, select the most meaningful information (the "active ingredient") that will make the most significant impact.

- *Share in the win:* Intervention with clients with autism can have its challenges so it is important to celebrate the wins. This is a time for everyone to see the progress, which helps the team forge ahead with intervention, especially in challenging cases.
- *Balance learning and teaching:* Equally value the opportunity to learn from other disciplines as you do the opportunity to teach others about your field. Often, learning about others' roles can help you perform your role better. Overall, good collaboration involves being both a student and a teacher.

SERVICE DELIVERY MODELS

Training Programs

Training programs may focus specifically on caregiver education. Despite varying content and inconsistent evaluation, such programs focus on teaching caregivers with the purpose of increasing support following a child's ASD diagnosis and promoting good practices to support the child's needs (Dawson-Squibb et al. 2019). Such programs have evidence of reducing parent stress, which can benefit the family as a whole (Kasari et al. 2015).

When developing a training program for parents of students with autism, goals should be directed at increasing parents' knowledge of autism and typical developmental milestones, as well as offering strategies to help parents better engage with their children to promote increased language, play, and engagement.

See a sample of unit topics for the Parent Professional Partnership Training developed at the Los Angeles Speech and Language Therapy Center, suggested topics include:

- What is autism?
- Typical speech and language development: What to expect from your child?
- Indirect language stimulation.
- Direct language stimulation.
- The importance of play.
- Understanding the individual education plan (IEP) process.
- Literacy as a communication tool.
- Music and movement to facilitate speech and language.
- Behavior management approaches.
- Augmentative and alternative communication.
- Parent advocacy.

Mediated Intervention Approaches

Mediated intervention approaches may be appropriate with caregivers who want to be actively involved in therapy and are available for direct coaching and training. Such approaches include the entire family, including parents and siblings, who are trained on evidenced-based approaches, which demonstrates some promising evidence for generalization of skills (Pacia et al. 2021). These caregivers then become interventionists, rather than observers. For toddlers with autism, evidence suggests that parent-mediated approaches positively impact joint engagement, particularly with increased parental buy-in, involvement, and application of intervention strategies (Gulsrud et al. 2015). For toddlers identified as at risk for autism from early screening tools, weekly coaching and parent-mediated intervention has been shown to increase social communication skills and to decrease autism symptomology and severity (Tanner and Dounavi 2020). With a wide array of parent-mediated approaches suggested in early intervention for children with autism, interventionists are encouraged to evaluate factors such as ASD severity, parent–child interaction style, and parental stress to determine whether parent mediated intervention would be appropriate and effective (Oono et al. 2013).

Research indicates that parent-mediated interventions for children and adolescents with ASD positively impact communication, cognition, and social emotional skills, noting overall improvements in both parent and child skills (Koly et al. 2021). Parent education alone is shown to reduce parent stress, while hands-on coaching and parent-mediated approaches appear to facilitate child social development and outcomes (Kasari et al. 2015). Considering the needs of your client's parents is an important aspect of delivering appropriate intervention that is responsive to the family's needs. Sometimes, parent education might mean a detailed 5- to 10-minute debriefing at the end of the session time. Other times, it might mean a handout or emailed video that the parent can review at a time that is best for their schedule.

So how do you determine which approach is best? You must evaluate each client and family circumstance individually and, most importantly, meet them where they are. Keep in mind that your approach with the same family could change over time as circumstances change. For example, imagine the case in the Active Learning Task below.

Active Learning Task

John is a four-year-old only child with ASD. He received early intervention services and his goals largely targeted increasing joint attention, play, and engagement. Since starting with you in therapy four months ago, John has made significant progress in his expressive language skills, expanding from single words to phrase-level speech. His mother, Jackie, is ecstatic about his progress. As a stay-at-home parent, she attends every session and actively participates.

(continued)

(continued)

- Given the background, what approach might be most appropriate for this family and why?

In the past three months, Jackie began uncharacteristically missing sessions or attending late. You learn that she has recently taken on care for her partner's father after a stroke. She is also expecting another child in the next few months.

- Given the changing circumstances noted above, what approach might be most appropriate for this family and why?

In addition to parent-mediated services, some settings may be ideal for sibling-mediated services. Considering that siblings, depending on the age gap, may be readily available peer models for children with autism, such approaches may be warranted, given an evaluation of family circumstances. These approaches have been used among children with other disabilities such as attention-deficit/hyperactivity disorder to teach positive behaviors and social skills (Daffner et al. 2019). Among children with autism, positive changes in joint attention and social behavior resulted from training typically developing siblings to engage with their autistic brothers (Tsao and Odom 2006). For young children with ASD, sibling-mediated intervention has been efficacious in training imitation skills, with both parents and siblings reporting high satisfaction following training (Walton and Ingersoll 2012). Among children with autism with limited spontaneous speech, training typical siblings on soliciting speech acts resulted in increased speech productions, indicating that sibling-mediated approaches and inclusion of siblings in interventions can have positive outcomes for children with ASD (Spector and Charlop 2018). Using video modeling showing an adult implementing strategies to promote appropriate play behaviors with the sibling with ASD resulted in typical siblings facilitating cooperative play with their autistic siblings by appropriately reinforcing play and engagement (Neff et al. 2017).

How can you know if it is appropriate to engage a sibling in intervention with a child with autism? When debating whether to employ a sibling mediated approach, consider if the neurotypical sibling has the temperament, aptitude, and patience to participate (Figure 11.2). If you believe the sibling has the temperament, aptitude, and patience to participate in a sibling-mediated approach, then proceed. If not, consider other ways to inform the typical sibling about ASD that might be a better fit, such as referring them to a support group for children with siblings with autism that can provide tips on relationship building while providing incidental learning (Lock and Finstein 2017). Alternatively, you might occasionally provide information to the sibling that might explain how to better engage at home or set boundaries.

Individual or Group Services

Services for students with autism can be delivered individually with just the client and the interventionist, or in a small group where the interventionist delivers treatment to two or more students with autism and/or other disorders simultaneously. Both formats

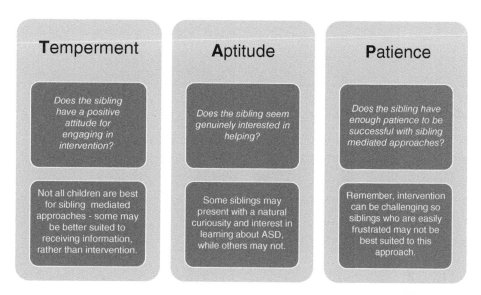

FIGURE 11.2 TAP: temperament, aptitude and patience.

have benefits. While *individual services* allow for direct treatment specifically tailored to the client's unique needs, *group services* may allow for an opportunity for students with autism to work on peer engagement and conversation, which can be helpful for those students with limited peer interaction skills.

Groups can be as small as a pair of two students or as large as groups of half a dozen in a cooperative task. How can you determine the appropriate group size? The students' profiles should be taken into consideration. This includes a combination of:

- *Language level:* Ideally, students will have similar expressive and receptive language skills. This helps to maximize the group time and creates the most opportunities for peer social interaction.
- *Behavior needs:* In considering behaviors, you want to be mindful to not include several children with significant behavior needs in the same group. Alternatively, you might decide to work in a smaller group, such as just two students, so you can better manage behavioral needs during intervention.
- *Attention skills:* You should also consider students' attention levels. Students with fewer skills to attend to long tasks might do better in smaller groups where they will have less time to wait for their turn.
- *Peer compatibility:* Lastly, you must keep student compatibility in mind. For example, you should be aware of students who might be adversarial in the classroom environment, so you do not opt to place them in a group together for intervention.

Ultimately, the decision on how to deliver services should be determined by the client's needs and the final determination may be subject to differences across clinicians, but use your clinical judgment and input from key stakeholders to make an appropriate determination on group placement.

Intervention Setting

Therapy Golden Nugget

Practical Tips for Effective Group Intervention Sessions

Practical Tips for Effective Group Intervention Sessions

Engaging Tasks	Popcorn Turn Taking	Peers as Teachers	Environmental Arrangement
• make sure your session activities are fun and interesting • materials should be engaging - large, colorful images and/or manipulatives if appropriate	• give all students opportunities to engage • randomize student turns, but make sure you divide time equally between students	• involve peers with each other when appropriate • have peers direct questions to each other, give each other directions, and offer each other reinforcement	• make sure all students have direct line of sight to you and the session materials being used • clients requiring more behavior management should be situated closer to you for easier support

Engaging clients effectively in a group setting allows for more productivity, while appropriately meeting client needs (Figure 11.3). There are a number of different options for intervention settings and modalities for individuals with autism.

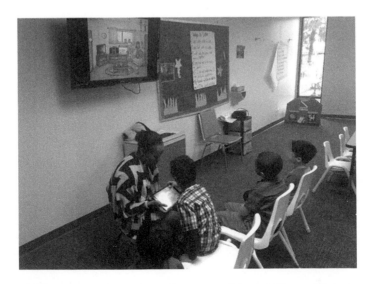

FIGURE 11.3   The interventionist works with a group of four children with autism who are working on similar goals of increasing use of verbs, turn taking with peers, and following simple directions. Children with more behavior needs are placed in the middle to help prevent elopement and promote active participation. Engaging clients effectively in a group setting allows for more productivity, while appropriately meeting client needs.

Pull-Out Services

Pull-out, individual services are often the most common, especially for new clinicians, who typically receive the most supervised training with this type of clinical approach. This type of service involves pulling the child out of the natural environment and conducting intervention in a traditional clinical office setting. This type of setting often gives the interventionist the most control – you decide where you work, exactly what materials you want to use, and usually there are minimal distractions. This setting is primed to be the most individualized to the client's unique needs.

Often, this kind of individuated, direct service is helpful for introducing and priming skills in a structured environment prior to venturing into natural settings to assess for generalization. For example, for students with autism working on social skills goals, you might work on target awareness and skill steps in the one-to-one clinic setting followed by role playing, which allows the student to practice the skills in a safe environment and receive targeted feedback. Later, you might opt to target skills outside of the clinic environment to target generalization and work on the fluency of the skill, so it is mastered across settings.

Push-In Services

Push-in services are often primed for collaboration with key stakeholders such as teachers, occupational therapists, and resource specialists. This push-in model is commonly used in the classroom setting in schools (Figure 11.4). Rather than pulling a child out of the classroom for services, interventionists in the school setting

Active Learning Task

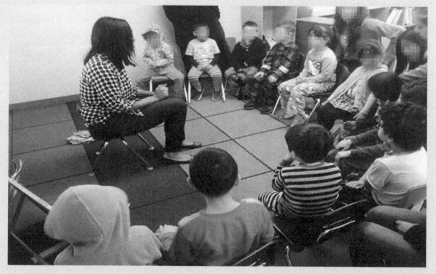

Interventionist delivers Push In Services in the whole group setting.

might go into the classroom to work with the child. This option may be ideal for creating opportunities to work directly with classroom teachers to support the student in the academic environment. Evidence indicates that paraprofessionals in school settings can effectively implement interventions with students with autism following targeted training (Walker et al. 2020). Such training might be particularly well suited for school settings where intervention is directed at the class as a whole. Push-in services also provide an opportunity to observe peer interaction and to seize opportunities to involve peers in intervention, if appropriate, while simultaneously destigmatizing the role of professionals who support individuals with autism.

SEVEN STEPS FOR SUCCESSFUL COLLABORATION IN THE SCHOOL SETTING

Collaboration is never an easy feat when you may be used to working independently. However, for a person with autism, we know collaborative practices are effective and much needed. Use these steps to create a well-planned and executed collaborative practice.

1. *Start small:* Often, interventionists are looking for a grand plan to put into place. It is critical to remember to start with a one-day project. Evaluate how it went and edit along the way.

2. *Start close:* Collaborate with a person who has similar complementary goals. In the school system, this may be the resource specialist or classroom teacher, whose primary role is to ensure a student's ability to succeed in academics.

3. *Share a goal:* Working in silos was discussed in Chapter 4. One way to break a silo is to report on the same goal. This can occur at a student's annual special education meeting or can even be amended to fit what you and your collaboration partner agree to target.

4. *Be innovative:* Thinking outside the box can lead to amazing outcomes when well thought out and executed.

5. *Be consistent and frequent:* Once you have trialed your effort to collaborate on a shared goal, activity, or assessment, remember to keep up the work. Change is never easy and may often take time. Rather than stop, stay the course to see your efforts pay off.

6. *Be inquisitive:* Take time to find out exactly what your colleague focuses on. While working with them, ask questions if you are unsure of why something is being done. It will help you to embrace possibilities when you better understand the roles of others on the team.

7. *Be respectful:* Simply put, there is no "I" in team. All the parts all have value.

In-Home Services

Some interventionists might go into the homes of children with autism and their families. This setting might permit for a naturalistic teaching approach and incidental learning in the natural environment, including strategies employed in behavioral interventions with autism (LeBlanc et al. 2006). This option may be particularly helpful to implement parent coaching and/or parent training. It may also allow those other key stakeholders, family members like siblings, grandparents, and other extended family members, to become more involved and informed about intervention approaches that can be carried into the home environment.

Active Learning Task

Reframe the statements into positives. How can you adapt in this situation to best serve your client and the family?

In-home "challenge"	In-home asset
The family dog is always bothering us during sessions.	Option 1: I can use the dog as a reinforcer by working for short breaks of "doggy time." Option 2 : I can use the dog to motivate the client to use words to complete tasks; e.g. Tell the dog what you see!
My client's twin always wants to get involved during sessions but "takes over" therapy.	
My client's parent observes, but does not join in.	
The family always eats dinner when I come over.	
Student choice:	

Therapy Golden Nugget

Many interventionists are accustomed to bringing in their therapy bag filled with toys and engaging intervention materials. Essentially, they attempt to recreate a clinic setting by isolating the child in a one-to-one setting. In an in-home intervention setting, we challenge you not to do that! Instead, assess the child's environment, note the "distractions" as assets and try to work distinctly in the environment, rather than in spite of it. In this home setting, collaborating with primary caregivers is key.

Tip: Interventionists may only consider the client–clinician dynamic.

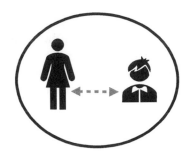

Traditional Therapy in clinic

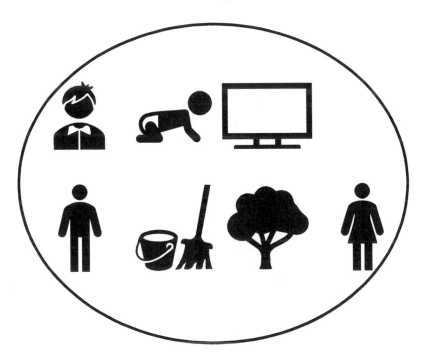

FIGURE 11.4   In Home Therapy Considerations.

With in-home settings, that circle may include siblings watching TV, parents cleaning and cooking, or time outside. EXPAND the circle and widen the possibilities (Figure 11.4)!

How can you use the variables with in-home sessions to your advantage? **EXPAND** your intervention:

E   *Encourage* family members to get involved with you. Invite them to join you during intervention sessions. You can do this by being warm and personable. Set the tone that the intervention session is not "your time" with the client, but the client and family's time with you.

X *Expect* the unexpected! Working in homes can be unpredictable so it is important to be flexible in your approach rather than being inconvenienced. If a parent has to walk to the corner to the mailbox, go with them to show how even short walks can be language rich opportunities. Embrace opportunities to integrate your intervention into the environment.

P *Prioritize* progress over perfection. Intervention may always have an ebb and flow status. Helping families to recognize the small wins in every session is critical to promoting buy-in and keeping caregivers motivated in supporting intervention.

A *Anticipate* using items in the natural environment such as the child's own toys, books, or common items in the home being used during daily tasks. Maximize learning moments like folding laundry as language rich opportunities.

N *Navigate* questions throughout the session by repeatedly asking parents to voice their concerns and by thoughtfully explaining your practices while you model your approaches.

D *Decrease* the emphasis on perfect treatment adherence when using evidenced-based interventions in favor of using evidenced-based approaches that take the client's natural environment into account and allow for flexibility, which increases the chance that caregivers will continue to use such approaches in your absence to encourage goal progress.

Telepractice

Telepractice, or remote delivery, can offer not only services to those in rural or under-served areas with less access to interventions and practitioners, but also cost saving advantages with reduced commuting and loss of productive work time to reduce burden for caregivers (Cason and Cohn 2014; Tindall and Huebner 2009; Meadan et al. 2017). Findings indicate significantly fewer missed appointment sessions via teletherapy in comparison with in-person sessions, which may be particularly of interest for clients with complex needs like autism (Covert et al. 2018). Technology has proven specifically useful in helping to train interventionists to use targeted approaches in autism treatment. For example, findings comparing interventionists in traditional face-to-face training with their counterparts in remote training found no significant differences in treatment fidelity among interventionists or child responses, indicating that remote autism training programs can be as effective as those traditionally held in person (Shire et al. 2020).

For assessment, evidence suggests the use of computers for test administration did not prompt significant differences in standard scores or behavioral presentation for school-age children (Alt and Moreno 2012). Similar efficacy was determined with assessment for autistic adults (Parmanto et al. 2013).

Evidence suggests that telepractice can be a successful modality to provide treatment for individuals with autism across a variety of related disciplines involved in client and family care (Boisvert et al. 2010). Research has suggested that telepractice for individuals with autism can be as effective, or more effective, than traditional face-to-face intervention and consultation models, while also reducing the strain on available specialized services and trained professionals (Baharav and Reiser 2010; Ellison et al. 2021; Sutherland et al. 2018; Boisvert et al. 2012). Research findings also suggest that intervention success is more correlated to treatment fidelity, rather than modality (Hao et al. 2021). Not only does evidence show that treatment via telepractice is effective for children with autism, but findings also indicate improvements can maintain over time (Neely et al. 2016). Similar to positive outcomes with early intervention speech and language therapy and parent training, evidence suggests that behavior-based interventions such as applied behavior analysis via telehealth are as effective as in-person sessions (Marino et al. 2020). So how can you determine if telehealth is an appropriate modality for your client?

Critical Telepractice Needs:

1. Working Equipment
2. Stable Internet
3. An Available Helper

Points to evaluate when considering use of telepractice with clients with autism include:

- *Is the technology available?* Do you and your client have adequate lighting, a working computer or tablet, and consistently available stable internet connection?
- *Is the commute a burden?* Does the client lack consistent access to transportation or is the commute consuming more time than the actual service?
- *Is there a reliable telehelper?* Does the client have access to a caregiver who can provide assistance to help log in and navigate tasks as needed?

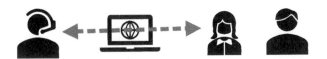

If the answer to all the above questions is *YES*, your client with autism may be an ideal candidate for intervention via telepractice. Remember, the device serves as a medium to connect you with your client. Interventionists should follow all applicable laws and licensure requirements as it pertains to providing services via telepractice to remain in compliance with their state and professional guidelines. As a note for effective documentation, we recommend making sure to include intervention modality in progress notes and assessment documents.

Therapy Golden Nugget

Consider clearly including the modality in writing up your documentation. For example:

"This evaluation/intervention was conducted online using live, interactive video conferencing on a HIPPA-compliant platform. Both parties met the minimum internet connection speeds to support the desired audio and video quality and assessment/intervention was performed in a quiet space with appropriate lighting and the full face of the student appeared in the video throughout the session. An adult accompanied the student for login assistance, camera and audio setup and basic technology support when needed. (*For evaluations*) The adult was directed to avoid any prompting or repeating of test items to the student unless explicitly instructed."

There are many existing resources to help plan engaging and interactive therapy sessions in a virtual setting that allow interventionists to either use existing materials or to create their own to individualize therapy materials to meet their client's needs (Figure 11.5).

We often suggest using YouTube to do book share activities, PowerPoint to create visual schedules and games, and a variety of websites and resources like Boom Cards (Boom Learning, wow.boomlearning.com), Kahoot! (`https://kahoot.com`), and other interactive applications or websites that are appropriate for your client to prepare active and engaging intervention. Like face-to-face intervention, the possibilities are endless, so get creative! All interventionists working with clients via telepractice should consistently evaluate progress to confirm that the modality is effective.

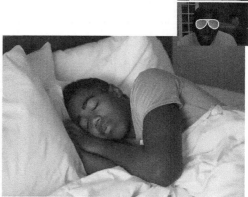

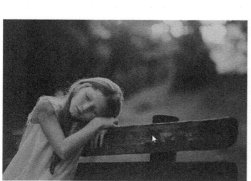

Matheus Bertelli/Pexels   digitalskillet1/Adobe Stock

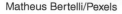

FIGURE 11.5 Example of a teletherapy session with a teen client with ASD using materials created in PowerPoint. Based on the materials above, what do you think the targeted goals are? What materials could you gather and/or develop to further target that intervention goal?

Tips for Engaging Clients with Autism in Telepractice

- Be proactive about behavior: Establish expectations and refer to them often to create clear guidelines.
- Create engaging tasks: Use tasks that are large and colorful enough to capture a client's interest, especially for clients who might be younger or have difficulty attending to structured tasks.
- You set the tone: Make sure you do not get so caught up in the materials that you lose sight of your role as the interventionist – your job is to bring the session to life and your high affect is what makes the session fun and engaging for the client.
- Set aside time for debriefing: Whether working with teachers, paraprofessionals, or parents, make sure to set aside time each session to debrief about the key takeaways from the session – what did the client improve on, are changes being noted in the natural environment, and what do you plan to do in the next meeting time? You can use the debriefing guide in Chapter 12 to help.

More Practical Intervention Suggestions

- What is "behavior" to older clients? Behavior does not have to mean a young child throwing tantrums. For older kids, it might mean setting expectations of doing their best during the session. We have said to clients, "Here is our schedule for the day. This activity might be boring so let's pick something fun for right after." This type of honesty can be refreshing for older clients, especially as tasks become increasingly more academic and complex if goals are targeting higher level language and social interaction skills.
- What if my client is not paying attention to me? Try asking the client about preferred tasks or asking a key stakeholder. Does the child have a favorite Marvel character? Add the character to your PowerPoint slides in animation so the client has to attend to the screen to find it. If repeated approaches are unsuccessful, it might be appropriate to discuss the efficacy of telepractice for your client's needs.
- Have a client with difficulty attending to structured tasks? Set timers for breaks! Have clients stretch, play a computer game, or share about their day to have a set time to release before returning to your planned session. "Break time" can be useful when planned and given in short increments to promote engagement. Also consider incorporating movement! There are several tablet applications to incorporate physical activity into intervention. Many are available free of charge. Some suggestions include:
  - Exercisebuddy Professional (for iPad only)
  - GoNoodle (www.gonoodle.com)

- Lazy Monster (https://www.f6s.com/lazymonster)
- NFL Play 60 (American Heart Association; https://www.heart.org/en/professional/educator/nfl-play-60)
- Sworkit (https://sworkit.com)/SworkitKids (https://www.educationalappstore.com/app/sworkit-kids)
- Super Stretch Yoga (https://adventuresofsuperstretch.com).

Active Learning Task

Create a 30-minute teletherapy session for a 10-year-old verbally fluent client with autism to target a goal of initiating and maintaining a conversation with a partner. You can create your own materials or use tools available online. After preparing your session, exchange lesson plans and materials with a peer to complete a peer evaluation. Make sure to note whether behavior needs are considered and assess whether the task and materials are age appropriate and engaging.

Hybrid Approach

Some interventionists might consider a hybrid approach for clients with autism, offering some intervention sessions via telepractice and some with face-to-face services. This might be an ideal compromise for clients who have significant commuting concerns, but still want to participate in face-to-face intervention sessions. For example, an interventionist might schedule in-person sessions every other week with teletherapy sessions focused on parent coaching and training in between. Problem-solving approaches like hybrid methods were successfully employed for intervention for children with autism during the COVID-19 pandemic, resulting in positive feedback from parents and a low dropout rate (Samadi et al. 2020).

Summary

When considering intervention for clients with autism, opportunities to collaborate across disciplines should be taken whenever possible. IPE and IPP elevates service provision among related professionals who serve individuals with autism. Various intervention settings and modalities should be considered to offer the most appropriate method to serve the complex needs of the client in the most effective manner. Interventionists should consistently evaluate client and family needs to determine appropriate care that meets the unique needs of all involved.

REFLECTIONS ALONG THE PATH

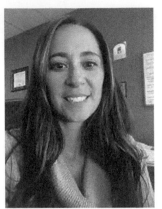

Melissa Bittner, PhD

My area of expertise is in adapted physical education (APE) and my research centers on APE as an evidence-based practice with students with autism. Literature indicates the value of engagement with other professionals on the interdisciplinary team and successful inclusion of students with disabilities in physical education (Bittner et al. 2021; Lieberman et al. 2017; Piletic and Davis 2010; Sato et al. 2017; Tripp et al. 2004). For example, interprofessional collaborative efforts between APE teachers, speech–language pathologists, and other professionals who work with students with autism employed in school settings can assist to increase generalization of skills, which can contribute to greater attainment of speech, language, and communication goals, ultimately helping students to demonstrate the skills needed to access their school curriculum.

Practical Collaboration Tips

1. Physical education has fun, kid-friendly equipment! This can be used to engage students in conversation (Bittner et al. 2021).

2. Most communication with students with disabilities takes place with adults (e.g. teacher, paraprofessional). Assist colleagues with how to initiate interaction with peers.

3. Help colleagues with considering how much a student can process at one time. For example, a teacher might give directions with too many chunks of information for a student to process. Encourage the teacher to provide instructions using only one or two bits of information at a time, and progress as developmentally appropriate (Winnick and Porretta 2022).

4. Open-ended questions may be very difficult for some students with ASD (e.g. "How are you feeling?"). Instead, collaborate to explain that some students may need choices (e.g. "Are you feeling happy or sad?").

5. Assist the APE teacher by adding physical education visual supports to the student's tablet if using an augmentative and alternative communication system; ask what upcoming units to expect and prepare the tablet accordingly to help prime the student.

6. Technology has been shown to have a positive effect on engagement of students with disabilities, especially when used concurrently with physical activity (Wong et al. 2015). The use of technology, an established

evidence-based practice on its own, is highly motivating and reinforcing (Takeo et al. 2007). Through the use of technology-aided instruction, students with disabilities may be able to engage in more on-task behaviors and learn physical activity skills at a faster rate than without technology-aided instruction (Case and Yun 2015).

Melissa Bittner PhD
Assistant Professor, Adapted Physical Education
California State University Long Beach

TEST QUESTIONS

1. Colleagues across related disciplines educating and learning from one another is called interprofessional practice. True or false?

2. When two or more professionals cooperate to improve outcomes and quality of care for their client without a preconceived professional hierarchy, it is called:
   A. IPE
   B. IPP
   C. Neither of the above

3. Colleagues across related disciplines educating and learning from one another is called interprofessional education. True or false?

4. Telepractice modalities should not be employed with individuals with autism due to poor efficacy. True or false?

5. Owing to the heterogeneity of ASD, group services are not best for intervention because sessions should be individualized for every client. True or false?

6. _____ involves colleagues in allied professions who educate and learn from each other.
   A. IPE
   B. IPP
   C. Neither of the above

7. All of the following are viable service delivery models for students with autism except:
   A. Push-in and consultative services
   B. Pull out individual and group services
   C. Teletherapy
   D. All of the above are viable service delivery modalities

REFERENCES

Alt, M. and Moreno, M. (2012). The effect of test presentation on children with autism spectrum disorders and neurotypical peers. *Language, Speech, and Hearing Services in Schools* 43 (2): 121–131.

Baharav, E. and Reiser, C. (2010). Using telepractice in parent training in early autism. *Telemedicine Journal and E-Health* 16 (6): 727–731.

Bittner, M., Daughrity, B., Ocampo, A. et al. (2021). Are adapted physical education teachers facilitating peer engagement and social communication? *Palaestra* 35 (1): 28–36.

Boisvert, M., Lang, R., Andrianopoulos, M., and Boscardin, M. (2010). Telepractice in the assessment and treatment of individuals with autism spectrum disorders: a systematic review. *Developmental Neurorehabilitation* 13 (6): 423–432.

Boisvert, M., Hall, N., Andrianopoulos, M., and Chaclas, J. (2012). The multi-faceted implementation of telepractice to service individuals with autism. *International Journal of Telerehabilitation* 4 (2): 11–24.

Case, L. and Yun, J. (2015). Visual practices for children with autism spectrum disorders in physical activity. *Palaestra* 29 (3): 21–25.

Cason, J. and Cohn, E. (2014). Telepractice: an overview and best practices. *Perspectives on Augmentative and Alternative Communication* 23 (1): 4–17.

Christopherson, T., Troseth, M., and Clingerman, E. (2015). Informatics-enabled interprofessional education and collaborative practice: a framework-driven approach. *Journal of Interprofessional Education and Practice* 1 (1): 10–15.

Covert, L., Slevin, J., and Hatterman, J. (2018). The effect of telerehabilitation on missed appointment rates. *International Journal of Telerehabilitation* 10 (2): 65–72.

Daffner, M., DuPaul, G., Kern, L. et al. (2019). Enhancing social skills of young children with ADHD: effects of a sibling-mediated intervention. *Behavior Modification* 44 (5): 698–726.

Dawson-Squibb, J., Davids, E., and Vries, P. (2019). Scoping the evidence for EarlyBird and EarlyBird plus, two United Kingdom-developed parent education training programmes for autism spectrum disorder. *Autism* 23 (3): 542–555.

Ellison, K., Guidry, J., Picou, P. et al. (2021). Telehealth and autism prior to and in the age of COVID-19: a systematic and critical review of the last decade. *Clinical Child and Family Psychology Review* 24 (3): 599–630.

Gulsrud, A., Hellemann, G., Shire, S., and Kasari, C. (2015). Isolating active ingredients in a parent-mediated social communication intervention for toddlers with autism spectrum disorder. *Journal of Child Psychology and Psychiatry* 57 (5): 606–613.

Hao, Y., Franco, J., Sundarrajan, M., and Chen, Y. (2021). A pilot study comparing tele-therapy and in-person therapy: perspectives from parent-mediated interventions for children with autism spectrum disorders. *Journal of Autism and Developmental Disorders* 51 (1): 129–143.

Johnson, A., Prelock, P., and Apel, K. (2016). IPE 101: introduction to interprofessional education and practice for speech-language pathology. In: *Interprofessional Education and Interprofessional Practice in Communication Sciences and Disorders: An Introduction and Case-Based Examples of Implementation in Education and Health Care Settings,* 2e (ed. A. Johnson). Rockville, MD: American Speech–Language–Hearing Association. Available at: `http://www.asha.org/uploadedFiles/IPE-IPP-Reader-eBook.pdf` (accessed 24 February 2022).

Kasari, C., Gulsrud, A., Paparella, T. et al. (2015). Randomized comparative efficacy study of parent-mediated interventions for toddlers with autism. *Journal of Consulting and Clinical Psychology* 83 (3): 554–563.

Koly, K., Martin-Hertz, S., Islam, S. et al. (2021). Parent mediated intervention programmes for children and adolescents with neurodevelopmental disorders in South Asia: a systematic review. *PLoS One* 16 (3): e0247432.

LeBlanc, L., Esch, J., Sidener, T., and Firth, A. (2006). Behavioral language interventions for children with autism: comparing applied verbal behavior and naturalistic teaching approaches. *Analysis of Verbal Behavior* 22 (1): 49–60.

Lieberman, L., Cavanaugh, L., Haegele, J. et al. (2017). The modified physical education class: an option for the least restrictive environment. *Journal of Physical Education, Recreation and Dance* 88 (7): 10–16.

Lock, R. and Finstein, R. (2017). Examining the need for autism sibling support groups in rural areas. *Rural Special Education Quarterly* 28 (4): 21–30.

Lytle, R., Lavay, B., Robinson, N., and Huettig, C. (2003). Teaching collaboration and consultation skills to preservice adapted physical education teachers. *Journal of Physical Education, Recreation and Dance* 74 (5): 49–53.

Marino, F., Chilá, P., Failla, C. et al. (2020). Tele-assisted behavioral intervention for families with children with autism Spectrum disorders: a randomized control trial. *Brain Sciences* 10 (9): 649.

Meadan, H., Meyer, L., Snodgrass, M., and Halle, J. (2017). Coaching parents of young children with autism in rural areas using internet-based technologies: a pilot program. *Rural Special Education Quarterly* 32 (3): 3–10.

Morrison, S., Lincoln, M., and Reed, V. (2011). How experienced speech-language pathologists learn to work on teams. *International Journal of Speech-Language Pathology* 13 (4): 369–377.

Neely, L., Rispoli, M., Gerow, S., and Hong, E. (2016). Preparing interventionists via telepractice in incidental teaching for children with autism. *Journal of Behavioral Education* 25: 393–416.

Neff, E., Betz, A., Saini, V., and Henry, E. (2017). Using video modeling to teach siblings of children with autism how to prompt and reinforce appropriate play. *Behavioral Interventions* 32 (3): 193–205.

Neubauer, N., Dayalu, V., Shulman, B., and Zipp, G. (2014). Interprofessional education at seton hall university. *Perspectives on Issues in Higher Education* 17 (2): 56.

Oono, I., Honey, E., and McConachie, H. (2013). Parent-mediated early intervention for young children with autism spectrum disorders (ASD). *Evidence-Based Child Health* 8 (6): 2380–2479.

Pacia, C., Holloway, J., Gunning, C., and Lee, H. (2021). A systematic review of family mediated social communication interventions for young children with autism. *Review Journal of Autism and Developmental Disorders* `https://doi.org/10.1007/s40489-021-00249-8`.

Parmanto, B., Pulantara, I., Schutte, J. et al. (2013). An integrated telehealth system for remote administration of an adult autism assessment. *Telemedicine and e-Health* 19 (2): 88–94.

Piletic, C. and Davis, R. (2010). A profile of the introduction to adapted physical education course within undergraduate physical education teacher education programs. *JOPERD: Journal of Physical Education, Recreation and Dance* 5 (2): 26–32.

Samadi, S., Bakhshalizadeh-Moradi, S., Khandani, F. et al. (2020). Using hybrid Telepractice for supporting parents of children with ASD during the COVID-19 lockdown: a feasibility study in Iran. *Brain Sciences* 10 (11): 892.

Sato, T., Haegele, J., and Foot, R. (2017). In-service physical educators' experiences of online adapted physical education endorsement courses. *Adapted Physical Activity Quarterly* 34 (2): 162–178.

Shire, S., Worthman, L., Shih, W., and Kasari, C. (2020). Comparison of face-to-face and remote support for interventionists learning to deliver JASPER intervention with children who have autism. *Journal of Behavioral Education* 29: 317–338.

Spector, V. and Charlop, M. (2018). A sibling-mediated intervention for children with autism Spectrum disorder: using the natural language paradigm (NLP). *Journal of Autism and Developmental Disorders* 48: 1508–1522.

Sutherland, R., Trembath, D., and Roberts, J. (2018). Telehealth and autism: a systematic search and review of the literature. *International Journal of Speech-Language Pathology* 20 (3): 324–336.

Takeo, T., Toshitaka, N., Daisuke, K. (2007). Development application softwares on PDA for autistic disorder children, IPSJ SIG Technical Reports 12, 31–38.

Tanner, A. and Dounavi, K. (2020). Maximizing the potential for infants at-risk for autism spectrum disorder through a parent-mediated verbal behavior intervention. *European Journal of Behavior Analysis* 21 (2): 271–291.

Tindall, L. and Huebner, R. (2009). The impact of an application of telerehabilitation technology on caregiver burden. *International Journal of Telerehabilitation* 1 (1): 3–8.

Tripp, A., Piletic, C., and Babcock, G. (2004). *A position statement on including students with disabilities in physical education*. Reston, VA: American Alliance for Health, Physical Education, Recreation and Dance.

Tsao, L. and Odom, S. (2006). Sibling-mediated social interaction intervention for young children with autism. *Topics in Early Childhood Special Education* 26 (2): 106–123.

Walker, V., Coogle, C., Lyon, K., and Turf, M. (2020). A meta-analytic review of paraprofessional-implemented interventions for students with autism spectrum disorder. *Psychology in the Schools* 58 (4): 686–701.

Walton, K. and Ingersoll, B. (2012). Evaluation of a sibling-mediated imitation intervention for young children with autism. *Journal of Positive Behavior Interventions* 14 (4): 241 253.

Winnick, J.P. and Porretta, D.L. (2022). *Adapted Physical Education and Sport*, 7e. Champaign, IL: Human Kinetics.

Wong, C., Odom, S.L., Hume, K. et al. (2015). *Evidence-Based Practices for Children, Youth, and Young Adults with Autism Spectrum Disorder*. Chapel Hill, NC: University of North Carolina, Frank Porter Graham Child Development Institute, Autism Evidence-Based Practice Review Group.

World Health Organization (2010). *Framework for Action on Interprofessional Education and Collaborative Practice*. Geneva: WHO.

FURTHER READINGS

Buckley, P., Murza, K., and Cassel, T. (2020). Perceptions of a collaborative professional learning program: seeing the "bigger picture". *Perspectives of the ASHA Special Interest Groups* 5 (1): 290–303.

Denning, C. and Moody, A. (2013). Supporting students with autism Spectrum disorders in inclusive settings: rethinking instruction and design. *Electronic Journal for Inclusive Education* 3 (1).

Donaldson, A. and Stahmer, A. (2014). Team collaboration: the use of behavior principles for serving students with ASD. *Language, Speech, and Hearing Services in Schools* 45 (4): 261–276.

Friend, M., Cook, L., Hurley-Chamberlain, D., and Shamberger, C. (2010). Co-teaching: an illustration of the complexity of collaboration in special education. *Journal of Educational and Psychological Consultation* 20: 9–27.

CHAPTER 12

Autism and the Parent

Reaching Across the Table

Learning objectives

By reading this chapter, interventionists will be able to:

1. Describe the relationship with self-efficacy, mental health, and knowledge for parents of individuals with autism.
2. Identify at least three different topics of importance to parents of individuals with autism throughout the lifespan.
3. Develop plans to support and teach families most effectively in individual and group therapy sessions.
4. Demonstrate understanding of parent perspective and experience.

THE ROLE OF DISPARITY

One day, a group of parents participated in a 12-week training called Parent Professional Partnership taking place at a private speech–language pathology practice located in Southern California. During that time, parents covered various topics relevant to supporting parents to succeed in working with their child with

Autism Spectrum Disorders from Theory to Practice: Assessment and Intervention Tools Across the Lifespan,
First Edition. Edited by Belinda Daughrity and Ashley Wiley Johnson.
© 2023 John Wiley & Sons Ltd. Published 2023 by John Wiley & Sons Ltd.

special needs. In one session, parents were covering the topic titled: "Advocacy, the individual education plan and your child." A parent speaker said to the parents "Remember, you are the parent and you are the most important person at the table. Never give up your power." Parents shook their heads vigorously in agreement.

Interventionists may say it is a given that the parent would be the most important person at the table. However, it is often not what is occurring in many school districts, clinic settings, and healthcare companies around the globe. As a result, many parents are placed in a position where they feel they have to "fight" for the best possible services for their child. Alternatively, they may be completely lost in the healthcare process and disengage early on due to barriers they may be experiencing. This is especially true when it comes to decisions surrounding handling of families, qualification criteria, diagnosis, services offered, and service delivery for clients with autism.

One barrier that many families may encounter in the process of navigating and obtaining new services for their children with autism is a disparity in provision of services. For the purposes of this text, we will refer to the National Institute on Aging (2022) Health Disparities Framework. Disparity is defined as "biological, behavioral, sociocultural, and environmental factors that influence population-level health differences" (Hill et al., 2015). This is often influenced by social and economic disadvantages. Social disadvantage is best described as less opportunities for access because of a person's position such as race or gender. Economic disadvantages describe limited opportunities to purchase services or goods due to having a low income (Dallman et al., 2021).

A study by Dallman et al. (2021) acknowledged disparities and differences that directly impact the use of allied health services, such as parents with a higher socioeconomic status and education level are more likely to receive interventions (speech therapy, occupational therapy, physical therapy, applied behavior analysis) in comparison with less educated and lower socioeconomic status peers. Knowledge of services available and ability to advocate was indicated as a potential reason for this significant difference among groups, indicating that the interventionist may be in a unique position to help increase parent knowledge and awareness of available treatments.

More specifically, children from lower socioeconomic backgrounds received 13 fewer treatment hours a month in comparison to students from a higher socioeconomic background (Rubenstein and Bishop-Fitzpatrick, 2018; Dallman et al., 2021). As an interventionist, this may actualize as a client receiving one or two fewer services a week, one type of service not being offered at all, or maybe no other services being offered aside from what is given in one setting. Children with autism coming from higher socioeconomic backgrounds are shown to have access to an autism diagnosis earlier and are prescribed less medicine than their peers. Furthermore, children from lower socioeconomic backgrounds tend to have limited resources and often cannot access independent evaluations early. As a result, they have to wait until their inception in K-12 school, losing valuable time that could have been spent in treatment (Dallman et al., 2021; Rubenstein and Bishop-Fitzpatrick, 2018; Wiley, 2016).

Social disadvantages resulting in disparity of provision of services for clients with autism can often be more subtle or blatantly obvious. For example, African-American and LatinX children with autism experience a lag between diagnosis and treatment and receive fewer services specific to treating children with autism in comparison with white counterparts (Dallman et al., 2021; Bishop-Fitzpatrick et al., 2019; Wiley, 2016). In terms of intervention, this may result in a delayed diagnosis, which impacts the prognosis for the client solely because of the client's minority background.

There are also health disparities that impact individuals with autism more broadly. Studies suggest that individuals with autism have a decreased life expectancy, increased mortality rate, and increases in unmet health needs in comparison with their peers with other developmental delays (Rubenstein and Bishop-Fitzpatrick, 2018; Dallman et al., 2021; Wiley, 2016). The reason behind these health disparities is emerging. Researchers have pointed to limited access to services, behavioral and language-based challenges, and parent knowledge of what is available to support their child as possible reasons contributing to the health disparities (Dallman et al., 2021; Wiley, 2016).

Reading about the disparate treatment that many individuals with autism will experience in their lifetime may ignite feelings of surprise, anger, frustration, and general disbelief, right? Well, imagine how a parent may feel when they watch it happening to their helpless young child. Alternatively, imagine how a parent may feel when experiencing disparities throughout the life of their now young adult with autism.

Authors Angell and Solomon (2017) studied parents' experiences of accessing and navigating their child's autism diagnosis, concluding that some parents reported feelings of "fighting like a bear to protect [their] child and their interests." Others found that securing the necessary help for a child with autism can require waging a small war with the gatekeepers of state and school district services (Zarembo, 2011; Angell and Solomon, 2017). Of course, some parents armed with the right knowledge and supports, report their experience with navigating their child's autism journey to be positive and feeling like they have been involved and included along the way.

Regardless of the personal accounts and experiences, one commonality expressed by many parents is the feeling of receiving an autism diagnosis for their child and then being met with the reality that the odds may be stacked against them for the rest of their lives. This feeling can easily make a parent go into "fight or flight" mode.

As we consider the importance of shaping the practices of newly minted interventionists such as yourself, we place value and importance on understanding the role of disparities prior to working with the parents of individuals with autism. When you are more prepared to understand parents' and clients' experiences, you have the potential to shift the trajectory and outcomes for individuals who you treat in your practice. So dive in, take some time to put yourself in a parent's shoes, and you will be better equipped to truly serve the clients and families on your future caseload.

Active Learning Task

In terms of intervention, disparities may manifest themselves in different ways when working with a client. Understanding the full picture before reacting is critical for making the best clinical judgment. Partner with a peer or peers to do this activity. Individually complete the chart below. Once completed, take a moment to compare answers with your partner. Write a group reflection on the differences or similarities found and what was learned from the activity.

Disparity	Client presentation	How may a parent respond	Interventionist response
Late diagnosis		Frustrated, looking for answers, limited trust.	
	Meeting language goals, social loner, shies away from talking in class.	Unsatisfied but looking for more, several questions, not satisfied with child's progress despite ability to fully articulate. Closest therapy clinic is 40 miles away in the closest large city.	
	Severe gastrointestinal issues causing challenges with toileting which results in the client wanting to leave your therapy session frequently throughout.	Thinks everything is fine; thinks you may be just picking on the child.	
Access to services		Parent continues to say at IEP meetings that the teacher is "racist;" is very upset; wants more services. Parent is not feeling heard.	
	Child is added to your caseload, they have some services but need more. You have other similar clients who are currently receiving individual services but this client is not.	Parent works two jobs, does not attend the IEP meetings because she is unable to get off work and catch the bus in time to make it.	You hold a meeting and amend the services to reflect the actual needs of the client.

IEP, individual education plan.

THE ROLE OF MENTAL HEALTH

I know I need to be strong, I know I need to be strong. It's not an option, I have to be...
I was depressed for a month, and one day I was like, "What am I doing here?" I'm
not going to help my son, I'm not going to do anything for him. I don't know how I
did it, but I stood up and I started to make a call, to do a lot of stuff. It was all by
myself. Every time I do things, it was all by myself... So I went down to the therapy.
All the LatinXs think that you have to be crazy to go and it's not true (Wiley, 2016).

For families of children with autism spectrum disorder (ASD), coping with their child's current ability is often a challenge, and can be very stressful. Research findings have shown that one major challenge that parents face is their child's behaviors (Hall, 2012). These behaviors are often challenging, not only at home but particularly in an outside setting when interacting within the family's community. Despite occasionally aggressive and/or self-injurious behaviors, a difference between children with ASD and children with other disabilities is a "normal" outward appearance, which often makes it hard to identify them at first glance as having autism. For some parents, feelings of blame and stress are often experienced, due to limited knowledge about autism and pressure from outside people (Hall, 2012; Bebbington and Beecham, 2007).

As a result of these additional stressors and experiences, quality of life is often reduced for families of children with ASD (Hall, 2012; Goin-Kochel et al., 2009). Many aspects of life in the community are affected, with parents reporting loss of employment or underemployment, due to difficulty finding employment which fits the demands of their home life. Parents also reported limited ability to socialize in the community settings because of people's limited knowledge of the needs and differences of their child with ASD (Hall, 2012).

When a child in the family has ASD, parents are at a significantly higher risk of being diagnosed with mental health issues, most commonly depression (Meltzer, 2011). Stress levels are elevated for many parents of children with ASD (Clifford and Minnes, 2013) especially during the first five years of intervention, because this is considered the "critical learning period." Meltzer (2011), studied 34 families (17 with children with ASD, 17 with typically developing children) and found parents of children with ASD reported higher levels of depression due to limited sleep and the child's behavior.

Meltzer (2011) found parents of children with ASD, in comparison with several other special needs (e.g. Down syndrome, intellectual disability, fragile X syndrome, and developmental delay), reported the highest level of depression, making it imperative to develop targeted interventions and resources for this population. Furthermore, findings revealed that mothers reported higher levels of depression in comparison with fathers, primarily attributed to sleep differences (Meltzer, 2011).

When further examining stress levels in the parents of children with autism, Cohen et al. (2015) found that many parents with high stress levels are more harsh, controlling, and inconsistent when child rearing in comparison with parents with lower perceived stress levels. As interventionists working with a client with autism, it is important to take into consideration the stressors that may cause the behavior seen in parents. For example, did you know that parents of children with disabilities are more likely to have police called on them by a professional or neighbor. In fact, a 2020

Time magazine article (Abrams, 2020) acknowledged that people with disabilities, especially Black individuals, are more likely to have interactions with police than white individuals without disabilities (Haas and Gibbs, 2020). While it is our responsibility as interventionists to keep the wellbeing of our client at the forefront of our decision making, it is important to take into consideration the obstacles that parents may face surrounding an autism diagnosis. Here are six strategies that an interventionist can use in treatment that support a parent's mental health:

- *Provide opportunities for knowledge for parents to increase their confidence levels.* Parents with higher confidence levels, known as parent self-efficacy, are perceived as more consistent, contingent, and authoritative (Cohen et al., 2015; Alper et al., 2021), and are also perceived as more fit to help their children to overcome barriers and navigate obstacles along the way.
- *Incorporate therapy goals with the goal of decreasing the presence of maladaptive behaviors experienced by the parents in mind.* When greater prosocial behaviors are taught in therapy to children with ASD, parents report lowers stress levels (Huang et al., 2014; Bishop-Fitzpatrick et al., 2019).
- *Provide parents of children with autism with information* geared toward supporting them such as parent support groups (*PSGs*) that they can access, and possible services available to them, such as respite care services, that will increase the quality of life for the client and for the family.
- *Parents of mainstreamed students with autism will benefit from the interventionist facilitating networks with other parents* of mainstreamed children to assist their child in developing important social opportunities. (Daughrity, 2018).
- *Create a safe space and ask appropriate qualifying questions* during debriefing with parents in an effort to help them to feel comfortable to share current challenges and to celebrate success.
- *Take time to celebrate victories.* Many times, parents may not be able to see small victories when they have challenges and stressors in front of them. As interventionists, it can be easy to report the challenges that arise in therapy, but it should be easier to focus on the positives in treatment as well. This will help you put all challenges in perspective and, when shared with the parent, it will help them to put challenges in perspective as well.

A NOTE ON PARENT SUPPORT GROUPS (PSG)

Parent support groups (PSGs) are considered a critical component in helping parents to better help their children and themselves. Research has shown that PSGs are valuable in helping a parent to build supportive and meaningful friendships, and also to gather and receive critical information needed about their child's disability (Papageorgiou and Kalyva, 2010). Further, participating in PSGs help parents to have decreased stress levels and more positive moods (Clifford and Minnes, 2013; Papageorgiou and Kalyva, 2010; Wiley, 2016). Although parent participation in PSGs is limited (Clifford and Minnes, 2013), PSGs can serve as a safe, supportive environment where parents can learn to cope, and also regain the positive self-efficacy needed to properly care for and support their child with special needs (Wiley, 2016).

In the field of autism, the use of PSGs has been researched and found to be effective in helping parents of children with ASD to experience positive child outcomes and better managed stress levels (Clifford and Minnes, 2013; Keen et al., 2010; Keen, 2010; Hall, 2012). Clifford and Minnes (2013) surveyed 149 parents of children with ASD on their beliefs about PSGs, coping styles, social support, mood, and use of the PSG. They found a significant difference in the reported adaptive coping strategies used, indicating that parents in a PSG reported using more adaptive strategies in comparison with both parents who formerly but did not currently attend a PSG and parents who had never attended a PSG. They also noted that parents who were not enrolled in a PSG indicated that accessibility was the primary agent keeping them from being involved.

In 2016, a research study was completed with 30 Hispanic mothers of children with autism to explore the relationships between self-efficacy and mental health with enrollment in a PSG. Mothers in the study were in three groups: parents of children with an autism diagnosis and in a PSG for five years or more, parents who were in the PSG for less than five years, and parents who currently were not in a PSG. Data found that parents who were not in the PSG for any length of time had significant mental health risk factors in comparison with all other groups. Results were analyzed from scores obtained on various mental health and self-efficacy scales. These results may have wider implications. One implication was that when parents are in a PSG, regardless of length of time, they may show more positive mental health in comparison to parents not connected to a PSG (Wiley, 2016).

While it may not be feasible to create a support group in your setting, it is important for interventionists to be knowledgeable about supports that are available to families and to provide that information to them as we are able. The National Association of Autism (2020) recommends the Wrightslaw Yellow Pages For Kids with Disabilities to identify PSGs by state for parents of children with disabilities. Keeping such resources of available supports in your area that you can readily share with families are valuable items in your toolkit as your transform a child and strengthen a family.

For more information on resources for families in your state visit Wrightslaw Yellow Pages For Kids with Disabilities (www.yellowpagesforkids.com).

CULTURAL CONSIDERATIONS

When I first received an autism diagnosis I was scared. I didn't know what it meant or what to expect. I was in the room with a lot of therapists who didn't know my child like I did but they told me he would have a hard time for the rest of his life. I went home to my husband, closed my door, and just cried.

Mother, Spanish speaking, child with autism less than five years post-diagnosis.
(Wiley, 2016)

Increasing workforce diversity has continued to be a challenge for many allied health professions. For example, African-Americans make up less than 1% of speech pathologists licensed through the American Speech–Language–Hearing Association. Moreover, only 6% of the entire membership body identifies as bilingual and able to serve linguistically diverse clients. Similarly, in 2016, the American Community Survey found that about 84% of the active psychology workforce was white, an over-representation compared with the national population, which is 76% white (American Psychological Association, 2018; Pappas, 2019).

Both ASHA and the American Psychological Association (APA) has made it a priority to create and support legislation that focuses on workforce diversity and reten-tion of practitioners of color. Why is this so important you may ask? According to a US Government Accountability Office (2017) study, having a more diverse healthcare workforce is important because patients have better outcomes when their provider looks like them and shares a similar ethnic and cultural background. While these efforts to diversify practitioners in allied health professions are great, it also brings to the fore-front the need for all interventionists to take time to be **culturally responsive** when interacting with students of color. When focusing to ensure that interventionists are culturally responsive, we create a pathway toward success for our clients in the future.

The APA calls interventionists to be culturally responsive by recognizing that family and individual beliefs and values will vary based on culture, background, personal pref-erences, and individual variability (American Psychological Association, 2018). In terms of interacting with parents in the therapy setting, this may look like parental dif-ferences in beliefs about disabilities, variability in parenting styles, and variability in perceptions about acceptable practices. One thing interventionists are called to do is to keep up with literature on ethnic and racial disparities in an effort to understand what is happening around us. Furthermore, interventionists are called to reflect and under-stand their own positionality which is their awareness and understanding of statuses and identities given the context of systematic power differences (Papoudi et al., 2021; American Speech–Language–Hearing Association, 2017; Perry and Evans, 2021a,b). The following is a list of appropriate culturally responsive practices for interventionists who interact with culturally and linguistically diverse clients and families:

- Become familiar with cultural difference and appreciate and celebrate diversity.
- Consider how racial and ethnocultural norms may shape your own behavior in practice.
- Evaluate how the values, norms and behaviors associated with one's own ethnic or racial identities influence your treatment process.
- Display **cultural humility** by employing the art of questioning parents about their preferences, beliefs, and attitudes to learn how to best interact with their child.
- Do not dismiss but validate the concerns of culturally and linguistically diverse families.
- Be cognizant of intragroup differences among ethnicities to ensure you do not typecast the parent or the child.

Autism and Cultural Experience

As an interventionist, we know that each client presents with unique circumstances and skill sets. We urge practitioners to not generalize these findings and apply them to all parents of clients within this ethnicity. Rather, spend time learning about trends, findings, and arguments. Keep this information in your toolkit to pull out as needed. The following information is a brief summary of data regarding parent findings organized by different minority groups.

African-American, Black

African-American parenting often is driven by Afrocentric beliefs and cultural heritage. The historical influence of slavery continues to be relevant in modern parenting patterns of African-American parents. During this time, parents placed extreme emphasis on keeping their child safe and as close to them as possible to protect their child. In terms of having a child with autism, African-American parents are often characterized by interventionists as more harsh or controlling when interacting with their children (Keefe et al., 2017).

It is important for interventionists to consider the unique familial concerns surrounding fathering when a child presents with developmental differences. For African-Americans, this is particularly concerning, given the disproportionate outcomes in occupation, education, and incarceration (Pearson et al., 2021; Hannon et al., 2017; Sue et al. 2008). In a study conducted by Hanon et al. (2018), six Black fathers of children with autism shared their experience with fathering. Patience was a common act that all men identified as having increased as a result of the challenge of having a child on the spectrum. Before casting judgment or making assumptions, it is critical to acknowledge that you likely do not understand what the parent is going through. Provide support to empower in the process of acceptance of the diagnosis by providing literature and access to resources when able. Black parenting styles place a strong emphasis on a child's behavior, with the importance of not embarrassing the family. This same level of importance is also placed on the child presenting as clean and neat. Taking this information into consideration, one may better understand why having a child with autism may be especially challenging for Black parents to cope with because behavioral challenges and personal care difficulties is a common challenge.

Dr. WILEY JOHNSON'S THERAPY VIEWPOINT

In practice, this may look like observing a Black parent spank a child to avoid embarrassment in public or being noticeably bothered if a child is returned unkempt after a messy sensory focused treatment session.

When debriefing or meeting with the child, this could look like a parent being more guarded. Remember, it is not because the parent does not like the interventionist. It likely could be a parents desire to protect their child and keep them safe at all times. As interventionists, there have been many times where we see that fear of the unknown makes a parent seem more difficult than they really may be. With the goal of gaining trust and getting results, we notice interactions improve greatly over time.

Asian-American

Asian culture is a more collectivistic culture than many Western cultures. Perceptions of others, communication styles, and values on education are important when considering Asian parents of children with autism. Post diagnosis, feelings of shame and isolation from extended family is a common experience of many members of this culture (Diep et al., 2016; Seung, 2013).

Asian culture often uses high-context communication styles, with an emphasis on silence, emotion, and inference. There is also an authoritarian hierarchy with an importance placed on education and respect of professionals.

> ### Dr. WILEY JOHNSON'S THERAPY VIEWPOINT
>
> In practice, this may look like a parent nodding in an individual education plan meeting and staying silent as you describe and plan for their child (Diep et al., 2016; Seung, 2013).

This nodding behavior may not be a sign of agreement, which can be interpreted by interventionists with European communication styles. Rather, it is sign of respect and a way to communicate. Asian parents also may not ask many questions because of the importance placed on education and deferring to the professional. It is important to educate yourself on these practices to make the parent feel comfortable to be involved in the process.

In terms of treatment, some Asian parents may be more likely to spend extra resources to have the child with an educational tutor instead of traditional therapies because enhancing academics is an area of importance in the Asian culture. In terms of treatment style, Asian parents of children with autism lean more toward structured methods like applied behavior analysis therapies over more qualitative methods such as play based interventions (Diep et al., 2016; Seung, 2013, 2017).

Hispanic

Of parents with children with ASD, LatinX families often are often at higher risk for mental health issues. They also have lower personal self-confidence levels, often because of external factors that can add to the challenges and obstacles of raising and being involved with a child with ASD. Some of these external factors for LatinX parents may include, but are not limited to, socioeconomic status, gender, family structure, immigration status, language barriers, and educational history (Lopez et al., 2019; Morales et al., 2011). Within the LatinX family unit, the mother usually assumes the responsibility of primary care provider for their child with ASD (Magaña et al., 2013; Iland et al., 2012). Interventionists should be sensitive to the potential influence of immigration status for families they serve. The parent may be more fearful to share due to current immigration status or may be the sole responsible person to care for all of the children in the household.

> ### Dr. WILEY JOHNSON'S THERAPY VIEWPOINT
>
> In practice, this may look like a parent being more hesitant to share biographical details regarding their child or even limited knowledge of their child's current skill sets. It is not because this mother is not involved.

Historically, Hispanic children have been disproportionately represented in special education, often being identified with ASD later then their non-Hispanic counterparts. In California, the California developmental system has shown that children with ASD who are born to poor, non-English speaking, single Latina mothers are least likely to receive state funding through the Regional Centers (Iland et al., 2012). When looking at the impact of both ethnic disparity and external contributing factors, Latina mothers of children with ASD can be considered an at-risk population, which deserves to be specially targeted to help mothers to develop the positive self-efficacy and strong mental health skills needed to champion services and support in working with their child with ASD. Taking time to connect the mother with resources that are linguistically important is critical to allow them to access as much information at possible.

While the above descriptions are not exhaustive, taking time to be culturally competent and responsive is a must when interacting with culturally, linguistically diverse families. When we keep these practices at the top of our interventionist toolkit, you will find parents will feel comfortable and hopefully will place value and importance in joining you in the process of planning the best care for their child. It is important to keep in mind that cultural groups are not a monolithic, and all families must be considered individually to appropriately address their needs.

CREATING OPPORTUNITIES TO PROVIDE KNOWLEDGE

> *Use the internet to do your homework, take a notebook when you meet with the individual education plan team. There is a lot of information and terms that people will use.*
>
> *Los Angeles Speech and Language Therapy Center, Parent Professional Partnership Training,* **Francis Gomez, 2020.**

Say the phrase "provide knowledge" to yourself. What type of picture comes to your head? You may see a picture of a person handing books to another person or even a teacher standing at the front of the class. While that does provide knowledge to another party in the general sense, that describes one piece of what is intended when we suggest providing knowledge to a parent of a person with autism.

Data has shown that when it comes to working with parents of young children with autism, the style has shifted from expert passing knowledge to *coaching a parent* and using *family involvement* to facilitate student achievement.

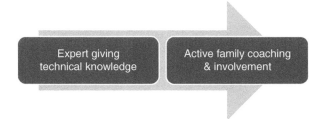

It has long been acknowledged by researchers that parent/family involvement is a critical component of a comprehensive program for a person with an autism diagnosis. It has also been acknowledged that the parent coaching component of an intervention session, when done mindfully, will provide the interventionist with the following (Siller et al., 2018):

- Intimate knowledge of the child's abilities, challenges, and typical performance.
- Better understanding of a family's daily routines, environments, and culture.
- Ideas of the goals the family would like to accomplish.

One of the first things to consider when engaging a parent is taking time to think of how your general communication style is received. While we all have our unique ways of communicating, we want to primarily create an environment or setting where a parent does not feel threatened and feels comfortable to share. When engaging a parent, it is critical to think of *how* you pose questions or make statements. The primary intent is to help a parent to feel comfortable engaging with you, open to receiving knowledge from you, and comfortable sharing their strengths and weaknesses. When creating an environment like this, you will have a critical channel of information and knowledge, while promoting family-centered care.

Active Learning Task

Take a moment to complete the following chart. Once completed, share your responses with your peers to engage them in conversations surrounding differences in how we ask and pose questions. After meeting with your group, write a reflection on the noted differences among peers and what you may or may not have learned in terms of how you may pose questions/make statements to a parent.

What do I need to know?	What will I ask or say?	Do you foresee this to be received negatively, positively, or neutrally? Why?
Language spoken in the home	You speak Spanish, right?	Negatively. Assuming someone's language can lead you down a road of trouble
How the child engages with siblings at home		
Share about the caregiver homework assignment from last week		
	I'm seeing Darrell being a little agitated recently. It is so different for him! Have you seen anything like that or maybe has something changed recently?	Positively
The client is no longer qualifying for service. You would like parent to buy in and share sentiment		
Student choice		

Sample Key

What do I need to know?	What will I ask or say?	Do you foresee this to be received negatively, positively, or neutrally? Why?
If the child speaks any other languages	You speak Spanish right?	Negatively
How the child engages with siblings at home	So, tell me more about Johnny and his brother! How does he interact and communicate with him?	Positively
Share about the caregiver homework assignment from last week	Did you have a chance to do last week's assignment? Can you tell me how it went?	Positively
Check if there have been any changes making the client agitated in the home	I'm seeing Darrell being a little agitated recently. It is so different for him! Have you seen anything like that or maybe has something changed recently?	Positively

What do I need to know?	What will I ask or say?	Do you foresee this to be received negatively, positively, or neutrally? Why?
The client is no longer qualifying for service. You would like parent to buy in and share sentiment	Wow it's amazing Johnny has met his goals! I am not seeing anything else I can work on with him currently and I was wondering what you are seeing at home?	Neutrally
Student choice		

While parent coaching is considered a reputable means of engaging a family and developing a parent's skill set, some interventionists, scientists, and even parents may argue that it does not work equally on all parents (Siller et al., 2018). We encourage interventionists to use various methods based on your parent base, the setting, and the style of interaction you can have with them. It may not be possible that you are able to see them face to face and share stories of what happened during the session. It may be that you only get to have a minute with them as a phone check-in as they are on their way from one therapy to another. Regardless of circumstance surrounding the opportunity, the primary emphasis should always be on sharing and imparting information. *Sharing information* will allow parents the opportunity to listen and/or respond to:

- methods of treatment
- strategies to help the parent to become the facilitator
- questions
- shared growth or challenge experiences.

Methods of Treatment

Sharing what occurred in therapy assists parents by increasing their knowledge base of *how* the interventionist is working with their child. When sharing therapeutic methods, it is important to prepare ahead of time and ensure that the description you are using can be understood by a professional and a parent alike. Some therapeutic terms or concepts may be hard for a caregiver to understand if they are not in the same discipline. Therefore, it is important to ensure that what you are saying is understandable in a layperson's terms, rather than only in professional jargon.

Active Learning Task

Jargon Made Simple
    Identify all the acronyms below frequently used in clinical treatment.

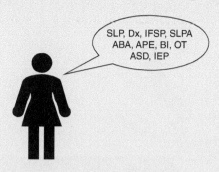

How many did you get correct out of 10? Now ask an individual outside of your major/department/professional field.

    How many did that person get correct? What are the implications for using jargon with caregivers?

When providing an example of therapeutic methods, it is equally important to share how the client responded to the treatment. The authors recommend providing the parent with an actual production (i.e. speech production or a sample of physical work) to help visualize what the interventionist is trying to describe. Another amazing way to share therapeutic methods is to include the use of video. Now we rely heavily on technology, we can use it to share with parents in a fun and interactive fashion.

While it may be challenging and time consuming to review each aspect of therapy and how the child responded, it is important to provide parents with a full picture of the treatment that occurred. One recommendation can be to give a brief synopsis of each task and provide one statement for how the child responded to the day's session.

Strategies can help the parent become a facilitator. A client has maximally met a goal when they are able to achieve success in the natural setting. For most interventionists, it is challenging to identify how a client does in the natural setting, since many support services for people with autism are provided in a therapeutic setting with limited access to the client's natural environment. Therefore, when engaging in sharing with a parent, it is important to share successful strategies used in the therapeutic setting. This will help parents to provide solutions to challenges and will teach parents how to support and empower their child. Remember, when clients show the behaviors learned in therapy everywhere, it results in a parent feeling less stressed when interacting with their child (Huang et al., 2014; Rubenstein and Bishop-Fitzpatrick, 2018).

When sharing strategies, it is recommended that you allow a parent an opportunity to practice the skills taught, as in Figure 12.1, which shows a method of developing a parent's confidence and ability to follow through using shared strategies.

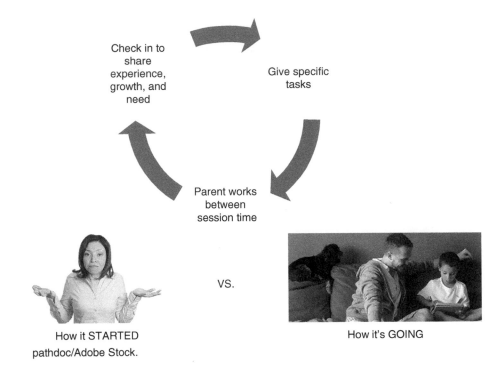

How it STARTED
pathdoc/Adobe Stock.

How it's GOING

FIGURE 12.1   Developing a parent's confidence.

Active Learning Task

Identify a parent activity to teach the following strategies:

- Establishing eye contact
- Naming items
- Answering "wh-" questions
- Having a three- to four-turn conversation
- Playing a simple game with rules
- Expressing wants and needs

Take some time to compare and contrast your activities with your peers. Compile your responses into parent handouts and create a guidebook of parent activities for various strategies. Think about parent demand, what is in the natural setting, and what may be "easy" for a parent to do given other demands they may have (jobs, other children, household tasks, etc.).

Questions and Sharing Growth and Experiences

The Individuals with Disabilities in Education Improvement Act states that services for individuals falling under that category should be family centered for early-intervention-age clients. Being able to ask questions and get answers from their service providers is not only their lawful right, but also helps them to better understand how to care for their child. However, for many families, culturally, they may not question persons of authority as they may see it as a sign of disrespect and or ignorance (Seung, 2017, Diep et al., 2016, Seung, 2013). It is important that you ensure that parents know that questions are encouraged and welcomed. One way to do that is to ask parents after each major point shared:

- Does that sound like your child?
- Do you have any questions about the information I just shared?
- Does that make sense to you?

While it seems counterintuitive, when an interventionist is tasked with seeing multiple clients in a day or overseeing a larger group, it is easy to forget to stop and ensure understanding. Therefore, make a habit of this early and often! When a family feels a sense of safety and security, they may be more willing to open and share about challenges and experiences they may have. Understanding the parent's perspective can assist an interventionist in making decisions on treatment direction, gain valuable insight with how the client is doing outside of the therapy setting, and better understand what is important to the parent (Siller et al., 2018).

ENGAGING PARENTS IN THE GROUP SETTING

Delay in social skills is a hallmark impairment of autism. As discussed in previous chapters, many services for students with autism may prove to be most effective in the group setting. This setting allows students to work on goals, especially in the area of social pragmatics. While there are several benefits from delivering group-based services, it comes as no easy task. As one may imagine, significant challenges may occur in the following areas:

- Managing the needs and behaviors of multiple clients at one time.
- Delegating to support staff.
- Working on multiple goals concurrently.
- Providing adequate oversight for the entire group.
- Engaging caregivers in the best possible way without burning yourself out.

Active Learning Task

Take a deeper look at the challenges commonly faced by interventionists in the group setting. Identify which deficit listed you may face in your current or future practice. Take time to identify two goals you want to achieve that focus on improvement in your known or anticipated "challenge" area.

For the purposes of this chapter, we take a closer look at engaging caregivers in the group setting. ASHA and the APA's position on parent coaching is that it is best practice to engage caregivers when you are able (Tambyraja, 2020, American Psychological Association, 2014). This includes engaging caregivers in group-based services. However, with multiple students, it may be a challenge to engage as many parents as possible. It is important to consider the amount of time, productivity, and carryover. When taking a moment to address parents thoroughly, you will demonstrate that you are a thoughtful and prepared interventionist. And, after all, who does not love a thoughtful person?

Sample Structure

Parent Debriefing

Ten minutes of a weekly two-hour social skills group.

- Share the day's agenda from a broad scale (one to two minutes).
- Have a report of each activity lead; share impressions of the session (one minute).
- Share some work samples or therapy examples (one minute).
- Check in on last week's assignment and allow families to share observations of child and experience (three to four minutes).
- Give assignment for the week to the family (one minute).
- Share any pertinent announcements for the week (one minute).
- Listen to parent questions (three to four minutes).

Notice the active verb highlighted in each point of the sample parent debriefing structure. The dominant active verb in this structure is "share." Sharing information is a critical component to a successful parent debriefing and will allow parents the opportunity to listen and respond to:

- Other parents: Simply put, parents identify with parents. Hearing successes and triumphs encourages parents who may be experiencing challenges as they navigate having a child with an autism diagnosis.
- Examples of work provided to the clients in the session.
- Individual experiences (when able) to assist families in understanding student achievement.

Once you have communicated with a family, ensure that you take time to listen to what they share or ask you. Parents of children with autism commonly report not being heard and feelings of being alone (Wiley, 2016). As an interventionist, you can decrease these feelings in a parent through allowing them to know they are heard. Using key phrases like "I hear what you are saying" or "Let me understand your question and restate what was said" will help to open the lines of communication for families in a positive direction.

Finally, take time to celebrate the small victories with parents. For some students, small victories may be all parents experience for some time. One strategy to use is to highlight a student who achieved a maximum level and one who achieved at the lowest level. Finding the positives in both students' performance encourages parents and helps them to see the positives amid many challenges.

Therapy Golden Nugget		

Parent and Interventionist Debrief Checklist
Client name/group: _____
Interventionist: _____ Date: _____

Key points	Timing (minutes)	Notes
Share each element of the session	1–2	
Report each activity lead. Share impressions of how the group and a few individuals did in the group after mentioned activity	1–2	
Show some work sample, video example, or therapy materials	1	
Give assignment for the week to the family to facilitate generalization	1	
Share any other pertinent announcement(s) for the week	1	
Ask and listen to parent questions, comments, or concerns	1–3	

CAREGIVER CENTERED EVIDENCE-BASED APPROACHES

The intent of this chapter is to stress the importance in understanding, engaging, and partnering with caregivers who have a child with autism. There are some approaches that are considered caregiver centered. These evidence-based approaches are acknowledged by professional organizations such as the ASHA and the APA. As an interventionist, if you decide that the emphasis of treatment should include a specific treatment approach which is parent centered, it is recommended to spend additional time researching the method and seeking further professional development in that area. Below you will find a number of commonly sited and referenced approaches for interventionists to use to support parents of individuals with autism.

- **Applied behavior analysis:** Parent training is one several principles of practice for applied behavior analysis. Parents are trained to learn how to facilitate interactions with your child, strategies to use, and are coached while practicing strategies with the interventionist. It creates the potential for a parent to learn effective techniques for behavior management and skill development.

- **Behavioral parent training** is a psychotherapeutic stand-alone or supplemental approach to work directly with parents to empower them to be the agent of change for their child (American Psychological Association, 2019). Parent training is known to specifically support families to reduce behavioral challenges like sleep difficulties, disruptive behaviors, bowel and bladder training, food sensitivity, and wandering and elopement.

- **Parent-mediated or parent-implemented intervention** consists of parents using direct, individualized intervention practices with their child to increase positive learning opportunities and acquisition of skills.

- **More Than Words – a Hanen Program**® that offers a parent-directed approach focusing on day-to-day life, taking advantage of everyday activities to help the child improve communication and social skills (Sussman, 1999). This program is typically used for early language intervention with young children with ASD.

- **Talkability**™ is a Hanen Program for parents of verbal children with ASD. The program teaches parents practical ways to help their child learn people skills, such as "tuning in" to others' feelings and thoughts by attending to nonverbal cues, such as body language, facial expressions, and tone of voice. The ability to consider others' point of view and to empathize are considered essential for successful conversation and for making friends (Sussman, 2006).

SHIFTING PARENT PERSPECTIVES: CREATING A WINNING MENTALITY

From the day her son was diagnosed with autism nine years ago, [mother's name] has made it her full-time job to find him the best possible help. Hiring lawyers and experts to press her case, she established herself as a mother whose demands could not easily be dismissed. The result has been a bounty of assistance for [child's name]: A behavioral therapist who works with him at home and comes along on family outings, a personal aide at school and specialists to design his curriculum, improve his speech and refine his motor skills. So far, the state of California and the Los Angeles Unified School District have spent at least $300 000 on specialized services for [child's name].

Angell and Solomon (2017).

The purpose of this chapter is to assist interventionists in the process of including and winning over parents. While there is no surefire way to achieve this and every parent is an individual, we hope that the information imparted will educate you and help you to focus on critical components of parent involvement.

Having a child with autism is a lifelong commitment and we are often are just one stop along the way in a family's journey. Parents of children with autism report that they initially approach interventionists with a "logic of care" mentality but are met with an "autism is a business" perspective from the schools and insurance companies. That disillusionment is often what causes parents to feel they must fight and treat us as adversaries rather than partners. Since we are not in the family's shoes day after day, the only thing we can truly focus on as interventionists is doing good WORK.

- ⚠ WORK to celebrate and share small victories.
- ⚠ WORK to educate and inform.
- ⚠ WORK to gain trust.
- ⚠ WORK to be empathetic.
- ⚠ WORK to be culturally competent.

When we WORK, we will WIN.

SUMMARY

Shifting parents to the center of service delivery is critical when an option. This chapter highlights strategies for engaging parent caregivers in the process of service delivery through providing personal accounts of what you saw their child do in the session and considering concrete strategies or evidence-based approaches to use in your own practice. Special emphasis is placed on cultural humility, the role of disparity, and important considerations for specific cultural and linguistically diverse populations.

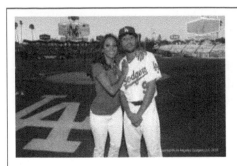

Holly Robinson Peete, celebrity, ADVOCATE, **RJ'S MOM.**

Congratulations on your decision to work with individuals with autism! My sincere hope is that your career brings you happiness, purpose, and makes an impact on countless individuals and their families for years to come. Autism is a deeply personal subject because my son, RJ, now 23 years old, is a brilliant young man who is thriving. He happens to be on the autism spectrum. In hindsight, I wish we were handed our "welcome to autism" packet. But we weren't. Instead, we went on a self-guided tour.

When RJ was diagnosed with autism in 2000 at age three, it was one of the hardest days of our lives. I call it the "never" day. We were told by a developmental pediatrician that he would *never* do much, would *never* live independently, and would *never* find meaningful employment. They even said that he would *never* say "I love you." Can you imagine the pain and confusion that we felt at that moment? It was tough on my entire family, especially my husband, Rodney Peete.

When we first found out, my husband, former NFL quarterback, super dad, our personal hero, didn't want to accept that his son was any different than any other child. He didn't want to believe his son was impacted by autism. Whatever this was, he believed he could "coach" it out of him. I would ask him to call certain people or read this piece of literature to teach him more about autism. Despite my attempts, the fact remained that this was just too hard to accept. As a unit, we had to have a "come to Jesus" moment. I asked him "Are you on team RJ or not? Make a choice because it's all hands on deck!"

His sentiments, shared by many fathers (and mothers) is one that I believe that all therapists should be aware of. If I could go back in time I would have had more patience with Rodney. I encourage you to use patience and to remember that many dads have high hopes for their children – especially their sons. Without being able to visualize all the potential that their child can have, they may feel confused, lost, or just plain mad. That's OK. Thankfully, with time, we encountered what I call our various *angels on the path*. People like Dr. Pamela Wiley or Mr. Tim Lee, who gave us hope and helped us to stay the sometimes-tiring course. I encourage you to become an "angel on the path" in the individuals lives that you reach. Be a hope peddler!

We are so grateful that where we started in 2000 is miles and miles away from where we are now. I like to tell people that autism is like a wall around your kid. You must be like Foxy Brown (one of my favorite film characters!) and kick that wall down and make cracks in that wall to get through to your child! You must get busy. The more cracks you make the more you have that opportunity to bring them into OUR world! Now, 20 years later, I can say with full certainty that continually kicking down that wall was worth it!

After being in the entertainment industry for several decades, I knew that my platform could be used to help so many more families who are struggling. That is why along with Rodney, I created HollyRod foundation, dedicated to providing help and hope to those living with autism and Parkinson's which my dad had.

We felt strongly that it was our duty to share what we learned to help other autism families to know there is light at the end of the tunnel. We didn't have that support initially.

Today, our son RJ who would "never" do much is a clubhouse attendant for the World Series Champion Los Angeles Dodgers, drives, and saves his hard-earned money! Who would have thought? I always say, I wouldn't change RJ for the world, but I *would* change the world for RJ. I inspire you to be that change.

Let's work together to change the "never" day so many families experience. We need to.

In gratitude,

Holly Robinson Peete
For more information about the efforts of Holly and
Rodney Peets, visit https://www.hollyrod.org.

Final Reflection

You have completed this book! At the start, you were prompted to think about the following questions below. How have your responses changed?

- What do I know about autism?
- How did I first learn about autism?
- What do I want to know about autism?

TEST QUESTIONS

1. In your own words, discuss cultural humility through the lens of working with parents of culturally and linguistically diverse children with autism. Be sure to include three realistic strategies found in the test to use in your own practice.

2. Take note of the sample structure provided for parent debriefing in the group setting. Create a sample script for a realistic group therapy session or one that you have created for a mock session.

3. In a parent debriefing session, once the interventionist has checked in with the parent to share specific strategies, growth, or need the interventionist will then be tasked to _____.
   A. Give the parent time to think about what was said.
   B. Give specific tasks for the parent to do between sessions.
   C. Allow the parent space to share their concerns.

4. Applied behavior analysis is an evidenced-based strategy intended for use with:
   A. The client
   B. The parent
   C. All of the above
   D. None of the above

5. One barrier that many families may encounter in the process of navigating and obtaining new services for their children with autism is:
   A. Disparity in provision of services
   B. Difficulties accepting a diagnosis
   C. Challenges with the child wanting to go to therapy

6. When a child in the family has ASD, parents are at a significantly higher risk of being diagnosed with:
   A. Autism as well
   B. Depression
   C. Bipolar disorder
   D. All of the above

7. Complete the following chart detailing disparity and its manifestation with clients and their parent caregivers:

Disparity	Client presentation	How may a parent respond	Interventionist response
Late diagnosis	Presence of significant behavioral challenges, limited language skills, difficulty engaging appropriately with toys.		
	Meeting language goals, social loner, shies away from talking in class.	Unsatisfied but looking for more, several questions, not satisfied with child's progress despite ability to fully articulate.	
	Severe gastrointestinal issues causing challenges with toileting, which results in the client wanting to leave your therapy session frequently throughout.	Thinks everything is fine; thinks you may be just picking on the child.	
Access to services		Parent continues to say at IEP meetings that the teacher is "racist," is very upset, and wants more services. Parent is not feeling heard.	

REFERENCES

Abrams, A. (2020). Black, disabled people at higher risk in police encounters. *Time*, 6 July. Available at `https://time.com/5857438/police-violence-black-disabled` (accessed 4 February 2022).

Alper, R.M., Beiting, M., Luo, R. et al. (2021). Change the things you can: modifiable parent characteristics predict high-quality early language interaction within socioeconomic status. *Journal of Speech, Language, and Hearing Research* 64 (6): 1992–2004.

American Psychological Association (2018). APA adopts new multicultural guidelines. *Monitor on Psychology* 49 (1): 47.

American Psychological Association. (2014). Parent engagement in schools. Available from `https://www.apa.org/pi/lgbt/programs/safe-supportive/parental-engagement` (accessed 24 February 2022).

American Speech–Language–Hearing Association. (2017). Issues in ethics: Cultural and linguistic competence. Available from `www.asha.org/Practice/ethics/Cultural-and-Linguistic-Competence` (accessed 24 February 2022).

Angell, A.M. and Solomon, O. (2017). 'If I was a different ethnicity, would she treat me the same?': Latino parents' experiences obtaining autism services. *Disability and Society* 32 (8): 1142–1164.

Bebbington, A. and Beecham, J. (2007). Social services support and expenditure for children with autism. *Autism* 11 (1): 43–61.

Bishop-Fitzpatrick, L., Dababnah, S., Baker-Ericzén, M.J. et al. (2019). Autism spectrum disorder and the science of social work: A grand challenge for social work research. *Social Work in Mental Health* 17 (1): 73–92.

Clifford, T. and Minnes, P. (2013). Logging on: evaluating an online support group for parents of children with autism spectrum disorders. *Journal of Autism and Developmental Disorders* 43 (7): 1662–1675.

Cohen, S.R., Holloway, S.D., Domínguez-Pareto, I., and Kuppermann, M. (2015). Support and self-efficacy among Latino and white parents of children with ID. *American Journal on Intellectual and Developmental Disabilities* 120 (1): 16–31.

Dallman, A.R., Artis, J., Watson, L. et al. (2021). Systematic review of disparities and differences in the access and use of allied health services amongst children with autism spectrum disorders. *Journal of Autism and Developmental Disorders* 51: 1316–1330.

Daughrity, B.L. (2018). Parent perceptions of barriers to friendship development for children with autism spectrum disorders. *Communication Disorders Quarterly* 40 (3): 142–151.

Goin-Kochel, R.P., Mackintosh, V.H., and Myers, B.J. (2009). Parental reports on the efficacy of treatments and therapies for their children with autism spectrum disorders. *Research in Autism Spectrum Disorders* 3 (2): 528–537.

Haas, K. and Gibbs, V. (2020). Does a Person's AUTISM play a role in their interactions WITH police: the perceptions of autistic adults and parent/xarers. *Journal of Autism and Developmental Disorders* 51 (5): 1628–1640.

Hall, H.R. (2012). Families of children with autism: behaviors of children, community support and coping. *Issues in Comprehensive Pediatric Nursing* 35 (2): 111–132.

Hannon, M.D., White, E.E., and Nadrich, T. (2017). Influence of autism on fathering style among Black American fathers: a narrative inquiry. *Journal of Family Therapy* 40 (2): 224–246.

Hill, C.V., Pérez-Stable, E.J., Anderson, N.A., and Bernard, M.A. (2015). The national institute on AGING health disparities research framework. *Ethnicity and Disease* 25 (3): 245–254.

Huang, C.Y., Yen, H.C., Tseng, M.H. et al. (2014). Impacts of autistic behaviors, emotional and behavioral problems on parenting stress in caregivers of children with autism. *Journal of Autism and Developmental Disorders* 44 (6): 1383–1390.

Iland, E.D., Weiner, I., and Murawski, W.W. (2012). Obstacles faced by Latina mothers of children with autism. *Californian Journal of. Health Promotion* 10 (SI-Latino): 25–36.

Keen, D., Couzens, D., Muspratt, S., and Rodger, S. (2010). The effects of a parent-focused intervention for children with a recent diagnosis of autism spectrum disorder on parenting stress and competence. *Research in Autism Spectrum Disorders* 4 (2): 229–241.

Keefe, R.H., Lane, S.D., Rubinstein, R.A. et al. (2017). African American fathers: Disproportionate incarceration and the meaning of involvement. *Families in Society* 98 (2): 89–96.

Lopez, K., Magaña, S., Morales, M., and Iland, E. (2019). Parents taking ACTION: reducing DISPARITIES through a culturally informed intervention for LATINX parents of children with autism. *Journal of Ethnic and Cultural Diversity in Social Work* 28 (1): 31–49.

Magaña, S., Lopez, K., Aguinaga, A., and Morton, H. (2013). Access to diagnosis and treatment services among Latino children with autism spectrum disorders. *Intellectual and Developmental Disabilities* 51 (3): 141–153.

Meltzer, L.J. (2011). Factors associated with depressive symptoms in parents of children with autism spectrum disorders. *Research in Autism Spectrum Disorders* 5 (1): 361–367.

Morales, A., Yakushko, O.F., and Castro, A.J. (2011). Language brokering among Mexican-immigrant families in the Midwest. *The Counseling Psychologist* 40 (4): 520–553.

National Institute of Aging. (2022). Health Disparities Framework. Available at https://www.nia.nih.gov/research/osp/framework (accessed 3 February 2022).

Papageorgiou, V. and Kalyva, E. (2010). Self-reported needs and expectations of parents of children with autism spectrum disorders who participate in support groups. *Research in Autism Spectrum Disorders* 4 (4): 653–660.

Papoudi, D., Jørgensen, C.R., Guldberg, K., and Meadan, H. (2021). Perceptions, experiences, and needs of parents of culturally and linguistically diverse children with autism: a SCOPING review. *Review Journal of Autism and Developmental Disorders* 8: 195–212.

Pappas, S. (2019). New guidance on race and ethnicity for psychologists. *Monitor on Psychology* 50 (11): 38.

Pearson, J.N. and Meadan, H. (2021). FACES: An advocacy intervention for African American parents of children with autism. *Intellectual and Developmental Disabilities* 59 (2): 155–171.

Perry, V., and Evans, M. (2021a). Expanding our views on behavior and black students: A call to action. *LeaderLive*, 22 February. Available from `https://leader.pubs.asha.org/do/10.1044/2021-0222-expanding-views-black-students/full` (accessed 4 February 2022).

Perry, V., and Evans, M. (2021b). Shifting the paradigm from disciplining black students to cultural responsiveness. *LeaderLive*, February 24. Available from https://leader.pubs.asha.org/do/10.1044/2021-0223-cultural-responsiveness (accessed 4 February 2022).

Rubenstein, E. and Bishop-Fitzpatrick, L. (2018). A matter of time: the necessity of temporal language in research on health conditions that present with autism spectrum disorder. *Autism Research* 12 (1): 20–25.

Seung, H. (2013). Cultural considerations in serving children with asd and their families: Asian american perspective. *Perspectives on Language Learning and Education* 20 (1): 14–19.

Seung, H.K. (2017). How to handle bilingual children with autism spectrum disorder. *CSHA Magazine* 46 (3): 10–13.

Siller, M., Hotez, E., Swanson, M. et al. (2018). Parent coaching increases the parents' capacity for reflection and self-evaluation: results from a clinical trial in autism. *Attachment & Human Development* 20 (3): 287–308.

Sue, D.W., Capodilupo, C.M., and Holder, A. (2008). Racial microaggressions in the life experience of Black Americans. *Professional Psychology Research and Practice* 39 (3): 329.

Sussman, F. (2006). *TalkAbility: People skills for verbal children on the autism spectrum; a guide for parents*. Toronto, ON: Hanen Centre.

Sussman, F. and Lewis, R.B. (1999). *More Than Words: A guide to helping parents promote communication and social skills in children with autism spectrum disorder*. Toronto, ON: Hanen Centre.

Tambyraja, S.R. (2020). Facilitating parental involvement in speech therapy for children with speech sound disorders: a survey of speech-language pathologists' practices, perspectives, and strategies. *American Journal of Speech–Language Pathology* 29 (4): 1987–1996.

US Government Office of Accountability. (2017). *Health Care Workforce: Comprehensive planning by HSS needed to meet national needs*. GAO Report GAO-16-17. Washington, DC: USGAO.

Wiley, A.D. (2016). Unlocking disparity of services for Latino children with autism spectrum disorder: Are mothers the answer? Doctoral dissertation, Claremont Graduate University. Emeryville, CA: ProQuest Dissertations. doi:10143608.

Zarembo, A. (2011). Warrior parents fare best in securing autism services. *Los Angeles Times*, 13 December. Available at `https://www.latimes.com/local/autism/la-me-autism-day-two-html-htmlstory.html` (accessed 4 February 2022).

FURTHER READINGS

Corcoran, J., Berry, A., and Hill, S. (2015). The lived experience of us parents of children with autism spectrum disorders. *Journal of Intellectual Disabilities* 19 (4): 356–366.

Gallagher, S., Phillips, A.C., and Carroll, D. (2009). Parental stress is associated with poor sleep quality in parents caring for children with developmental disabilities. *Journal of Pediatric Psychology* 35 (7): 728–737.

Shorey, S., Ng, E.D., Haugan, G., and Law, E. (2019). The parenting experiences and needs of Asian primary caregivers of children with autism: a meta-synthesis. *Autism* 24 (3): 591–604.

Glossary

Term	Definition
Ableism	Attitudes that discriminate and devalue people with disabilities.
Asperger's syndrome	Diagnosis in the DSM-VI used for individuals with autism with low symptomology.
Camouflaging	Masking autism behaviors to appear neurotypical.
Comorbid	Other disorders in addition to a primary diagnosis.
Community-based outing	Opportunities for clients to apply intervention targets in the community setting.
Community integration tasks	Tasks that involve the client in the community to integrate skill in a natural setting.
Critical learning period	A period in early childhood when children are highly capable of acquiring new languages with near native proficiency.
Cultural humility	A commitment to self-evaluation and critique in learning about diverse cultural groups.
Culturally responsive	Applying assessment and/or intervention approaches that incorporate the client's cultural values and beliefs.
Daily living skills	Department of Labor's O*NET database
Disparity	significant difference as in economic, social, and/or health disparity
Double empathy problem	Autistic people relate to each other much in the same way that neurotypical people relate to each other, despite intergroup challenges.
Elopers	A client who runs away or escapes during intervention.
Emotional regulation	The ability to calm and regulate one's response to stress and anxiety.
Ethnographic interviewing	Includes asking the right questions in the right way to obtain accurate information.
Executive functioning	Cognitive skills needed to facilitate goal attainment including planning, organization, attention, and memory among other skills

Autism Spectrum Disorders from Theory to Practice: Assessment and Intervention Tools Across the Lifespan, First Edition. Edited by Belinda Daughrity and Ashley Wiley Johnson.
© 2023 John Wiley & Sons Ltd. Published 2023 by John Wiley & Sons Ltd.

Term	Definition
Functional play	An early play milestone that includes simple play acts to play with toys as intended, such as puzzles and cars; this stage generally correlates with first words.
Identity-first language	Includes using autistic person rather than person with autism.
Integrated employment opportunities	The individual with a disability works and interacts with a range of individuals, most of whom are considered neurotypical.
Interdependent group-oriented contingencies	A reward system where success of the group is dependent on each individual.
Interpreter	A trained individual who serves to bridge communication and/or culture between a clinician and client/family who speak different languages.
Interprofessional Practice (IPP)	Allied health professionals across related disciplines working together to serve clients with needs across multiple domains of functioning
Interprofessional Education (IPE)	Colleagues across related disciplines educating and learning from one another to generate shared decisions
Joint attention	Attending to an object or event with another person.
Language use	Pragmatics.
Masking	see camouflaging; includes hiding autistic behaviors to appear neurotypical.
Mastery	Includes a quantitative marker of attaining a skill, such as demonstrating it in at least 80% of obligatory contexts.
Medical model of disability	Approaches disability as a problem of the individual who needs to be assisted to be more "typical."
Neurodiversity movement	Asserts there is a range of presentations in neurological function without a hierarchy given to neurotypical individuals over those presenting with autism or other disorders.
Neurotypical	Not presenting with any neurologically atypical patterns of thought or behavior.
Oh goodness! plan	The plan you have in your therapy toolkit to quickly access if you find that your original plan is not working well.
Onlooker behavior	A child looking at other children playing, but not engaged in play themselves.
Parallel play	A child playing next to another child and engaged in a similar activity without direct social overtures.
Parent-mediated interventions	Interventions that are carried out directly via the parent instead of the interventionist.
Parent support groups (PSGs)	Groups for parents to offer emotional and/or other support for caregivers of neurodiverse children
Person-first language	Includes putting the person before the disability, as in person with autism.

Term	Definition
Plateau	When a client is no longer demonstrating measurable progress on an observed skill.
Pull-out services	Services where the client is taken out of the natural environment into a private intervention service with a clinician.
Push-in services	Services where the clinician goes into the natural environment with the client and provides intervention services in that setting.
Regression	Includes the loss of previously acquired skills.
RIASEC test Script	A rehearsed approach with planned responses and/or behaviors to address social scenarios.
Segregated job setting	An employment setting where the employee is working with other individuals who have disabilities.
Self-determination	Process by which a person takes control over their own life.
Self-stimulatory behaviors	Restricted and/or repetitive behaviors that serve as a calming function to self-soothe.
Self-reports	Include the client's direct reports of their own level of functioning and/or areas of difficulty.
Social skill steps	Intervention approach to teach competence in verbal and nonverbal skills required for effective communication with others.
Social targets	Intervention goal targeting an aspect of social behavior.
Soft skills	Unlike hard skills, which include concrete facts about information, soft skills include emotional intelligence and appropriate counseling techniques to reflect appropriate flexibility in applying learned skills in natural contexts.
Solitary play	A child playing alone or only with an adult.
Symbolic play	Play that involves using an object to represent something else.
Suprasegmental	Include intonation, timing and stress of words, phrases and sentences that carry meaning.
Tailor day workers	Assisting students with autism and/or other disabilities with their daily living skills and needs.
Theory of mind	The ability to discern others' mental states.
Token economy	Used in positive behavior support, where tokens are given in response to a child demonstrating a desired behavior and those tokens are exchanged for a reward.
Typical developmental norms	Include a range of times when most typically developing children will master a particular skill/milestone.
Verbal reprimands	A verbal warning regarding an undesired behavior.
Video modeling	An evidenced-based practice that uses video recordings to offer a visual model of a targeted skill or behavior.
Vocational readiness Vocal stereotypy	Can be a diagnostic feature of autism spectrum disorder where a client uses a feature of sound in a distinct and/or repetitive fashion.

Answers to Test Questions

CHAPTER 1

1. (B) 3
2. (C) Social interaction
3. (A) 2
4. (A) Boys are diagnosed more than girls
5. (D) 1943
6. (D) Difficulty maintaining eye gaze
7. True
8. Masking

CHAPTER 2

1. (C) The presence of restricted and/or repetitive behaviors
2. True
3. (D) All of the above
4. False
5. True
6. True
7. False
8. False
9. (B) Specific, measurable, attainable, realistic, time bound
10. (D) A and B only

CHAPTER 3

1. (B) Conventional gesture
2. (A) Descriptive gesture
3. False
4. True
5. (C) Facebook group

Autism Spectrum Disorders from Theory to Practice: Assessment and Intervention Tools Across the Lifespan,
First Edition. Edited by Belinda Daughrity and Ashley Wiley Johnson.
© 2023 John Wiley & Sons Ltd. Published 2023 by John Wiley & Sons Ltd.

6. (C) Four years
7. (A), (B), (C), (D)
8. Personal answer
9. True
10. True

CHAPTER 4

1. True
2. False
3. True
4. False
5. False
6. True
7. False
8. (C) Regression
9. (B) Symbolic play
10. (B) Onlooking

CHAPTER 5

1. (D) All of the above
2. False
3. True
4. False
5. True
6. (A) Recess
7. False
8. False

CHAPTER 6

1. True
2. False
3. True
4. True

CHAPTER 7

1. False
2. (D) All of the above
3. False

4. (C)
5. True
6. (A, B, C, D) All answers apply

CHAPTER 8

1. Personal answer
2. Personal answer
3. Personal answer
4. (B) Gestalt language
5. (A) "Wh" questions
6. (A) 85%
7. (E) All of the above
8. (A) Within two conversational turns of the exchange
9.

Key strategy	Therapeutic presentation
Facilitate verbal initiations	Focus on opportunities for the client initiate language production rather than responding to questions and prompts.
Elicit careful and continual observations	Make sure to track nonverbal indicators of comprehension like gaze, body language, and changes in facial expression. Note changes in types and frequency of echolalia to credit progress.
Facilitate low constraint interactions	Avoid using high constraint utterances like questions or commands.
Map language contents into known contexts	Use language the child already uses and change aspects to increase language diversity.
Model useful gestalts	Model carefully selected, individualized, age-appropriate, high-frequency, socially communicative utterances for the client to add to their current repertoire. In treatment, target smaller more flexible units as a means to help generate more creative and meaningful utterances.
Provide practice opportunities	Offer multiple repetitions to help the client learn the desired skill.
Identify, preserve, and strengthen patterns of social closeness	Facilitate opportunities for social engagement.
Develop opportunities to teach quiet behavior in specific settings	In certain settings, it is highly disruptive or not appropriate to use echolalia. Teach the client to pause or to remain quiet to best cope with the demands of the environment. This is a useful tip that can lead to successful social skills.

CHAPTER 9

1. Personal answer
2. Personal answer
3. Personal answer
4. Personal answer

CHAPTER 10

1. False
2. (A) Operational competence
3. (D) Strategic competence
4. False
5. True
6. (D) All of the above
7. (B) Augmentative alternative communication

CHAPTER 11

1. False
2. (B) Interprofessional practice (IPP)
3. True
4. False
5. False
6. (A) Interprofessional education (IPE)
7. (D) All of the above are viable service delivery modalities

CHAPTER 12

1. Personal answer
2. Personal answer
3. (B) Give specific tasks for the parent to do between sessions
4. (A) The client
5. (D) All or one of the above
6. (B) Depression

7.

Disparity	Client presentation	How may a parent respond	Interventionist response
Disparity resulting in a Late diagnosis	Presence of significant behavioral challenges, limited language skills, difficulty engaging appropriately with toys.		Connect parent with resources, evaluate client, follow up, identify PSG.
Disparity in provision of services	Meeting language goals, social loner, shies away from talking in class.	Unsatisfied but looking for more, several questions, not satisfied with child's progress despite ability to fully articulate.	
Disparity in access to knowledge surrounding diagnosis	Severe gastrointestinal issues causing challenges with toileting, which results in the client wanting to leave your therapy session frequently throughout.	Thinks everything is fine; thinks you may be just picking on the child.	
Disparity in access to competent service providers.		Parent continues to say at IEP meetings that the teacher is "racist," is very upset, and wants more services. Parent is not feeling heard.	Amend goals to ensure it reflects high but realistic expectations, Continue to build trust with family to break down barriers.

Index

Autism Spectrum Disorders from Theory to Practice: Assessment and Intervention Tools Across the Lifespan,
First Edition. Edited by Belinda Daughrity and Ashley Wiley Johnson.
© 2023 John Wiley & Sons Ltd. Published 2023 by John Wiley & Sons Ltd.